PEDRO CASTRO
PCASTRO.ECON@GMAIL.COM

APPLIED SURVIVAL ANALYSIS

Regression Modeling of Time-to-Event Data

Second Edition

DAVID W. HOSMER
University of Massachusetts
School of Public Health and Health Sciences
Department of Public Health
Division of Biostatistics and Epidemiology
Amherst, MA

STANLEY LEMESHOW
The Ohio State University
College of Public Health
Center for Biostatistics
Columbus, OH

SUSANNE MAY
University of California, San Diego
Department of Family & Preventative Medicine
Division of Biostatistics and Bioinformatics
La Jolla, CA

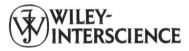
WILEY-
INTERSCIENCE

A John Wiley & Sons, Inc., Publication

Library of Congress Cataloging-in-Publication Data:

Hosmer, David W.
   Applied survival analysis : regression modeling of time-to-event data /
David W. Hosmer, Stanley Lemeshow, Susanne May. — 2nd ed.
      p. cm.
   Includes bibliographical references and index.
   ISBN 978-0-471-75499-2 (cloth : alk. paper)
   1. Medicine—Research—Statistical methods.   2. Medical
sciences—Statistical methods—Computer programs.   3. Regression
analysis—Data processing.   4. Prognosis—Statistical methods.   5. Logistic
distribution.   I. Lemeshow, Stanley.   II. May, Susanne.   III. Title.
   [DNLM: 1. Survival Analysis.   2. Logistic Models.   3. Mathematical
Computing.   4. Prognosis.   5. Regression Analysis.   WA 950 H827a 2008]
   R853.S7H67 2008
   610.72'7—dc22   2007035523

10 9 8 7 6 5 4 3 2 1

To Trina: Wife, Mother, Athlete, and
Companion in Life's Adventures
D. W. H.

To Elaine: with respect and admiration for her compassion, generosity and
appreciation of what is important in our lives and in our world
S. L.

To Bruce: Husband, Friend and Partner
S. M.

Contents

Preface to the Second Edition

Since the publication of the first edition nine years ago, analyses using time-to-event methods have increased considerably in all areas of scientific inquiry. We believe that two important reasons for the increase are: (1) the statistical methods for the analysis of time-to-event data are now taught in many intermediate level methods courses and not just advanced courses and (2) the software to perform most of the methods is now available and easy to use in all the major software packages.

The approach taken in the second edition has not changed from the first edition, where the goal was to provide a focused text on regression modeling for the time-to-event data typically encountered in health related studies. As in the first edition, we assume that the reader has had a course in linear regression at the level of Kleinbaum, Kupper, Muller and Nizam (1998) and one in logistic regression at the level of Hosmer and Lemeshow (2000). Emphasis is placed on the modeling of data and the interpretation of the results. Crucial to this is an understanding of the nature of the "incomplete" or "censored" data encountered. Understanding the censoring mechanism is important as it may influence model selection and interpretation. Yet, once understood and accounted for, censoring is often just another technical detail handled by the computer software, allowing emphasis to return to model building, assessment of model fit, and assumptions and interpretation of the results.

In the second edition, we have replaced the HMO–HIV data as the main data set for illustrating methods with a sample of 100 observations from the Worcester Heart Attack Study. We have kept the data from the UMARU Impact Study (UIS), but only use it occasionally. The main modeling data set is a sample of 500 observations from the Worcester Heart Attack Study. Data from the German Breast Cancer Study and the ACTG320 Study are used to demonstrate various modeling and analysis techniques and methods. In short, most of the examples in the text and exercises are new or use new data.

A reading of the Table of Contents for the first four chapters will look as if nothing much has changed. However, the actual text has many changes and additions. For example, the discussions of interactions and the covariate-adjusted survival functions in Chapter Four are greatly expanded. In Chapter Five, we have added variable selection by multivariable fractional polynomials. Changes in Chapter Six follow from a new model based on data from the Worcester Heart

Attack Study studied in Chapter Five. The major change to Chapter Seven is a greatly expanded discussion of time varying covariates with examples. In Chapter Eight we, again, focus on the exponential, Weibull, and log-logistic parametric regression models but have expanded the discussion of each. In Chapter Nine, we have taken advantage of the addition of the capability to fit frailty/random effects models in Stata. Examples are used to compare fitting stratified models to frailty models. The last sections of Chapter Nine contain new material on competing risk models, sample size and power, and using multiple imputation methods to analyze data with missing values.

As we noted, we believe that the increase in the use of statistical methods for time-to-event data is directly related to their incorporation into the major statistical software packages. There are some differences in the capabilities of the various software packages and, when a particular approach is available in a limited number of packages, we note this in the text. Analyses have, for the most part, been performed in Stata Version 9 [Stata Corp. (2005)]. This easy-to-use package combines good graphics and excellent analysis routines, is fast, is compatible across Macintosh, Windows, and UNIX platforms, and interacts well with Microsoft Word 2004 for Mac. Just as we were going to press, Stata Version 10 was released. Among the enhancements in this version is the ability to perform time to event analysis of survey data. Unfortunately we were not able to incorporate that capability into this text. The only other major statistical package employed at various points during the preparation of this text is SAS Version 9.1 [SAS Institute Inc. (2003)].

This text was prepared in camera-ready format using Microsoft Word 2004 for Mac Version 11.3.5 on a PowerBook G4 using Mac OS X Version 10.4.9. Mathematical equations and symbols were built using Math Type Version 5.1 [MathType[5] Mathematical Equation Editor (2004)].

All data may be obtained from the John Wiley & Sons, Inc. ftp site,

ftp://ftp.wiley.com/public/sci_tech_med/survival.

They may also be obtained from the a web site at the University of Massachusetts / Amherst by going the following link and then the section for survival analysis,

http://www.umass.edu/statdata/statdata.

As was the case with the first edition we will have a link at the John Wiley & Sons, Inc. ftp site listed above for errata and corrections.

As in any project with the scope and magnitude of this text, there are many who have contributed directly or indirectly to its content and style and we feel quite fortunate to be able to acknowledge the contributions of others. We thank Rob Goldberg for providing us with a subset of the Worcester Heart Attack Study that we used to create further subsets of 100 and 500 observations. These are used extensively in the text. We thank Fred Anderson and Gordon FitzGerald for providing a subset of data from the GRACE registry containing time-varying covariates. We thank former faculty colleagues Jane McCusker, Anne Stoddard, and Carol Bigelow for the use and insights into the data from the Project IMPACT Study. We thank the AIDS Clinical Trials Group for making the ACTG 320 data available. We appreciate Ohio State Provost Barbara Snyder's agreeing to allow SL to take a special research assignment (SRA) so that he had the time necessary to work on this book. Not only did Annick Alpérovitch, Carole Dufouil and Christophe Tzourio at INSERM Unit 708 in Paris, France provide an office and an environment conducive for working on this book during the SRA, but they also facilitated obtaining data from the 3C Study Investigators that we were able to use as an exercise in Chapter 7.

We express special thanks to Patrick Royston and Willi Sauerbrei for their helpful suggestions on the text describing fractional polynomials and for comments on numerous other sections of the text. They generously shared with us data from the German Breast Cancer Study that they have analyzed extensively in their publications.

We would like to thank Janice Jones for pointing out the 5731 commas that were missing in the initial draft and for many suggestions that made the text much easier to read. We also thank Charisse Darrell-Fields for inserting Janice's commas into the manuscript. Finally, we thank Tracy McHone for coordinating the printing and organization of the final manuscript.

Over the last nine years we have used the first edition in semester-long course offerings at the University of Massachusetts as well as numerous short courses to audiences around the world. We thank collectively the students in these courses for their comments and insights on how to make things clearer. We hope we have done so in this edition.

DAVID W. HOSMER
STANLEY LEMESHOW
SUSANNE MAY

Stowe, Vermont
Columbus, Ohio
San Diego, California
August, 2007

CHAPTER 1

Introduction to Regression Modeling of Survival Data

1.1 INTRODUCTION

Regression modeling of the relationship between an outcome variable and one or more independent (predictor) variable(s) is commonly employed in virtually all fields. The popularity of this approach is due to the fact that plausible models may be easily fit, evaluated, and interpreted. Statistically, the specification of a model requires choosing both systematic and error components. The choice of the systematic component involves an assessment of the relationship among the "average" of the outcome variable relative to specific levels of the independent variable(s). This may be guided by an exploratory analysis of the current data and/or past experience. The choice of an error component involves specifying the statistical distribution of what remains to be explained after the model is fit.

In an applied setting, the task of model selection is, to a large extent, based on the goals of the analysis and on the measurement scale of the outcome variable. For example, a clinician may wish to model the relationship among body mass index (BMI, kg/m^2) and caloric intake and gender among teenagers seen in the clinics of a large health maintenance organization (HMO). A good place to start would be to use a model with a linear systematic component and normally distributed errors (i.e., the usual linear regression model). Suppose, instead, that the clinician decides to convert BMI into a 0 – 1 dichotomous variable (taking on the value 1 if BMI > 30) and assess its association with caloric intake and gender. In this case, the logistic regression model would be a good choice. The logistic regression model has a systematic component that is linear in the log-odds and has binomial/Bernoulli distributed errors. While there are many issues involved in the fitting, refinement, evaluation, and interpretation of each of these models, the same basic modeling paradigm would be followed in each scenario.

This basic modeling paradigm is commonly used in texts taking a data-based approach to either linear or logistic regression [e.g., Kleinbaum, Kupper, Muller and Nizam (1998) and Hosmer and Lemeshow (2000)]. In general we follow this same modeling paradigm in this text to motivate our study of regression models where the dependent variable measures the time to the occurrence of an event of interest. However, as we will see shortly, the fact that *time* to an event is the outcome of interest requires us to think carefully about what actually has been measured. Also the fact that time is a dynamic process provides challenges in formulating a model that are not present in settings where a typical linear or logistic regression model might be applied. In this spirit, we begin with an example.

Example

Throughout this book, we use a number of different data sets to illustrate the methods and provide grist for the exercises at the end of each chapter. Some, but not all, of these are described in Section 1.3. One is a subset of the data from the Worcester Heart Attack Study (WHAS) provided to us by its principal investigator, Dr. Robert J. Goldberg. Briefly, the goal of the WHAS is to study factors and time trends associated with long-term survival following acute myocardial infarction (MI) among residents of the Worcester, Massachusetts, Standard Metropolitan Statistical Area (SMSA). The study began in 1975 and has collected data approximately every other year, with the most recent cohort being subjects who experienced an MI in 2001. The main study has data on over 11,000 subjects, and we will focus our analyses on two samples from the main study. We present one such sample of 100 subjects in Table 1.1. These data are referred to as the WHAS100 data in this text. Suppose our goal for the data in Table 1.1 is to study the effects of gender, age, and body mass index (kg/m^2) at time of hospitalization for the MI on length of survival. Typical regression modeling questions might include: (1) Do women have a more favorable survival experience over time than men? (2) In what way do the age and BMI at admission affect survival over time? (3) Are the effects of age and BMI the same for men and women? Before we can discuss a regression model to address these questions, we need to consider what outcome variable we are going to model. If the outcome is time to an event, then what is the event and how do we define time to it? Suppose we consider the event of interest to be death from any cause following hospitalization for an MI and we define the time to it as the number of days from admission to the hospital until death. The next step in the regression modeling paradigm is to specify the systematic component. Because we have followed subjects over time, it seems logical that the systematic component should be the "mean" of this dynamic process and how it changes as a function of covariates. Prior experience in linear and logistic regression provides little guidance on how to do this. The first few chapters of this book are devoted to providing the necessary background and methods to begin to address this question as well as specification of the error component. The remainder of the text considers application of the methods to different time-to-event scenarios.

Returning to our outcome variable, each subject in Table 1.1 has a date recorded for when the last follow up occurred. Vital status reports whether the subject was dead or alive on that date. For those subjects who died, the reported date of death and the value presented for follow-up time is the actual value of the outcome of interest: survival time following hospitalization for an MI.   For example, subject 5 in Table 1.1 was admitted to the hospital on February 9, 1995, and, 1205 days later, died on May 29, 1998. Subject 10 was admitted to the hospital on July 22, 1995, and was still alive at the time of his last follow up, December 31, 2001. For this subject, all we know is that his survival time exceeds the follow up time of 2719 days.   Hence the observation of survival time is incomplete. The statistical term used to describe the process producing this type of incomplete observation is called "censoring" and the observation is referred to as being "censored." In general, incomplete observation of time to an event can occur in several ways and we provide an overview of them in the next section. Methods for handling incompletely observed time-to-event data in regression models is a central theme in this text.

1.2 TYPICAL CENSORING MECHANISMS

We cannot discuss a censored observation until we have carefully defined an uncensored observation. This point may seem rather obvious, but in applied settings confusion, about censoring may not be due to the fact that some observations are incomplete but may instead be the result of an unclear definition of survival time.[1] The observation of survival time has two components that must be unambiguously defined: a beginning point (i.e., when the "clock starts") and an endpoint that is reached when the event of interest occurs (i.e., when the "clock stops"). The point where analysis time, t, is zero is denoted $t = 0$. In the WHAS example, observation began on the day a subject was admitted to the hospital following an MI. In a randomized clinical trial, observation of survival time usually begins on the day a subject is randomized to receive one of the treatment protocols.   In an occupational exposure study, $t = 0$ may be the day a subject began work at a particular plant. In some applications, the best $t = 0$ point may not be obvious. For example, in the WHAS study, other beginning points might be the date of discharge from the hospital or the actual moment that the MI occurred. Observation may end at the time when a subject literally "dies" from the disease of interest, or it may end upon the occurrence of some other non-fatal, well-defined, condition such as meeting clinical criteria for remission of a cancer. The survival time is the distance on the time scale between these two points.

---

[1] In this text, we use interchangeably the terms time to event, survival time, and life length to describe the outcome variable. In any example, we choose the one that seems most appropriate but we have a preference for survival time.

Table 1.1 Study ID, Admission Date, Follow Up Date, Length of Hospital Stay, Follow Up Time (Days), Vital Status at Follow Up, Age at Admission (Years), Gender, and Body Mass Index (kg/m^2) (BMI) for 100 Subjects in the Worcester Heart Attack Study

ID	Admission Date	Follow Up Date	Length of Stay	Follow Up Time	Vital Status	Age at Admission	Gender	BMI
1	3/13/95	3/19/95	4	6	Dead	65	Male	31.4
2	1/14/95	1/23/96	5	374	Dead	88	Female	22.7
3	2/17/95	10/4/01	5	2421	Dead	77	Male	27.9
4	4/7/95	7/14/95	9	98	Dead	81	Female	21.5
5	2/9/95	5/29/98	4	1205	Dead	78	Male	30.7
6	1/16/95	9/11/00	7	2065	Dead	82	Female	26.5
7	1/17/95	10/15/97	3	1002	Dead	66	Female	35.7
8	11/15/94	11/24/00	56	2201	Dead	81	Female	28.3
9	8/18/95	2/23/96	5	189	Dead	76	Male	27.1
10	7/22/95	12/31/02	9	2719	Alive	40	Male	21.8
11	10/11/95	12/31/02	6	2638	Alive	73	Female	28.4
12	5/26/95	9/29/96	11	492	Dead	83	Male	24.7
13	5/21/95	3/18/96	6	302	Dead	64	Female	27.5
14	12/14/95	12/31/02	10	2574	Alive	58	Male	29.8
15	11/8/95	12/31/02	7	2610	Alive	43	Male	23.0
16	10/8/95	12/31/02	5	2641	Alive	39	Male	30.1
17	10/17/95	5/12/00	6	1669	Dead	66	Male	32.0
18	10/30/95	1/5/03	9	2624	Dead	61	Male	30.7
19	12/10/95	12/31/02	6	2578	Alive	49	Male	25.7
20	11/23/95	12/31/02	5	2595	Alive	53	Female	30.1
21	10/5/95	2/5/96	6	123	Dead	85	Male	18.4
22	11/5/95	12/31/02	8	2613	Alive	69	Female	37.6
23	9/9/95	10/22/97	4	774	Dead	54	Male	29.0
24	9/9/95	3/13/01	14	2012	Dead	82	Male	19.9
25	12/15/95	12/31/02	4	2573	Alive	67	Female	28.3
26	12/3/95	1/19/01	11	1874	Dead	89	Female	23.4
27	10/18/95	12/31/02	2	2631	Alive	68	Male	26.4
28	3/16/95	6/4/00	7	1907	Dead	78	Male	28.2
29	10/25/95	4/15/97	5	538	Dead	56	Male	24.1
30	10/6/95	1/18/96	4	104	Dead	85	Female	36.7
31	9/3/95	9/9/95	4	6	Dead	72	Male	28.0
32	6/30/95	5/1/99	5	1401	Dead	50	Male	20.4
33	7/22/95	12/22/02	8	2710	Dead	81	Female	28.6
34	9/17/95	1/5/98	4	841	Dead	85	Female	20.2
35	3/21/97	8/16/97	6	148	Dead	84	Female	23.6
36	2/23/97	12/31/02	12	2137	Alive	75	Male	23.7
37	1/1/97	12/31/02	16	2190	Alive	61	Male	23.4
38	1/18/97	12/31/02	5	2173	Alive	48	Male	33.5
39	1/19/97	4/25/98	8	461	Dead	83	Female	19.6
40	3/18/97	12/31/02	10	2114	Alive	82	Male	25.8
41	2/3/97	12/31/02	4	2157	Alive	62	Male	30.9
42	5/17/97	12/31/02	5	2054	Alive	39	Male	24.2
43	3/8/97	12/31/02	5	2124	Alive	45	Male	31.7
44	2/23/97	12/31/02	4	2137	Alive	65	Male	26.2
45	6/14/97	1/5/03	18	2031	Dead	76	Female	32.4
46	7/7/97	12/31/02	9	2003	Alive	77	Female	24.6
47	4/27/97	12/31/02	9	2074	Alive	68	Male	21.3
48	5/15/97	2/13/98	7	274	Dead	73	Male	26.5
49	7/26/97	12/31/02	4	1984	Alive	64	Male	28.0
50	7/17/97	12/31/02	6	1993	Alive	80	Male	36.0
51	9/9/97	12/31/02	7	1939	Alive	84	Female	22.3

Table 1.1 Continued

ID	Admission Date	Follow Up Date	Length of Stay	Follow Up Time	Vital Status	Age at Admission	Gender	BMI
52	6/19/97	9/3/00	4	1172	Dead	43	Female	25.3
53	8/20/97	11/17/97	3	89	Dead	87	Female	18.8
54	8/28/97	1/3/98	7	128	Dead	70	Female	18.6
55	9/9/97	12/31/02	17	1939	Alive	80	Male	25.5
56	9/1/97	9/15/97	11	14	Dead	64	Female	24.4
57	9/3/97	6/10/00	5	1011	Dead	59	Female	29.9
58	9/24/97	10/30/01	6	1497	Dead	92	Male	24.4
59	9/19/97	12/31/02	3	1929	Alive	51	Male	34.8
60	4/17/97	12/31/02	1	2084	Alive	41	Male	27.3
61	10/21/97	2/5/98	6	107	Dead	90	Male	24.8
62	10/2/97	12/27/98	4	451	Dead	83	Male	21.8
63	1/8/97	12/31/02	3	2183	Alive	61	Male	27.4
64	11/11/97	12/31/02	7	1876	Alive	64	Male	26.2
65	11/7/97	5/31/00	3	936	Dead	82	Male	26.9
66	4/20/97	4/18/98	5	363	Dead	91	Female	27.6
67	6/18/97	5/1/00	5	1048	Dead	48	Male	31.6
68	10/29/97	12/31/02	12	1889	Alive	63	Male	23.3
69	4/29/97	12/31/02	5	2072	Alive	81	Male	28.4
70	11/8/97	12/31/02	7	1879	Alive	52	Male	32.6
71	11/17/97	12/31/02	4	1870	Alive	65	Male	32.0
72	11/28/97	12/31/02	5	1859	Alive	74	Male	25.0
73	5/19/97	12/31/02	5	2052	Alive	62	Male	30.2
74	12/11/97	12/31/02	4	1846	Alive	60	Female	29.3
75	5/10/97	12/31/02	7	2061	Alive	71	Male	32.3
76	10/6/97	12/31/02	3	1912	Alive	73	Male	31.5
77	12/21/97	12/31/02	5	1836	Alive	43	Male	28.6
78	11/22/97	3/16/98	7	114	Dead	80	Male	33.4
79	10/31/97	2/4/02	7	1557	Dead	72	Male	21.8
80	6/28/97	12/27/00	5	1278	Dead	57	Male	23.6
81	12/21/97	12/31/02	3	1836	Alive	80	Female	28.4
82	10/2/97	12/31/02	6	1916	Alive	76	Male	28.0
83	9/14/97	12/31/02	3	1934	Alive	53	Male	24.2
84	9/25/97	12/31/02	10	1923	Alive	44	Male	32.6
85	12/2/97	1/15/98	3	44	Dead	71	Male	23.1
86	9/26/97	12/31/02	6	1922	Alive	64	Male	31.8
87	10/24/97	7/25/98	5	274	Dead	86	Male	21.1
88	11/27/97	12/31/02	7	1860	Alive	72	Female	25.2
89	4/12/97	3/23/02	4	1806	Dead	73	Female	22.9
90	2/15/97	12/31/02	6	2145	Alive	85	Female	26.1
91	10/22/97	4/22/98	5	182	Dead	60	Male	23.2
92	6/27/97	12/31/02	4	2013	Alive	63	Male	35.5
93	1/17/97	12/31/02	5	2174	Alive	80	Female	20.6
94	12/12/97	5/24/02	4	1624	Dead	74	Male	30.1
95	11/4/97	5/10/98	10	187	Dead	79	Female	16.8
96	11/4/97	12/31/02	4	1883	Alive	48	Female	32.1
97	12/24/97	4/19/02	3	1577	Dead	32	Female	39.9
98	11/26/97	1/27/98	8	62	Dead	86	Female	14.9
99	8/10/97	12/31/02	16	1969	Alive	56	Male	29.1
100	3/26/97	2/13/00	7	1054	Dead	74	Male	32.9

In practice, a value of time is obtained by calculating the number of days (or months, or years, etc.) between two calendar dates. Table 1.1 shows the admission date and the follow up date for the subjects in this sample from the WHAS study. Most statistical software packages have functions that allow the user to manipulate calendar dates in a manner similar to other numeric variables. They do this by creating a numeric value for each calendar date, which is defined as the number of days from some predetermined reference date. For example, the reference date used by most, if not all, packages is January 1, 1960. Subject 5 entered the study on February 9, 1995, which is 12,823 days after the reference date, and died May 29, 1998, which is 14,028 days after the reference date. The interval between these two dates is $14,028 - 12,823 = 1,205$ days. The number of days can be converted into the number of months by dividing by $30.4375 = (365.25 / 12)$. Thus, the survival time in months for subject 5 is $39.589 = (1,205 / 30.4375)$. It is common, when reporting results in tabular form, to round months to the nearest whole number, e.g., 40 months. The level of precision used in reporting and analyzing survival time should depend on the particular application.

Two mechanisms can lead to incomplete observation of time: censoring and truncation. A censored observation is one whose value is incomplete due to factors that are random for each subject. A truncated observation is incomplete due to a selection process inherent in the study design. The most commonly encountered form of a censored observation is one where observation begins at the defined time $t = 0$ and terminates before the outcome of interest is observed. Because the incomplete nature of the observation occurs in the right tail of the time axis, such observations are said to be *right censored*. For example, in the WHAS study, a subject could move out of town or still be alive at the last follow up. In a study where right censoring is the only type of censoring possible, observation on subjects may begin at the same time or at varying times. For example, in a test of computer life length, we may begin with all computers started at exactly the same time. In a randomized clinical trial or in an observational study, such as the WHAS study, patients may enter the study over several years. As we see in Table 1.1, subject 2 entered the study on January 14, 1995, while subject 50 entered on July 17, 1997. In this type of study, regardless of calendar time, each subject's time of enrollment is assumed to define the $t = 0$ point.

For obvious practical reasons, all studies have a point when observation ends on all subjects; therefore subjects entering at different times will have variable lengths of maximum follow-up time. In the WHAS study, the last follow up date is December 31, 2002. Subject 13 entered the study on May 21, 1995. Thus the longest this subject could have been followed is 7 years, 7 months, and 10 days. However, this subject was not followed for the maximum length of time because the subject died on March 18, 1996, yielding a survival time of 302 days. Incomplete observation of a survival time due to the end of the study or follow-up is considered a right censored observation because the process by which subjects entered the study is random at the subject level.

A typical pattern of entry into a follow-up study is shown in Figure 1.1. This is a hypothetical 2-year study in which patients are enrolled during the first year. We see that subject 1 entered the study on January 1, 1990, and died on March 1, 1991. Subject 2 entered the study on February 1, 1990, and was lost to follow-up on February 1, 1991. Subject 3 entered the study on June 1, 1990, and was still alive on December 31, 1991, the end of the study. Subject 4 entered the study on September 1, 1990, and died on April 1, 1991. Subjects 2 and 3 have survival times that are right-censored. These data are plotted on the analysis time scale, in months, in Figure 1.2. Note that each subject's time is plotted as if he or she were enrolled at exactly the same calendar time and were followed until his or her respective end point. The two figures illustrate the difference between collecting data in calendar time and then converting it to analysis time.

In some studies, there may be a clear definition of the beginning time point; but subjects may not come under actual observation until after this point has passed. For example, in modeling age at menarche, suppose we define the zero value of time as 8 years. Suppose a subject enters the study at age 10, still not having experienced menarche. We know that this subject could have experienced menarche after age 8 but, due to the study design, was not enrolled in the study until age 10. This subject would not enter the analysis until time 10. This type of incomplete observation of time is called *left truncation* or *delayed entry*. Another example would be to study survival time in the WHAS among those discharged from the hospital alive. Here subjects stay in the hospital for varying lengths of time but we do not begin to study them until they "leave the front door."

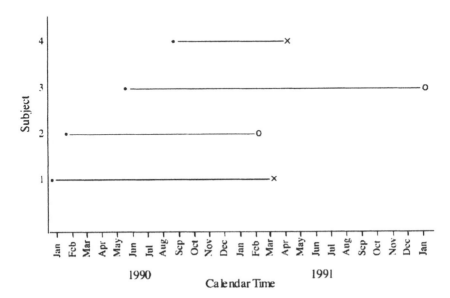

Figure 1.1 Line plot in calendar time for four subjects in a hypothetical follow-up study.

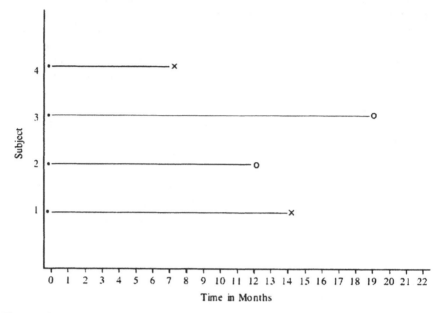

Figure 1.2 Line plot in the time scale for four subjects in a hypothetical follow-up study.

Another censoring mechanism that sometimes occurs in practice is *left censoring*. An observation is left censored if the event of interest has already occurred when observation begins. For example, in the study of age at menarche, if a subject enrolls in the study at age 10 and has already experienced menarche, this subject's time is left censored. In the WHAS study, if we begin observation at seven days post admission then subjects who die in the first week are left censored.

A less common form of incomplete observation occurs when the entire study population has experienced the event of interest before the study begins (i.e., subjects have been selected because they have experienced the event of interest). This is sometimes referred to as *length biased sampling* and it must be accounted for in the analysis. An example would be a study of risk factors for time to diagnosis of colorectal cancer among subjects in a cancer registry with this diagnosis. In this study, being in the cancer registry represents a selection process assuring that time to the event is known for each subject. This type of incomplete observation of time is called *right truncation*. Because this type of data occurs relatively infrequently in practice, we do not consider it further in this text. Readers interested in learning more about the analysis of right truncated data are referred to Klein and Moeschberger (2003).

In some practical settings, one may not be able to observe time continuously. For example, in a study of educational interventions to prevent IV drug use, the protocol may specify that subjects, after completion of their "treatment," will be contacted every 3 months for a period of 2 years. In this study, the outcome might be time of first relapse to IV drug use. Because subjects are contacted every 3 months, time is only accurately measured to multiples of 3 months. Given the discrete nature of the observed time variable, it would be inappropriate to use a statistical model that assumed the observed values of time were continuous. Thus, if a subject reports at the 12-month follow-up that she has returned to drug use, we know only that her time is between 9 and 12 months. Data of this type are said to be *interval censored*.

We consider methods for the analysis of right censored data throughout this text because this is the most commonly occurring type of censoring. The next most common forms of incomplete observation are left truncation and interval censoring. Modifications of the methods to handle these mechanisms are discussed in Chapter 7.

Prior to considering any regression modeling, the first step in the analysis of survival time, or for that matter any set of data, should be a thorough univariate analysis. In the absence of censoring and truncation, this analysis would use the techniques covered in an introductory course on statistical methods. The exact combination of statistics used would depend on the application. It might include graphical descriptors such as histograms, box and whisker plots, cumulative percentage distribution polygons or other methods. It would also include a table of descriptive statistics containing point estimates and confidence intervals for the mean, median, standard deviation, and various percentiles of the distribution of survival time. The presence of censored data in the sample complicates the calculations but not the fundamental goal of univariate analysis. In the next chapter we present methods for univariate analysis of right censored survival time.

1.3 EXAMPLE DATA SETS

In addition to the data from the WHAS study presented in Table 1.1, data are available from a larger sample from the entire WHAS study. These data are new to this revision and not the same data used from the WHAS in the first edition. Three additional studies are used throughout the text to illustrate methods and provide data for exercises presented at the end of each chapter. All data may be obtained from the John Wiley & Sons web site,

ftp://ftp.wiley.com/public/sci_tech_med/survival.

They may also be obtained from the web site for statistical services at the University of Massachusetts at Amherst by going to the datasets link and then the section on survival data,

http://www.umass.edu/statdata/statdata.

As noted previously, the data from the WHAS study have been provided to us by Dr. Robert J. Goldberg of the Department of Cardiology at the University of Massachusetts Medical School. The main goal of this study is to describe factors associated with trends over time in the incidence and survival rates following hospital admission for acute myocardial infarction (MI). Data have been collected during 13 one-year periods beginning in 1975 and extending through 2001 on all MI patients admitted to hospitals in the Worcester, Massachusetts Standard Metropolitan Statistical Area. The main data set has information on more than 11,000 admissions.   Several variables that provide us the opportunity to demonstrate and discuss various aspects of modeling time-to-event data were added to the data collection in the later three cohorts. The data in this text were obtained by taking an approximately 23 percent random sample from the cohort years 1997, 1999, and 2001, yielding 500 subjects. This data set is called the WHAS500 study in this text. In addition, only a small subset of the variables from the main study is included in our data set. Dr. Goldberg and his colleagues have published more than 30 papers reporting the results of various analyses from the WHAS.   For an example of a recent publication from the study see Goldberg et al. (2005) as well as Goldberg et. al. (1986, 1988, 1989, 1991, 1993) and Chiriboga et al. (1994).

Table 1.2 describes the subset of variables used, with their codes and values. One should not infer that results reported and/or obtained in exercises in this text are comparable in any way to analyses of the complete data from the WHAS.

Our colleagues, Drs. Jane McCusker, Carol Bigelow and Anne Stoddard, provided a data set used extensively in the first edition of this text. It is a subset of data from the University of Massachusetts AIDS Research Unit (UMARU) IMPACT Study (UIS).   This was a 5-year (1989–1994) collaborative research project (Benjamin F. Lewis, P.I., National Institute on Drug Abuse Grant #R18-DA06151) comprised of two concurrent randomized trials of residential treatment for drug abuse. The purpose of the study was to compare treatment programs of different planned durations designed to reduce drug abuse and to prevent high-risk HIV behavior.   The UIS sought to determine whether alternative residential treatment approaches are variable in effectiveness and whether efficacy depends on planned program duration. These data were used to illustrate model building in the first edition of this book and are being retained for use in the second edition primarily for end of chapter exercises. The small subset of variables from the main study we use in this text is described in Table 1.3.

Because the analyses we report in this text are based on this small subset of variables, the results reported here should not be considered as being in any way comparable to results from the main study. In addition, we have taken the liberty of simplifying the study design by representing the planned duration as short versus long.   Thus, short versus long represents 3 months versus 6 months planned duration at site A, and 6 months versus 12 months planned duration at site B. The time variable considered in this text is defined as the number of days from admission to one of the two sites to self-reported return to drug use. The censoring variable is coded 1 for return to drug or lost to follow-up and 0 otherwise. The

Table 1.2 Description of the Variables Obtained from the Worcester Heart Attack Study (WHAS), 500 Subjects

Variable	Description	Codes / Values
id	Identification Code	1 – 500
age	Age at Hospital Admission	Years
gender	Gender	0 = Male, 1 = Female
hr	Initial Heart Rate	Beats per minute
sysbp	Initial Systolic Blood Pressure	mmHg
diasbp	Initial Diastolic Blood Pressure	mmHg
bmi	Body Mass Index	kg/m^2
cvd	History of Cardiovascular Disease	0 = No, 1 = Yes
afb	Atrial Fibrillation	0 = No, 1 = Yes
sho	Cardiogenic Shock	0 = No, 1 = Yes
chf	Congestive Heart Complications	0 = No, 1 = Yes
av3	Complete Heart Block	0 = No, 1 = Yes
miord	MI Order	0 = First, 1 = Recurrent
mitype	MI Type	0 = non Q-wave, 1 = Q-wave
year	Cohort Year	1 = 1997, 2 = 1999, 3 = 2001
admitdate	Hospital Admission Date	mm/dd/yy
disdate	Hospital Discharge Date	mm/dd/yy
fdate	Date of last Follow Up	mm/dd/yy
los	Length of Hospital Stay	Days between Hospital Discharge and Hospital Admission
dstat	Discharge Status from Hospital	0 = Alive, 1 = Dead
lenfol	Total Length of Follow-up	Days between Date of Last Follow-up and Hospital Admission Date
fstat	Vital Status at Last Follow-up	0 = Alive 1 = Dead

study team felt that a subject who was lost to follow-up was likely to have returned to drug use. The original data have been modified to preserve subject confidentiality.

Cancer clinical trials are a rich source for examples of applications of methods for the analysis of time to event. Willi Sauerbrei and Patrick Royston have graciously provided us with data obtained from the German Breast Cancer Study Group, which they used to illustrate methods for building prognostic models (Sauerbrei and Royston, 1999). In the main study, a total of 720 patients with primary node positive breast cancer were recruited between July 1984, and December 1989, (see Schmoor, Olschweski and Schumacher M. 1996 and Schumacher et al. (1994)). Data used in this text are for 686 subjects with complete data on the covariates in Table 1.4.

Table 1.3 Description of Variables in the UMARU IMPACT Study (UIS), 628 Subjects

Variable	Description	Codes/Values
id	Identification Code	1–628
age	Age at Enrollment	Years
beck	Beck Depression Score at Admission	0.000–54.000
hercoc	Heroin/Cocaine Use During 3 Months Prior to Admission	1 = Heroin & Cocaine 2 = Heroin Only 3 = Cocaine Only 4 = Neither Heroin nor Cocaine
ivhx	IV Drug Use History at Admission	1 = Never 2 = Previous 3 = Recent
ndrugtx	Number of Prior Drug Treatments	0 – 40
race	Subject's Race	0 = White 1 = Other
treat	Treatment Randomization Assignment	0 = Short 1 = Long
site	Treatment Site	0 = A 1 = B
lot	Length of Treatment (Measured from Admission)	Days
time	Time to Return to Drug Use (Measured from Admission)	Days
censor	Returned to Drug Use	1 = Returned to Drug Use 0 = Otherwise

Another clinical trial data set used in this text was provided by the AIDS Clinical Trials Group (ACTG 320). The data come from a double-blind, placebo-controlled trial that compared the three-drug regimen of indinavir (IDV), open label zidovudine (ZDV) or stavudine (d4T), and lamivudine (3TC) with the two-drug regimen of zidovudine or stavudine and lamivudine in HIV-infected patients (Hammer et al., 1997). Patients were eligible for the trial if they had no more than 200 CD4 cells per cubic millimeter and at least three months of prior zidovudine therapy. Randomization was stratified by CD4 cell count at the time of screening. The primary outc ome measure was time to AIDS defining event or death. Because efficacy results met a pre-specified level of significance at an interim analysis, the trial was stopped early. Variables and codes for these data are provided in Table 1.5.

Table 1.4 Description of Variables in the German Breast Cancer Study (GBCS), 686 Subjects

Variable	Description	Codes/Values/ Range
id	Study ID	1 – 686
diagdate	Date of Diagnosis	ddMonthyyyy
recdate	Date of Recurrence Free Survival	ddMonthyyyy
deathdate	Date of Death	ddMonthyyyy
age	Age at Diagnosis	Years
menopause	Menopausal Status	0 = No, 1 = Yes
hormone	Hormone Therapy	0 = No, 1 = Yes
size	Tumor Size	mm
grade	Tumor Grade	1 – 3
nodes	Number of Nodes involved	1 – 51
prog_recp	Number of Progesterone Receptors	1 – 2380
estrg_recp	Number of Estrogen Receptors	1 – 1144
rectime	Time to Recurrence	Days
censrec	Recurrence Censoring	0 = Censored 1 = Recurrence
survtime	Time to Death	Days
censdead	Death Censoring	0 = Censored 1 = Death

EXERCISES

One of the most effective graphical tools that can be employed in regression modeling is a scatter plot of the outcome versus continuous covariates. For example, in linear regression, such a plot can provide guidance as to the plausibility of a linear relationship between the mean of the outcome and the covariate as well as the distribution about the line (i.e., the error component).

1. Using the data from the Worcester Heart Attack Study in Table 1.1, obtain a scatter plot of follow up time versus age. If possible, use the value of the vital status variable as the plotting symbol.
   (a) In what ways is the visual appearance of this plot different from a scatter plot in a typical linear regression setting?
   (b) By eye, draw on the scatter plot from problem 1(a) what you feel is the best regression function for a survival time regression model.

Table 1.5 Description of Variables in the AIDS Clinical Trials Group Study (ACTG 320), 1151 Subjects

Variable	Description	Codes/Values
id	Identification Code	1–1156
time	Time to AIDS diagnosis or death	Days
censor	Event indicator for AIDS defining diagnosis or death	1 = AIDS defining diagnosis or death 0 = Otherwise
time_d	Time to death	Days
censor_d	Event indicator for death (only)	1 = Death 0 = Otherwise
tx	Treatment indicator	1 = Treatment includes IDV 0 = Control group (treatment regimen without IDV)
txgrp	Treatment group indicator	1 = ZDV + 3TC 2 = ZDV + 3TC + IDV 3 = d4T + 3TC 4 = d4T + 3TC + IDV
strat2	CD4 stratum at screening	0 = CD4 ≤ 50 1 = CD4 > 50
sex	Sex	1 = Male 2 = Female
raceth	Race/Ethnicity	1 = White Non-Hispanic 2 = Black Non-Hispanic 3 = Hispanic (regardless of race) 4 = Asian, Pacific Islander 5 = American Indian, Alaskan Native 6 = Other/unknown
ivdrug	IV drug use history	1 = Never 2 = Currently 3 = Previously
hemophil	Hemophiliac	1 = Yes 0 = No
karnof	Karnofsky Performance Scale	100 = Normal; no complaint; no evidence of disease 90 = Normal activity possible; minor signs/symptoms of disease 80 = Normal activity with effort; some signs/symptoms of disease 70 = Cares for self; normal activity/ active work not possible
cd4	Baseline CD4 count (derived from multiple measurements)	Cells/milliliter
priorzdv	Months of prior ZDV use	Months
age	Age at Enrollment	Years

      (c) Is the regression function drawn in 1(b) a straight line? If not, then what function of age would you use to describe it?

      (d) Is it possible to fit this model in your favorite software package with censored data?

2.   What key characteristics about the observations of total length of follow-up must be kept in mind when considering computing sample univariate descriptive statistics?

3.   The investigator of a large clinical trial would like to assess factors that might be associated with drop-out over the course of the trial. Describe what would be the event and which observations would be considered censored for such a study.

CHAPTER 2

Descriptive Methods for Survival Data

2.1 INTRODUCTION

In any applied setting, a statistical analysis should begin with a thoughtful and thorough univariate description of the data. The fundamental building block of this analysis is an estimate of the cumulative distribution function. Typically, little attention is paid to this fact in an introductory course on statistical methods, where directly computed estimators of measures of central tendency and variability are more easily explained and understood. However, routine application of standard formulas for estimators of the sample mean, variance, median, etc., will not yield estimates of the desired parameters when the data include censored or truncated observations. In this situation, we must first obtain an estimator of the cumulative distribution function to obtain statistics that do, in fact, provide estimates the parameters of interest.

In the WHAS100 study described in Chapter 1, we saw that the recorded data are continuous and are only subject to right censoring. Remember that time itself is always continuous, but we must deal with our inability to measure it precisely. The cumulative distribution function of the random variable survival time, denoted T, is the probability that a subject selected at random will have a survival time less than or equal some stated value, t. This is denoted as $F(t) = \Pr(T \leq t)$. The survival function is the probability of observing a survival time greater than some stated value t, denoted $S(t) = \Pr(T > t)$. Note that the sum of the two functions is 1.0 at any value of t (i.e., $S(t) = 1 - F(t)$). In most applied settings, we are typically, though not always, more interested in describing how long the study subjects live, rather than how quickly they die. Thus we focus attention on estimation (and inference) of the survival function.

In this chapter we present methods for: (1) obtaining univariable descriptive statistics for right censored time-to-event data; (2) comparing the survival experience of two or more groups and (3) obtaining estimators of other functions unique to the study of time-to-event data.

16

2.2 ESTIMATING THE SURVIVAL FUNCTION

The Kaplan-Meier estimator of the survival function [Kaplan and Meier (1958)], also called *the product limit* estimator, is the default estimator used by most software packages. This estimator incorporates information from all the observations available, both uncensored (event times) and censored, by considering survival to any point in time as a series of steps defined at the observed survival and censored times. We use the observed data to estimate the conditional probability of confirmed survival at each observed survival time and then multiply them to obtain an estimate of the overall survival function.

To illustrate these ideas, we describe estimation of the survival function in detail using data for four subjects (ID's 1, 56, 85, and 98) from the WHAS100 data and one hypothetical subject with a censored survival time. The data are given in Table 2.1, where the subject identifiers are changed for convenience in the example.

The "steps" are intervals defined by the rank ordering of the observed times. Each interval begins at an observed time and ends just before the next ordered time and is indexed by the rank order of the time point defining its beginning. Subject 1's survival time of 6 days is the shortest and is used to define the interval $I_0 = \{t : 0 \le t < 6\} = [0,6)$. The expression in curly brackets, { }, defines a collection or set of values that includes all times beginning with and including 0 and up to, but not including, 6. This is more concisely denoted using the mathematical notation of a left square bracket to mean the value is included, a right parenthesis to mean the value is not included, and the comma to mean including all values in between. We use both notations in this text. The second rank-ordered time is subject 4's survival time of 14 days. This survival time, in conjunction with the ordered survival time of subject 1, defines interval $I_1 = \{t : 6 \le t < 14\} = [6,14)$. The next ordered time is subject 3's time of 21 days and, in conjunction with subject 4's value of 14 days, defines interval $I_2 = \{t : 14 \le t < 21\} = [14,21)$. The next interval uses subject 2's value of 44 days and the previous value of 21 days and defines interval $I_3 = \{t : 21 \le t < 44\} = [21,44)$. Subject 5's value of 62 days and subject 2's value of 44 days are used to define the next-to-last interval $I_4 = \{t : 44 \le t < 62\} = [44,62)$. The last interval defines the remainder of the possible values of time, $I_5 = \{t : t \ge 62\} = [62,\infty)$.

Table 2.1 Survival Times and Vital Status (Censor=1 for deaths) for Five Subjects from the WHAS Study

Subject	Time	Censor
1	6	1
2	44	1
3	21	0
4	14	1
5	62	1

All subjects were alive at time $t = 0$ and remained so until subject 1 died at 6 days. Thus, the estimate of the probability of surviving through interval I_0 is 1.0. The estimate of the survival function is $\hat{S}(t) = 1.0$ at each t in I_0. Just before time 6 days, five subjects were alive, and at 6 days one subject died. To describe the value of the estimator at 6 days, consider a small interval beginning just before 6 days and ending at 6 days. We designate such an interval as $(6-\delta, 6]$. The estimated conditional probability of dying in this small interval is $1/5$ and the probability of surviving it is $1 - 1/5 = 4/5$. At any specified time point, the number of subjects alive is called the number at risk of dying or simply the number at risk. At time 6 days, this number is denoted as n_1, the 1 referring to the fact that 6 days is the shortest observed time. The number of deaths observed at 6 days is 1 but, with a larger sample, more than one could have been observed. To allow for this, we denote the number of deaths observed at the first failure time as d_1. In this more general notation, the estimated probability of dying in the small interval around 6 is d_1/n_1 and the estimated probability of surviving is $(n_1 - d_1)/n_1$. The probability that a subject survives to 6 days is estimated as the probability of surviving through interval I_0 times the conditional probability of surviving through the small interval around 6. Throughout the discussion of the Kaplan-Meier estimator, the word "conditional" refers to the fact that the probability applies to those who survived to the point or interval under consideration. Because we observed the death at exactly 6 days, this estimated probability would be the same no matter how small a value of δ we use to define the interval around 6 days. Thus, we consider the estimate of the survival probability to be at exactly 6 days. The value of this estimate is $\hat{S}(6) = 1.0 \times (4/5) = 0.8$.

Next we consider estimating the survival function at each time point in the remainder of interval I_1. No other failure times (deaths) were observed, hence the estimated conditional probability of survival through small intervals about every time point in the interval is 1.0. Cumulative multiplication of these values of 1.0 times the estimated survival function leaves it unchanged from its value at 6 days.

The next observed failure time is 14 days. At 14 days the number at risk is $n_2 = 4$ and the number of deaths is $d_2 = 1$. The estimated conditional probability of surviving through a similarly defined small interval at 14 days, $(14-\delta, 14]$, is $(4-1)/4 = 0.75$. By the same argument used at 6 days, the estimate of the survival function at 14 days is the product of the respective estimated conditional probabilities

$$\hat{S}(14) = 1.0 \times (4/5) \times (3/4) = 0.6 .$$

No other failure times were observed in I_2, thus the estimate remains at 0.6 through the interval.

The number at risk at the next observed time, 21 days, is $n_3 = 3$ and the number of deaths is zero because subject 3 was lost to follow-up at 21 days. The estimated conditional probability of survival through a small interval at 21 days is $(3-0)/3 = 1.0$. Again, the estimated survival function is obtained by successive multiplication of the estimated conditional probabilities and is

$$\hat{S}(21) = 1.0 \times (4/5) \times (3/4) \times (3/3) = 0.6 .$$

No failure times were observed in I_3 and the estimate remains the same until the next observed failure time.

The number at risk 44 days after the beginning of the study is $n_4 = 2$ and the number of deaths is $d_4 = 1$. The estimated conditional probability of survival through a small interval at 44 days is $(2-1)/2 = 0.5$. Hence, by the same argument used at 6, 14 and 21 days, the estimated survival function at 44 days after the beginning of the study is

$$\hat{S}(44) = 1.0 \times (4/5) \times (3/4) \times (3/3) \times (1/2) = 0.3 .$$

No other failure times were observed in I_4, thus the estimated survival function remains constant and equal to 0.3 throughout the interval.

The last observed failure time was 62 days. There was a single subject at risk and this subject died, hence $n_5 = 1$ and $d_5 = 1$. The estimated conditional probability of surviving through a small interval at 62 days is $(1-1)/1 = 0.0$. The estimated survival function at 62 days is

$$\hat{S}(62) = 1.0 \times (4/5) \times (3/4) \times (3/3) \times (1/2) \times (0/1) = 0.0 .$$

No subjects were alive after 62 days; thus the estimated survival function is equal to zero after that point.

Through this example, we have demonstrated the essential features of the Kaplan-Meier estimator of the survival function. The estimator at any point in time is obtained by multiplying a sequence of conditional survival probability estimators. Each conditional probability estimator is obtained from the observed number at risk of dying and the observed number of deaths and is equal to "$(n-d)/n$." This estimator allows each subject to contribute information to the calculations as long as he/she is known to be alive. Subjects who die contribute to the number at risk until their time of death, at which point they also contribute to the number of deaths. Subjects who are censored contribute to the number at risk until they are lost to follow-up.

The estimate obtained from the data in Table 2.1 is presented in tabular form in Table 2.2. Computer software packages often present an abbreviated version of this table containing only the observed failure times and estimates of the survival function at these times with the implicit understanding that it is constant between failure times.

A graph is an effective way to display an estimate of a survival function. The graph shown in Figure 2.1 is obtained from the survival function in Table 2.2. The graph shows the decreasing step function defined by the estimated survival function. It drops at the values of the observed failure times and is constant between observed failure times.

In our example, no two subjects shared an observation time, and the longest observed time was a failure. Simple modifications to the method described above are required when either of these conditions is not met. Consider a case where a failure and a censored observation have the same recorded value. We assume that, because the censored observation was known to be alive when last seen, its survival time is longer than the recorded time. Thus a censored subject contributes to the number at risk at the recorded time but is not among those at risk immediately after that time. Along the same lines, suppose we have multiple failures, $d > 0$, at some time t. It is unlikely that each subject died at the exact same time t; however, we were unable to record the data with any more accuracy. One way to break these ties artificially would be to order the d tied failure times randomly by subtracting a tiny random value from each. For example, if we had observed three values at 8 days we could subtract from each failure time the value of a uniformly distributed random variable on the interval (0, 0.01). This would artificially order the values, yet not change their respective positions relative to the rest of the observed failure times. We would estimate the survival function with $d = 1$ at each of the randomly ordered times. The resulting estimate of the survival function at the last of the d times turns out to be identical to that obtained using $(n - d)/n$ as the estimate of the conditional probability of survival for all d considered simultaneously. Thus, as far as the Kaplan-Meier estimator is concerned, it is unnecessary to make adjustments for ties when estimating the survival function. However, if there are extensive numbers of tied failure times, then a discrete time model may be a more appropriate choice (see Chapter 7).

Table 2.2 Estimated Survival Function Computed from the Survival Times for the Four Subjects from the WHAS100 Study and One Hypothetical Subject Shown in Table 2.1

Interval	Conditional probability	$\hat{S}(t)$
$0 \le t < 6$	1.0	1.0
$6 \le t < 14$	$1.0 \times (4/5) = 0.8$	0.8
$14 \le t < 21$	$1.0 \times (4/5) \times (3/4) = 0.6$	0.6
$21 \le t < 44$	$1.0 \times (4/5) \times (3/4) \times (3/3) = 0.6$	0.6
$44 \le t < 62$	$1.0 \times (4/5) \times (3/4) \times (3/3) \times (1/2) = 0.3$	0.3
$t \ge 62$	$1.0 \times (4/5) \times (3/4) \times (3/3) \times (1/2) \times (0/1) = 0$	0.0

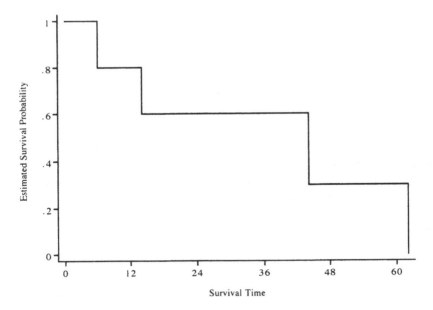

Figure 2.1 Graph of the Kaplan-Meier estimate of the survival function in Table 2.2.

If the last observed time corresponds to a censored observation, then the estimate of the survival function does not go to zero. Its smallest value is that estimated at the last observed survival time. In this case the estimate is considered to be undefined beyond the last observed time. If both censored and non-censored values occur at the longest observed time, then the protocol of assuming that censoring takes place after failures dictates that $(n-d)/n$ is used to estimate the conditional survival probability at this time. The estimated survival function does not go to zero and is undefined after this point. When ties occur, software packages, which provide a tabular listing of the observed survival times and estimated survival function, list the censored observations after the survival time, with the value of the estimated survival function at the survival time.

To use the Kaplan–Meier estimator in other contexts, we need a more general formulation. Assume we have a sample of n independent observations denoted (t_i, c_i), $i = 1, 2, \ldots, n$ of the underlying survival time variable T and the censoring indicator variable C.[1] Assume that, among the n observations, there are $m \leq n$ recorded times of failure and $n - m$ censored values. We denote the rank-ordered survival times as $t_{(1)} < t_{(2)} < \cdots < t_{(m)}$. In this text, when quantities are placed in rank order, we use the same variable notation but place subscripts in parentheses. Let

---

[1] Unless stated otherwise, we assume recorded values of time are continuous and subject only to right censoring.

the number at risk of dying at $t_{(i)}$ be denoted n_i and the observed number of deaths be denoted d_i. The Kaplan–Meier estimator of the survival function at time t is

$$\hat{S}(t) = \prod_{t_{(i)} \le t} \frac{n_i - d_i}{n_i} \qquad (2.1)$$

with the convention that $\hat{S}(t) = 1$ if $t < t_{(1)}$. This formulation differs slightly from that described using the data in Table 2.1 in that intervals defined by censored observations are not considered. We saw in the example that conditional survival probabilities are equal to one at censored observations and that the estimate of the survival function is unchanged from the value at the previous survival time. Thus the general formula in (2.1) uses only the points at which the value of the estimator changes.

Figure 2.2 presents the graph of the Kaplan–Meier estimate of the survival function in (2.1), using all 100 subjects in WHAS100 data where follow up time is shown in years rather than days. The data, along with calculations for the beginning and end of the survival function, are presented in Table 2.3. The columns in Table 2.3 present the time interval, the number at risk of dying (n), the number of deaths (d), the number of subjects lost to follow up (i.e., censored) (c),

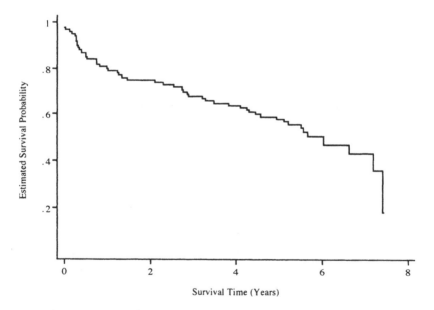

Figure 2.2 Kaplan-Meier estimate of the survival function for the WHAS100 data.

Table 2.3 Partial Calculations for the Kaplan–Meier Estimate Shown in Figure 2.2

Interval	n	d	c	$(n-d)/n$	$\hat{S}$
[0,6)	100	0	0	1.0	1.000
[6,14)	100	2	0	0.98	0.980
[14,44)	98	1	0	0.9899	0.970
[44,62)	97	1	0	0.9897	0.960
[62,89)	96		0	0.9896	0.950
⋮	⋮	⋮	⋮		⋮
[2641, 2710)	3	0	1	1.0	0.361
[2710, 2719)	2	1	0	0.5	0.180
[2719, 2719]	1	0	1	1.0	0.180

the estimate of the conditional survival probability $[(n-d)/n]$, and the estimate of the survival function, $\hat{S}(t)$. All quantities are evaluated at the time point defined by the end of the previous interval and the beginning of the current interval.

The first observed survival time is 6 days; thus the value of the estimated survival function at each point in the interval [0,6) is 1.0. At 6 days there were 100 subjects at risk. Of these, 2 died and 0 were lost to follow-up (censored), yielding an estimate of the conditional survival probability of $0.98 = (100-2)/100$. The estimate of the survival function at 6 days is $0.98 = (1.0) \times 0.98$. The estimate remains at this value at each point in the interval [6,14). At the next observed survival time, 14 days, there were 98 subjects at risk because 2 died and 0 were lost to follow-up at 6 days. At 14 days, 1 subject died and 0 were lost to follow-up; thus the estimate of the conditional survival probability is $0.9899 = (98-1)/98$. The estimate of the survival function is obtained as the product of the value of the survival function just prior to 14 days and the conditional survival probability at 14 days and is $0.97 = 0.98 \times 0.9899$. The estimate remains at this value throughout the interval [14,44). At the next observed survival time, 44 days, there were 97 subjects at risk, because 1 died and 0 were censored at 14 days. The estimate of the conditional survival probability is $0.9897 = (97-1)/97$ and the estimate of the survival function is $0.96 = 0.97 \times 0.9897$. The estimate remains at this value until the next observed survival time, 62 days, at which time 96 subjects are at risk. This process continues, sequentially, considering each observed survival time, until the last observed survival time, which was 2710 days or 7.42 years. At that time, 2 subjects were at risk, 1 died, and 0 were censored. The estimate of the conditional survival probability is $0.5 = (2-1)/2$. The estimate of the survival function is $0.180 = 0.5 \times 0.361$. The largest observed time is 2719 days or 7.44 years, when 1 subject remained at risk and was censored. Thus, the estimate of the conditional survival probability is $1.0 = (1-0)/1$ and the estimate of the survival function remains at the value 0.180. The function is undefined beyond 2719 days, which is denoted in Table 2.3 by recording the last interval as [2719, 2719].

When we have a large study whose mortality experience is presented in calendar time units (such as quarterly, semi-annually, etc.), the life-table estimator of the survival function may be used as an alternative to the Kaplan–Meier estimator. The life-table estimator has been used for more than 100 years to describe human mortality experience and is among the earliest examples of the application of statistical methods. It will not play a large role in the analysis of survival data in this text, but we present it because of its historical importance and the fact that it is a grouped-data analog of the Kaplan–Meier estimator. More detail on the various types of life-table estimators may be found in Lee and Wang (2003).

In some applied settings, the data may be quite extensive, with sample sizes in the many hundreds or thousands of subjects. For example, the entire WHAS study has more than 11,000 subjects. In these situations, it can be quite cumbersome to tabulate or graph the Kaplan–Meier estimator of the survival function. In a sense, the problem faced is similar to one addressed in a first course on statistical methods: how best to reduce the volume of data but not the statistical information that can be gleaned from it. To this end the histogram is usually introduced as an estimator of the density function and the resulting cumulative percentage distribution polygon as an estimator of the cumulative distribution function. This process could be reversed. That is, we might first derive the estimator of the cumulative distribution and, afterwards, compute the histogram as a function of the cumulative distribution. When the data contain censored observations, using the second approach and deriving an estimator of the survival function (instead of the cumulative distribution function) is the more feasible option. The first step is to define the intervals used to group the data. The goal in the choice of intervals is the same as for the construction of a histogram—the intervals should be clinically meaningful, yield an adequate description of the data and, if convenient, be of equal width. However, the most meaningful unit will likely be some multiple of a year.

Once a set of intervals has been chosen, the construction of the estimator follows the basic idea used for the Kaplan–Meier estimator. Suppose we decide to use 6-month intervals. A typical interval will be of the form $[t, t+6)$. As before,

Table 2.4 Life-Table Estimator of the Survival Function for the WHAS100 data

Interval	Enter	Die	Censored	$\hat{S}$
$[0,1)$	100	20	0	0.80
$[1,2)$	80	5	0	0.75
$[2,3)$	75	7	0	0.68
$[3,4)$	68	4	0	0.64
$[4,5)$	64	6	0	0.58
$[5,6)$	58	5	38	0.51
$[6,7)$	15	2	1	0.44
$[7,8)$	12	2	10	0.31

let n denote the number of subjects at risk of dying at time t. These subjects are often described as the number who enter the interval alive. As we follow these subjects across the interval, d subjects have survival times and c subjects have censored times in this interval. Thus, not all subjects were at risk of dying for the entire interval. A modification typically employed is to reduce the size of the risk set by one-half of those censored in the interval. The rationale behind this adjustment is that, if we assume the censored observations were uniformly distributed over the interval, then the average size of the risk set in the interval is $n-(c/2)$. This average risk set size is used to calculate the estimate of the conditional   probability   of   survival   through   the   interval   as $(n-(c/2)-d)/(n-(c/2))$. These estimates of the conditional probabilities are multiplied to obtain the life-table estimator of the survival function.

The life-table estimator of the survival function for the WHAS100 data using 1-year intervals is shown in Table 2.4. The estimated value of the survival function in the first interval is $0.80 = (100-(0/2)-20)/(100-(0/2))$. We note that, because no observations were censored in the first interval, the life table estimate is the same as the Kaplan-Meier estimate. The first interval with censored data is in

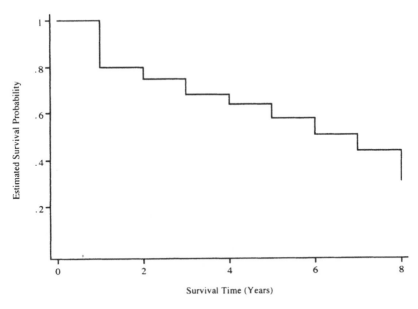

Figure 2.3 Step function representation of life-table estimate of the survival function for the WHAS100 data in Table 2.4.

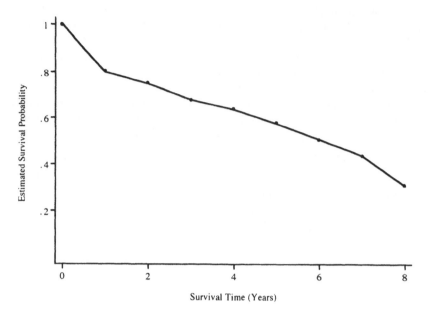

Figure 2.4 Polygon representation of life-table estimate of the survival function for the WHAS100 data in Table 2.4.

the sixth year of follow up when 58 enter at risk, 38 are censored and 5 die. The estimate in the interval $[5, 6)$ is

$$0.505 = 0.51 \times \left(58 - (38/2) - 5\right)\big/\left(58 - (38/2)\right).$$

The remaining values are calculated in a similar fashion.

When we graph the estimate, we have to decide how to represent the actual values. Consider the first interval $[0, 1)$, where the value of the estimated survival function is reported in Table 2.4 as 0.80. If, as in Figure 2.3, we were to represent the graph as a step function, then this interval would be represented by a horizontal straight line of height 1 until 1 year, when it would drop to 0.80. Other intervals would be represented in a similar manner. An alternative representation, used by some software packages, is a polygon connecting the value of the estimator drawn at the end of the interval. The first interval would be represented by a point of height 0.80 plotted at 1 year, the second by a point of height 0.75 at 2 years, the third by a point of height 0.68 at 3 years, and so on. Straight lines connect these points. The polygon better represents the assumed underlying continuous distribution of survival time. Some, but not all, programs will plot a point equal to 1.0 at time zero because, by definition, that is the value of the survival function at zero. This point is then connected to the point representing the first interval. The polygonal representation of the life-table estimator from Table 2.4 is shown in

Table 2.4 is shown in Figure 2.4. One problem with using a polygon is that it imparts an artificial smoothness to the estimate and, as such, we prefer the step function. Also as a grouped-data statistic the life table estimator is not as precise as the Kaplan–Meier estimator, since the latter uses the individual values.

In the next section we discuss using the Kaplan-Meier estimator to obtain point and interval estimators of descriptive statistics.

2.3   USING THE ESTIMATED SURVIVAL FUNCTION

In Section 2.2, we described in detail how to calculate the Kaplan–Meier and lifetable estimators of the survival function with little discussion of how to interpret the resulting estimate or how it may be used to derive point estimates of quantiles of the distribution. One of the biggest challenges in survival analysis is becoming accustomed to using the survival function as a descriptive statistic. This function describes the complement of what we typically describe in a set of data. The change from thinking about the percentage of observations less than a value to the percentage greater than that value becomes easier with practice.

The survival function estimate in Figure 2.2 descends sharply for approximately the first year and then descends slowly for the second year. The descent is then even more gradual and approximately constant from year 2 to year 6, at which point only 15 of the original 100 subjects are still being followed. From years 6 to 7.5, the larger drops in the steps in the figure are due to the small number of subjects still at risk and the fact that many of these have censored follow up times. The initial steep descent is a result of a relatively higher mortality rate in the first year following an MI. The mortality rate then decreases and remains at about the same level for the remainder of the follow up period in these 100 subjects. The minimum value of the survival function is not zero because the largest observed time was a censored observation. The shape of the curve depends on the observed survival times and the proportion of censored observations. If many subjects in the WHAS100 study had longer survival times with the same pattern of censored observations, then the curve would descend slowly at first and then more rapidly until the minimum is reached. If the survival times were more evenly distributed over the 7.5 years, then the curve would descend at a constant rate to its minimum value. The pattern of enrollment in a follow-up study can influence the shape of the curve. A study with a 2-year enrollment period and 5 years overall length with many late entries is likely to have more censored observations and thus a different looking estimated survival function than the same study with many early entries. Many factors influence the shape of the estimator of the survival function, and thus it is difficult to make accurate statements about what a "typical" estimated survival function will look like.

In most, if not all, applied settings, we will need a confidence interval estimate of the survival function as well as point and confidence interval estimates of key quantiles of the survival time distribution. We begin by discussing confidence interval estimation of the survival function itself.

Several different approaches may be taken to derive an estimator for the variance of the Kaplan–Meier estimator. We derive it from a technique that is often referred to as the *delta method* and is based on a first-order Taylor series expansion. This method is presented in general terms in Appendix 1. The Kaplan–Meier estimator at any time t may be viewed as a product of proportions. Rather than derive a variance estimator of this product, we derive one for its log because the variance of a sum is easier to calculate than the variance of a product. The log of the Kaplan–Meier estimator is

$$\ln\left(\hat{S}(t)\right) = \sum_{t_{(i)} \le t} \ln\left(\frac{n_i - d_i}{n_i}\right)$$
$$= \sum_{t_{(i)} \le t} \ln\left(\hat{p}_i\right),$$

where

$$\hat{p}_i = \left(n_i - d_i\right)/n_i .$$

If we consider the observations in the risk set at time $t_{(i)}$ to be independent Bernoulli observations with constant probability, then $\hat{p}_i$ is an estimator of this probability and an estimator of its variance is the familiar expression $\left(\hat{p}_i(1 - \hat{p}_i)\right)/n_i$. As shown in Appendix 1, the variance of the log of a variable, X, is approximately

$$\text{Var}\left[\ln(X)\right] \cong \frac{1}{\mu_X^2} \sigma_X^2, \tag{2.2}$$

where the mean and variance of X are denoted by μ_X and σ_X^2, respectively. An estimator for the variance is obtained by replacing μ_X and σ_X^2 in (2.2) with estimators of their respective values. Applying this result to $\ln\left(\hat{p}_i\right)$ yields the estimator

$$\widehat{\text{Var}}\left[\ln(\hat{p}_i)\right] \cong \frac{1}{\hat{p}_i^2} \frac{\hat{p}_i(1 - \hat{p}_i)}{n_i}$$
$$\cong \frac{d_i}{n_i(n_i - d_i)} .$$

If we assume that observations at each time are independent, then the estimator of the variance of the log of the survival function is

$$\hat{\text{Var}}\left[\ln\left(\hat{S}(t)\right)\right] = \sum_{t_{(i)} \leq t} \hat{\text{Var}}\left[\ln\left(\hat{p}_i\right)\right]$$

$$= \sum_{t_{(i)} \leq t} \frac{d_i}{n_i(n_i - d_i)} . \tag{2.3}$$

An estimator of the variance of the survival function is obtained by another application of the delta method shown in Appendix 1. This time an approximation is applied to find the variance of an exponentiated variable and is

$$\text{Var}(e^X) \cong \left(e^{\mu_X}\right)^2 \sigma_X^2 . \tag{2.4}$$

Using the fact that $\hat{S}(t) = \exp\left\{\ln\left[\hat{S}(t)\right]\right\}$, if we let X denote $\ln\left[\hat{S}(t)\right]$, σ_X^2 represent the variance estimator in (2.3) and if we approximate μ_X by $\ln\left[\hat{S}(t)\right]$ in expression (2.4) then we obtain Greenwood's formula [Greenwood (1926)] for the variance of the survival function

$$\hat{\text{Var}}\left(\hat{S}(t)\right) = \left(\hat{S}(t)\right)^2 \sum_{t_{(i)} \leq t} \frac{d_i}{n_i(n_i - d_i)} . \tag{2.5}$$

The method shown to derive the estimator in (2.5) is, in some sense, the "traditional" approach in that it may be found in most textbooks on survival analysis published prior to 1990. In contrast, the texts by Fleming and Harrington (1991) and Andersen, Borgan, Gill and Keiding (1993) consolidate a large number of results derived from applications of theory based on counting processes and martingales. This theory is well beyond the scope of this text, but we mention it here as it has allowed development of many useful tools and techniques for the analysis of survival time data. The current thrust in the development of software is based on the counting process paradigm because its methods and tools may be used to analyze, in a relatively uncomplicated manner, some rather complex problems. The estimator in (2.5) may also be obtained from the counting process approach.

The counting process approach to the analysis of survival time plays a central role in many of the methods discussed in this text. A brief presentation of the central ideas behind the counting process formulation of survival analysis is given in Appendix 2. We will use results from this theory to provide justification for estimators, confidence interval estimators and hypothesis testing methods.

After obtaining the estimated survival function, we may wish to obtain pointwise confidence interval estimates. The counting process theory has been used to prove that the Kaplan–Meier estimator and functions of it are asymptotically normally distributed [Kalbfleisch and Prentice (2002, Section 5.6), Andersen, Borgan, Gill and Keiding (1993, Chapter IV) or Fleming and Harrington (1991, Chapter 6)]. Thus, we may obtain pointwise confidence interval estimates for the survival function or functions thereof by adding and subtracting the product of the estimated standard error times a quantile of the standard normal distribution. We could apply this theory directly to the Kaplan–Meier estimator using the variance estimator in (2.5). However, this approach could easily lead to confidence interval endpoints less than zero or greater than one. In addition, the assumption of normality implicit in the use of the procedure may not hold for the small to moderate sample sizes often seen in typical problems. To address these problems, Kalbfleisch and Prentice (2002, page 18) suggest that confidence interval estimation should be based on the function $\ln\left\{-\ln\left[\hat{S}(t)\right]\right\}$, called the *log-log survival function*. One advantage of this function over the survival function is that its possible range is from minus to plus infinity. The expression for the variance of the log-log survival function is obtained from a second application of the delta method for a log-transformed variable shown in (2.2). The estimator of the variance of the log-log survival function is

$$\hat{\text{Var}}\left\{\ln\left[-\ln\left(\hat{S}(t)\right)\right]\right\} = \frac{1}{\left[\ln\left(\hat{S}(t)\right)\right]^2} \sum_{t_{(i)} \leq t} \frac{d_i}{n_i(n_i - d_i)}. \tag{2.6}$$

The endpoints of a $100(1-\alpha)$ percent confidence interval for the log-log survival function are given by the expression

$$\ln\left[-\ln\left(\hat{S}(t)\right)\right] \pm z_{1-\alpha/2}\hat{\text{SE}}\left\{\ln\left[-\ln\left(\hat{S}(t)\right)\right]\right\}, \tag{2.7}$$

where $z_{1-\alpha/2}$ is the upper $\alpha/2$ percentile of the standard normal distribution and $\hat{\text{SE}}(\cdot)$ represents the estimated standard error of the argument, which in this case, is the positive square root of (2.6). If we denote the lower and upper endpoints of this confidence interval as $\hat{c}_l$ and $\hat{c}_u$, it follows that the lower and upper endpoints of the confidence interval for the survival function are, respectively

$$\exp\left[-\exp(\hat{c}_u)\right] \text{ and } \exp\left[-\exp(\hat{c}_l)\right]. \tag{2.8}$$

That is, the lower endpoint from (2.7) yields the upper endpoint in (2.8). These are the endpoints reported by most, if not all, software packages for each observed survival time. The confidence interval is valid only for values of time over which the Kaplan–Meier estimator is defined, which is basically the observed range of survival times. Borgan and Leistøl (1990) studied this confidence interval and found that it performed well for sample sizes as small as 25 with up to 50 percent right-censored observations.

Figure 2.5 presents the Kaplan–Meier estimator of the survival function for the WHAS100 study and the upper and lower pointwise 95 percent confidence bands computed using (2.8). The endpoints of the pointwise confidence intervals are connected to form a "confidence band." (Recall that for a collection of individual 95 percent confidence interval estimates, the probability that they all contain their respective parameters is much less than 95 percent.) An alternative presentation used by some software packages connects the endpoints of the confidence intervals with vertical lines. This is useful for small data sets, but for large data sets, the resulting graph becomes cluttered with too many lines, and we lose the visual conciseness seen in Figure 2.5. This figure demonstrates some of the properties of the log-log-based confidence interval estimator. The intervals are skewed for large and, though harder to see in Figure 2.5, small values of the estimated survival function and are fairly symmetric around 0.5. The direction of skewness is opposite for the two tails, toward zero for values of the estimated survival function near one and toward one for values near zero. In all cases, the endpoints lie between zero and one.

As we noted, the rationale for basing confidence intervals on the log-log transformation of the survival function is that its possible range is minus to plus infinity,

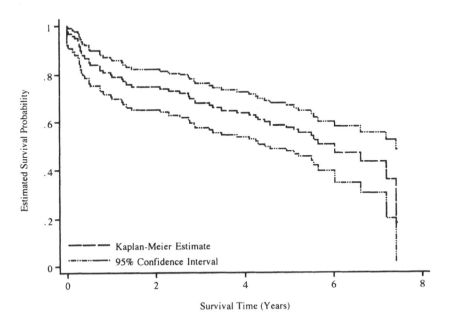

Figure 2.5 Kaplan-Meier estimate and pointwise 95 percent confidence intervals of the survival function for the WHAS100 data.

thus agreeing with that of a normal distribution and also assuring that the limits lie between zero and one. Other transformations have been suggested, and several of these are available in the SAS statistical package version 9 and higher. For comparison purposes, we show in Figure 2.6 plots of the confidence limits based on the log-log transformation, $\ln\left\{-\ln\left[\hat{S}(t)\right]\right\}$, the log transformation, $\ln\left[\hat{S}(t)\right]$, the logit transformation, $\ln\left\{\hat{S}(t)\big/\left[1-\hat{S}(t)\right]\right\}$ and the arcsine transformation, $\arcsin\left[\sqrt{\hat{S}(t)}\right]$. The confidence bands in Figure 2.6 are all quite close to each other over the first 6 years of follow up. Between 6 and 7.5 years, when the sizes of the risk sets become quite small, the limits based on the arcsine transformation are noticeably wider than the others, thus suggesting that: (1) the arcsine transformation is not recommended for use with small risk sets and (2) there is little practical difference between confidence bands of the other three transformations. Hence if a software package's default is one of these, there is little practical reason the switch to another transformation.

Simultaneous confidence bands for the entire survival function are not as readily available as the pointwise estimates, because they require percentiles for a

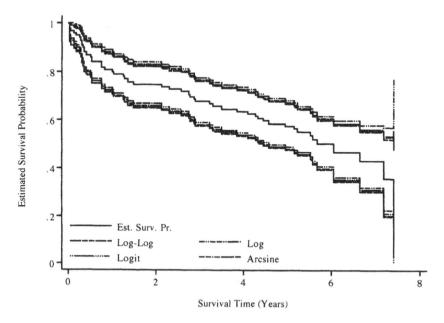

Figure 2.6 Kaplan-Meier estimate and pointwise 95 percent confidence intervals based on the log-log, log, logit and arcsine transformations of the survival function for the WHAS100 data.

statistical distribution not typically computed by software packages. The confidence band proposed by Hall and Wellner (1980) is discussed in some detail in Andersen, Borgan, Gill and Keiding (1993) and Fleming and Harrington (1991). It is also discussed in Marubini and Valsecchi (1995). The Hall and Wellner limits may be obtained in the SAS version 9 software package. To assist users of other packages, we include a table of percentiles obtained from Hall and Wellner (1980) in Appendix 3. Given the tabled percentiles, confidence bands based on the estimated survival function itself, or its log-log transformation, are not difficult to calculate. Borgan and Leistøl (1990) show that the performance of the Hall and Wellner confidence bands is comparable for both functions (survival function and log-log transformation) and is adequate for samples as small as 25 with up to 50 percent censoring. To maintain consistency with the pointwise intervals calculated in (2.8), which are based on the log-log transformation, we present the Hall and Wellner bands for the transformed function. Hall and Wellner, as well as Borgan and Leistøl, recommend that these confidence bands be restricted to values of time smaller than or equal to the largest observed survival time, i.e., the largest non-censored value of time denoted $t_{(m)}$. The endpoints of the $100(1-\alpha)$ percent confidence bands in the interval $[0, t_{(m)}]$ for the log-log transformation are

$$\ln\left[-\ln\left(\hat{S}(t)\right)\right] \pm H_{\hat{a},\alpha} \frac{\left(1 + n\hat{\sigma}^2(t)\right)}{\sqrt{n}\left|\ln\left(\hat{S}(t)\right)\right|}, \qquad (2.9)$$

where

$$\hat{\sigma}^2(t) = \sum_{t_{(i)} \le t} \frac{d_i}{n_i(n_i - d_i)},$$

the estimator of the variance of the log of the Kaplan–Meier estimator from (2.3), and $H_{\hat{a},\alpha}$ is a percentile from Appendix 3, where

$$\hat{a} = n\hat{\sigma}^2(t_{(m)}) / \left[1 + n\hat{\sigma}^2(t_{(m)})\right].$$

If we denote the lower and upper endpoints of this confidence band as $\hat{b}_l$ and $\hat{b}_u$, then the lower and upper endpoints of the confidence band for the survival function are

$$\exp\left[-\exp\left(\hat{b}_u\right)\right] \text{ and } \exp\left[-\exp\left(\hat{b}_l\right)\right]. \qquad (2.10)$$

To obtain the bands for the survival function from the WHAS100 study, we note that the largest observed survival time is 2710 days or 7.42 years and

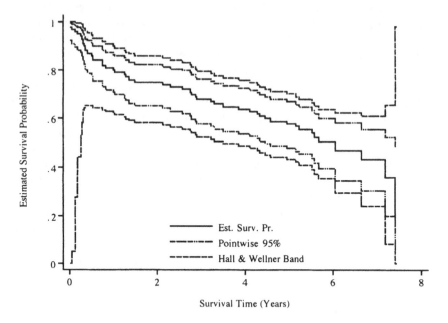

Figure 2.7 Kaplan–Meier estimate, pointwise 95% confidence intervals, and Hall and Wellner 95% confidence bands for the survival function for the WHAS100 study.

$\hat{\sigma}^2(2710) = 0.557$. Most software packages will provide values of either the estimated variance of the log of the Kaplan–Meier estimator or the Greenwood estimator of the variance of the survival function. The values of $\hat{\sigma}^2(t)$ are easily obtained by dividing the Greenwood estimator by the square of the Kaplan–Meier estimator. To obtain the percentile from Appendix 3 we compute

$$\hat{a} = (100 \times 0.557)/(1 + 100 \times 0.557) = 0.98$$

and note that, since both $H_{0.9,0.95}$ and $H_{1.0,0.95}$ equal 1.358, linear interpolation of tabled values is not necessary and we use 1.358. In cases when $\hat{a} < 0.9$, linear interpolation between two tabled values may be required to obtain the most accurate value. To obtain the confidence bands, we compute the endpoints in (2.9) and (2.10) for each observed event time. We can ignore censored times because the estimated survival function and its variance are constant between observed failure times. These endpoints may be plotted, along with the estimated survival function, restricting the plot to the interval |0, 7.425|. This plot is shown in Figure 2.7; which also shows the increased width of the confidence bands relative to the pointwise confidence intervals. The increased width is needed to assure that the probability is 95 percent that each of the individual 95 percent confidence interval estimates simultaneously covers its respective parameter. In particular, we note the lack of precision in the band for times at the maximum of 7.425 years. The somewhat anomalous result of wide bands at the first two observed survival times, when we know that the estimated survival function must be just slightly less than 1.0, is due to the fact that in (2.9) the absolute value of $\ln\left[\hat{S}(t)\right]$ is quite small relative to the value of $\hat{\sigma}^2(t)$.

The estimated survival function, its confidence intervals and perhaps its confidence bands can provide a useful descriptive measure of the overall survival experience. However, it is often useful to supplement the presentation with point and interval estimates of key quantiles. The estimated survival function may be used to estimate quantiles of the survival time distribution in the same way that the estimated cumulative distribution of height or weight may be used to estimate quantiles of its distribution. This may be done graphically, and the graphical procedure can be codified into a formula for analytic calculations based on the tabular form of the estimate.

The quantiles most frequently reported by software packages are the three quartiles of the survival time distribution. To obtain graphical estimates, begin on the survival probability or percentage (*y*) axis at the quartile of interest and draw a horizontal line until it first touches the estimated survival function. A vertical line

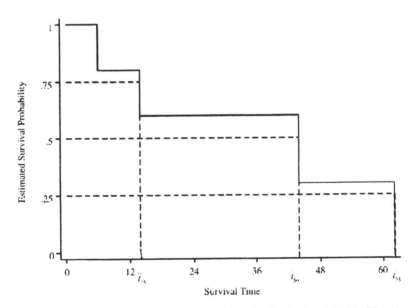

Figure 2.8 Kaplan–Meier estimate of the survival function for the data in Table 2.1 and graphically determined estimates of the quartiles.

is drawn down to the time axis to obtain the estimated quartile. For the estimate to be finite, the horizontal line must hit the survival function. Thus, the minimum possible estimated quantile that has a finite value is the minimum of the estimated survival function, and only quantiles within the observed range of the estimated survival function may be estimated. For example, if the range was from 1.0 to 0.38 then we could estimate the 75th and 50th percentiles but not the 25th percentile. Graphically determined estimates of the three quartiles, denoted $\hat{t}_{75}$, $\hat{t}_{50}$ and $\hat{t}_{25}$, based on the Kaplan–Meier estimate of the survival function in Figure 2.1 are shown in Figure 2.8.

The graphical method is easy to use, but it is not especially precise. The method may be described in a formula, from which a more accurate numerical value may be determined from a tabular presentation of the estimated survival function. We illustrate the method by estimating the median or second quartile, $\hat{t}_{50}$, and we then generalize it into a formula that may be used for any quantile. We see that the horizontal dashed line hits the survival function at the riser connecting steps ending somewhere between 36 and 48 months. By referring back to Table 2.2, we see that this is at survival time 44 months. Thus the estimated median survival time in this example is $\hat{t}_{50} = 44$. A formula that describes this estimator is

$$\hat{t}_{50} = \min\{t : \hat{S}(t) \leq 0.50\} \,.$$

In words, the formula says to proceed as if you are walking up a set of stairs from the right to the riser where the horizontal line hits. The estimate is the time value defining the left-most point of the step on which you are standing. If we assume that the riser is attached at the top and bottom, then the description also works when the horizontal line hits one of the steps. The estimate is, again, the value of time defining the left-most point of the step. In general, the estimate of the pth percentile is

$$\hat{t}_{p} = \min\{t : \hat{S}(t) \leq (p/100)\} \,. \tag{2.11}$$

The estimates of the other quartiles from Table 2.2 are $\hat{t}_{75} = 14$ and $\hat{t}_{25} = 62$.

For the full WHAS100 data set, the estimates of the three quartiles are (in days) $\hat{t}_{75} = 538$, $\hat{t}_{50} = 2201$, and $\hat{t}_{25} = 2710$. Expressed in years, the estimates are $\hat{t}_{75} = 1.47$, $\hat{t}_{50} = 6.03$, and $\hat{t}_{25} = 7.42$. To interpret these values, we estimate that 75 percent will live at least 538 days (or 1.47 years), half are estimated to live at least 2201 days (or 6.03 years), and only 25 percent are estimated to live at least 2710 days (or 7.42 years).

We have defined the quantiles in terms of the proportion or percentage surviving more than the stated values. Many software packages provide estimates of the proportion not surviving. For example, SAS and STATA label the value of 538 days as the 25th percentile and the value of 2710 days as the 75th percentile. It all depends on whether one wishes to count the living or the dead.

The estimator in (2.11) is used by most software packages. However some packages, for example SAS, use an estimator that yields a different value when $\hat{S}(t) = p$ for an observed survival time. In this case the estimator in (2.11) is equal to the survival time defining the step. The estimated survival function remains constant and equal to p until the next largest observed survival time. Because each value of time between these two times could technically be an estimator of t_p the two survival times are averaged. As an example, in the WHAS100 data $\hat{S}(1.473) = 0.75$, $\hat{S}(2.119) = 0.74$ and the estimate reported by SAS is the average of the two, $1.796 = (1.473 + 2.119)/2$.

A confidence interval estimate for the quantiles can add further understanding about possible values for the parameter being estimated. Approximate confidence intervals may be obtained by appealing to the theory that, for large samples, the quantile estimator is normally distributed with mean equal to the quantile being estimated. An estimator of the variance of this distribution may be obtained from an application of the delta method, as outlined in Collett (2003) and discussed in greater detail using the counting process approach in Andersen, Borgan, Gill and Keiding (1993). The suggested estimator for the variance of the estimator of the pth percentile is

$$\hat{\text{Var}}\left(\hat{t}_p\right) = \frac{\hat{\text{Var}}\left(\hat{S}(\hat{t}_p)\right)}{\left[\hat{f}(\hat{t}_p)\right]^2}.$$

(2.12)

The numerator of (2.12) is Greenwood's estimator and the denominator is an estimator of the density function of the distribution of survival time. The estimator of the density function used by many software packages is

$$\hat{f}(\hat{t}_p) = \frac{\hat{S}(\hat{u}_p) - \hat{S}(\hat{l}_p)}{\hat{l}_p - \hat{u}_p}.$$

(2.13)

The values $\hat{u}_p$ and $\hat{l}_p$ are chosen such that $\hat{u}_p < \hat{t}_p < \hat{l}_p$ and most often are obtained from the equations shown below:

$$\hat{u}_p = \max\left\{t : \hat{S}(t) \geq (p/100) + 0.05\right\}$$

and

(2.14)

$$\hat{l}_p = \min\left\{t : \hat{S}(t) \leq (p/100) - 0.05\right\}.$$

While values other than 0.05 could have been used in (2.14), 0.05 seems to work well in practice and is used by a number of statistical packages. The endpoints of a $100(1-\alpha)$ percentage confidence interval are

$$\hat{t}_p \pm z_{1-\alpha/2}\hat{SE}(\hat{t}_p),\qquad(2.15)$$

where $\hat{SE}(\hat{t}_p) = \sqrt{\hat{Var}(\hat{t}_p)}$.

Evaluation of (2.12) through (2.15) is most easily illustrated with an example. In the WHAS100 study, the estimated median survival time is $\hat{t}_{50} = 2201$ days or 6.03 years. At this point, we may continue to use days as the unit of time or to switch to years (days/365.25). Because years are generally easier to understand than days, we continue the presentation using years as the unit of time. The value of $\hat{u}_{50}$ is the largest value of time, t, such that $\hat{S}(t) \geq 0.5 + 0.05 = 0.55$. After sorting on survival time and listing the values of the Kaplan–Meier estimator, we find that $\hat{S}(5.221) = 0.5567$ and $\hat{S}(5.509) = 0.5404$, hence $\hat{u}_{50} = 5.221$. The value of $\hat{l}_{50}$ is the smallest value of time, t, such that $\hat{S}(t) \leq 0.5 - 0.05 = 0.45$. From the same listing, we find that $\hat{S}(6.026) = 0.4687$ and $\hat{S}(6.628) = 0.4327$, hence $\hat{l}_{50} = 6.628$. Thus the estimate of the density function in (2.13) is

$$\hat{f}(\hat{t}_{50}) = \frac{\hat{S}(5.221) - \hat{S}(6.628)}{6.628 - 5.221} = \frac{0.5567 - 0.4327}{6.628 - 5.221} = 0.0881.$$

The value of Greenwood's estimator at $t = 6.03$ years is

$$\hat{Var}\left(\hat{S}(6.03)\right) = 0.00368$$

and evaluation of (2.12) yields

$$\hat{Var}\left(\hat{t}_{50}\right) = \frac{0.00368}{[0.0881]^2} = 0.4741.$$

The end points of the 95 percent confidence interval for median survival time are

$$6.03 \pm 1.96 \times \sqrt{0.4741} = (4.68, 7.38).$$

Table 2.5 presents the estimated survival times for the quartiles, their estimated

Table 2.5 Estimated Quartiles, Estimated Standard Errors, and 95% Confidence Interval Estimates for Survival Time (years) in the WHAS100 Study

Quantile	Estimate	Std. Err.	95% CIE
75	1.47	0.77	. , 2.98
50	6.03	0.69	4.68, 7.38
25	7.42	0.18	7.08, .

standard errors, and 95 percent confidence intervals. The results illustrate some of the strengths as well as the limitations of these confidence intervals. The right-hand endpoint of the confidence interval from (2.15) for the 25th percentile of the survival time distribution is approximately 7.77, which lies outside the range of times where the Kaplan-Meier estimator is defined. In this case, it is common practice to report the value as undefined, as indicated by a "." in Table 2.5. The left-hand endpoint of the confidence interval from (2.15) for the 75th percentile of the survival distribution is approximately -0.04, again outside the observed range of time. Again we report this value as undefined. One might be tempted to report the lower endpoint as 0.0. From a practical point of view, this makes no sense as it implies that 25 percent of the study population could experience the event before the study even begins. For this reason, it is better to leave it as undefined. The conclusion we draw from these two examples are that the confidence intervals based on (2.14) may not yield well-defined intervals when the estimated survival function does not go well below the smallest quantile of the survival distribution we wish to estimate. Also if the estimated survival distribution drops too quickly, lower confidence limits for larger quantiles of the distribution may not be well determined. The estimate of the median survival time illustrates the conditions that must occur to obtain both upper and lower endpoints, e.g., the point estimate of the quantile must lie well within the observed range of the estimated survival distribution.

The confidence interval estimator in (2.15) requires that we compute an estimator of the density function at the estimator of the quantile. Brookmeyer and Crowley (1982) proposed an alternative method that does not require estimation of the density function [this is discussed in general terms in Andersen, Borgan, Gill and Keiding (1993)]. In this method, the confidence interval for a quantile consists of the values t such that

$$z_{t_p} = \frac{\left| \ln\left\{ -\ln\left[\hat{S}(t) \right] \right\} - \ln\left\{ -\ln\left[(p/100) \right] \right\} \right|}{\widehat{SE}\left(\ln\left\{ -\ln\left[\hat{S}(t) \right] \right\} \right)} \le z_{1-\alpha/2}. \qquad (2.16)$$

The expression on the left side of (2.16) is a test statistic for the hypothesis $H_o : S(t) = p/100$. The confidence interval is defined as the set of values of t for which we would fail to reject the hypothesis. In other words, it is the set of observed survival times for which the confidence interval estimates for the survival function contain the quantile. This interval may be determined graphically in a manner similar to that in Figure 2.6 by drawing a horizontal line from $p/100$ to where it intersects the step functions defining the upper and lower pointwise confidence intervals. By drawing vertical lines down to the time axis one obtains the endpoints of the interval. If the software package provides the capability to list the endpoints of the confidence intervals for the estimated survival function, then the upper and lower endpoints can be precisely determined. We note that z_{t_p} could be defined using other functions of the estimated survival function such as $\hat{S}(t)$ or $\ln\left[\hat{S}(t)\right]$. The procedures for determining the confidence limits are the same.

Table 2.6 gives an abbreviated list of the values of the estimated survival function, the calculated value of z_{t_p} from (2.16), and the endpoints of 95 percent confidence intervals for survival times around the median value of 6.03 years. We see that the confidence interval estimate at 4.318 years does not contain 0.5, and $|z| = 2.09$, while at 4.446 years, it does contain 0.5 and $|z| = 1.91$. Thus the lower endpoint of the Brookmeyer–Crowley interval is 4.446 years. We see that the confidence interval at 7.420 years does not contain 0.5 with $|z| = 2.08$, while the interval at 7.184 years does contain 0.5 and $|z| = 1.66$. Hence, we recommend using the upper limit of 7.184 years. We note that some packages (e.g., STATA) use 7.420 as the upper endpoint for this example. The rationale is that 7.184 may underestimate the right-hand endpoint because $|z| = 1.66 < 1.96$ and a wider interval will have better coverage. It is curious that the same logic is not applied to the lower end point where it also true that $|z| < 1.96$. Hence, we prefer using endpoints where the inequality in (2.16) is satisfied.

The Brookmeyer–Crowley confidence interval for the median (4.45, 7.18) is comparable to the interval (4.68, 7.38) from Table 2.5, which was based on the large sample distribution of the estimator of the median. The Brookmeyer–Crowley confidence interval for the 75th percentile of the survival distribution is (0.75, 3.21); for the 25th percentile it is (7.18). In this case, the interval is well defined for the 75th percentile, but not for the 25th percentile as the confidence interval at the largest time, 7.44 years, still contains 0.25 and the estimator is undefined beyond this point.

In the analysis of survival time, the sample mean is not as important a measure of central tendency as in other settings. (The exception is in fully parametric modeling of survival times when the estimator of the mean, or a function of it, provides an estimator of a parameter vital to the analysis and interpretation of the data. We discuss parametric modeling in Chapter 8.) This is due to the fact that censored survival time data are most often skewed to the right, a setting where the median usually provides a more intuitive measure of central tendency. For the sake of completeness, we describe how the estimator of the mean and the estimator of its

Table 2.6 Listing of Observed Survival Times (Years), the Estimated Survival Function, and Individual 95% Confidence Interval Estimate for Values of Time near the Estimated Median Survival Time of 6.03 Years for the WHAS100 Data

Time	Estimate	$|z|$	95% CIE
4.318	0.610	2.09	0.507, 0.698
4.446	0.600	1.91	0.497, 0.688
4.569	0.590	1.73	0.487, 0.679
$\vdots$	$\vdots$	$\vdots$	$\vdots$
5.654	0.505	0.09	0.396, 0.604
6.026	0.469	0.52	0.347, 0.582
6.628	0.433	1.04	0.302, 0.556
7.184	0.361	1.66	0.200. 0.524
7.420	0.180	2.08	0.018. 0.482

variance are calculated and illustrate their use with examples from the WHAS100 study.

The estimator used for the mean is obtained from a mathematical result stating that, for a positive continuous random variable, the mean is equal to the area under the survival function. From mathematical methods of calculus, this may be represented as the integral of the survival function over the range, that is

$$\mu = \int_0^\infty S(u)\, du \, .$$

If we restrict the variable to the interval $[0, t^*]$, then the mean of the variable in this interval is

$$\mu(t^*) = \int_0^{t^*} S(u)\, du \, .$$

The estimator is obtained by using the Kaplan–Meier estimator of the survival function. We restrict the range over which the mean is calculated because the Kaplan–Meier estimator may be undefined beyond the largest value of time. Computational questions arise when the largest observation is censored. In this case, two computational strategies are possible: (1) use only the observed survival times (in this case, the estimator is biased downward) or (2) use all observations (i.e., one "pretends" that the largest observation was actually a survival time). In either case, the estimator is interpreted conditionally on the observed range. In the absence of censoring, both approaches yield the usual arithmetic mean. The value of t^* used depends on which of the two approaches is chosen. Recall that the observed ordered survival times are denoted $t_{(i)}$, $i = 1, \ldots, m$. We denote the largest observed value of time in the sample as $t_{(n)}$. The two approaches to calculating the estimator of the mean correspond to defining $t^* = t_{(m)}$, that is, using the interval $[0, t_{(m)}]$, or defining $t^* = t_{(n)}$, i.e., using the interval $[0, t_{(n)}]$. Because most packages use the first method, we describe the calculations for this choice. The notation for the second approach is easily obtained by replacing $t_{(m)}$ with $t_{(n)}$.

The value of the estimator is the area under the step function defined by the Kaplan–Meier estimator. To illustrate the calculation, consider the data in Table 2.1 for which the estimated survival function is presented in Table 2.2 and is graphed in Figure 2.1. In this example, the largest observed value of time is 62 days, and it represents a survival time. Thus, the value of the estimated mean is the area under the step function shown in Figure 2.1. This area is the sum of the areas of four rectangles defined by the heights of the four steps and the four observed survival times. The actual calculation is performed as follows (refer to Table 2.2):

$$\hat{\mu}(62) = 1.0 \times |6 - 0| + 0.8 \times |14 - 6| + 0.6 \times |44 - 14| + 0.3 \times |62 - 44|$$
$$= 35.8.$$

For sake of illustration, suppose that the value recorded at 62 days was a censored observation. In this case, we use the interval $[0, 44]$ and the estimate is reported as $\hat{\mu}(44) = 30.4$. This is the area of the first three rectangles in Figure 2.1.

The equation defining the estimator based on the observed range of survival times is

$$\hat{\mu}(t_{(m)}) = \sum_{i=1}^{m} \hat{S}(t_{(i-1)})\left(t_{(i)} - t_{(i-1)}\right), \tag{2.17}$$

where $\hat{S}(t_{(0)}) = 1.0$ and $t_{(0)} = 0.0$. Each term in the summation in (2.17) denotes the calculation of the area of one of the rectangles defined by the Kaplan–Meier estimator and two observed times.

The estimator of the variance of the sample mean is neither particularly intuitive nor easy to motivate, so we simply provide it and demonstrate the calculation. Andersen, Borgan, Gill and Keiding (1993) present a mathematical derivation of the estimator of the mean and its variance, as well as results that show that the standard normal distribution may be used to form a confidence interval estimator. The equation defining the estimator of the variance of the sample mean computed using (2.17) is as follows:

$$\widehat{\text{Var}}\left(\hat{\mu}(t_{(m)})\right) = \frac{n_d}{n_d - 1} \sum_{i=1}^{m-1} \frac{A_i^2 d_i}{n_i\left(n_i - d_i\right)}, \tag{2.18}$$

where $n_d = \sum_{i=1}^{m} d_i$ denotes the total number of subjects with an observed survival time and A_i is the area under the Kaplan-Meier estimator to the right of $t_{(i)}$, namely

$$A_i = \sum_{j=i}^{m-1} \hat{S}(t_{(j)})(t_{(j+1)} - t_{(j)}).$$

The multiplier of the sum in (2.18) is used to correct for the bias in an estimator based solely on the sum of terms. The data in Table 2.1 yields an estimated mean $\hat{\mu}(62) = 35.8$. Evaluation of the estimator in (2.18) yields

$$\widehat{Var}[\hat{\mu}(62)] = \frac{4}{4-1}\left[\frac{29.8^2}{5(5-1)} + \frac{23.4^2}{4(4-1)} + \frac{5.4^2}{2(2-1)}\right]$$

$$= 139.4827$$

where
$$A_1 = 0.8(14-6) + 0.6(44-14) + 0.3(62-44) = 29.8,$$
$$A_2 = 0.6(44-14) + 0.3(62-44) = 23.4,$$
and
$$A_3 = 0.3(62-44) = 5.4.$$

Approximate confidence intervals are obtained using percentiles from the standard normal distribution. Using the data in Table 2.1, the endpoints of the 95 percent confidence interval are $35.8 \pm 1.96\sqrt{139.4827}$. This is shown only for purposes of illustration because the sample size is only five with four survival times and any asymptotic theory will not hold. In practice, the estimated mean and its estimated standard error would typically be included in the table containing the estimates of the key quantiles and their estimated standard errors.

For the whole WHAS100 study, expressed in years, the estimate of the mean is $\hat{\mu}(7.42) = 4.78$ and the estimated variance from (2.18) is 0.292, yielding a 95 percent confidence interval of $(4.21, 5.35)$.

Before leaving the discussion of the estimator of the mean and the estimator of its standard error, we comment on some differences in software packages using the data from Table 2.1. In Table 2.7 we show the estimates obtained from SAS, SPSS and STATA using the data in Table 2.1 when the status at 62 days is either death or censored. These results show that SAS uses method 1, evaluating the mean over the range of observed survival times and uses the bias corrected estimator of the variance in (2.18). SPSS and STATA evaluate the mean over the observed range of time, and note if the largest time is a censored observation. For some unspecified reason, SPSS uses the bias-corrected estimator of the variance when the largest time is an event and the uncorrected estimator when the largest time is a censored

Table 2.7 Estimates of the Mean and Standard Error of the Mean from Data in Table 2.1

Package	SAS		SPSS		STATA	
Estimator	Death[*]	Censored[#]	Death[*]	Censored[#]	Death[*]	Censored[#]
Mean	35.8	30.4	35.8	35.8	35.8	35.8
SE	11.81	9.23	11.81	10.23	10.23	10.23
*Observation at 62 days is a death.						
#Observation at 62 days is censored.						

observation, with both being computed over the entire range of time. STATA uses the uncorrected estimator computed over the entire range of time. The same results hold, up to some round off, for the WHAS100 data. Based on these results, we urge caution when estimating the mean and recommend that one consult the documentation for the software package to check how the estimators are being calculated and verify the package's results with hand calculations.

2.4 COMPARISON OF SURVIVAL FUNCTIONS

After providing a description of the overall survival experience in the study, we turn our attention to a comparison of the survival experience in key subgroups. These groups are typically defined by covariates thought to be related to survival such as treatment arms in a clinical trial or other key factors. The goals in this analysis are identical to those of the two sample t–test, the non–parametric rank sum test, and the one-way analysis of variance. Namely, we wish to quantify differences between groups through point and interval estimates of key measures. Standard statistical procedures, such as those named above, may be used without modification when there are no censored observations.

Because survival data are typically right skewed, we would use rank-based non-parametric tests followed by estimates and confidence intervals of medians (and possibly other quantiles) within groups. Modifications of these procedures are required when censored observations are present in the data. These tests are described and illustrated with the WHAS100 study data beginning with methods for comparing two groups.

When comparing groups of subjects, we should begin with a graphical display of the data in each group. In studies of survival time, we should graph the Kaplan-Meier estimator of the survival function for each of the groups. In the WHAS100 study, gender is thought to be related to the survival experience. Figure 2.9 presents the graphs of the estimated survival functions for males and females.

Both groups show a similar pattern of survival: a rapidly descending estimated survival function for the first year followed by a relatively constant decrease thereafter. Because the estimated survival function for males does not go to zero, we know that the largest observation was a censored value. The figure also shows a separation of the functions for the two genders. The estimated survival function for males lies completely above that for females. In general, the pattern of one survival function lying above another means the group defined by the upper curve lived longer, or had a more favorable survival experience, than the group defined by the lower curve. In other words, at any point in time, the proportion of subjects estimated to be alive is greater for one group (represented by the upper curve) than for the other (represented by the lower curve). Estimates of the within-group statistics, such as the median, are computed using the methods described in Section 2.3. The statistical question is whether the observed difference seen in Figure 2.9 is statistically significant.

A number of statistical tests have been proposed to answer this question, and most software packages provide results from at least two of these tests. However, comparison of the results obtained by different packages can become confusing due to small but annoying differences in terminology and methods used to calculate the tests. The original developers of these tests sought ways to extend tests used with non-censored data to the censored data setting (Gehan (1965), Mantel (1966), Breslow (1970), Peto and Peto (1972)], Prentice (1978).

The derivation and algebraic representation of the tests can, at times, seem complex and confusing. Lawless (2003) presents a concise summary of the traditional approach to the development of these tests, based on the theory of non-parametric tests, using exponentially ordered scores. These tests have been examined from the counting process point of view and have been shown to be special cases of a more general class of counting process-based tests. These results are summarized in Andersen, Borgan, Gill and Keiding (1993).

The calculation of each test is based on a contingency table of group by status at each observed survival time, as shown in Table 2.8. In this table, the number at risk at observed survival time $t_{(i)}$ is denoted by n_{0i} in Group 0 and by n_{1i} in Group 1; the number of observed deaths in each of the these two groups is denoted by d_{0i} and d_{1i}, respectively; the total number at risk is denoted by n_i; and the total number

Table 2.8 Table Used for Test of Equality of the Survival Function in Two Groups at Observed Survival Time $t_{(i)}$

Event/Group	1	0	Total
Die	d_{1i}	d_{0i}	d_i
Not Die	$n_{1i} - d_{1i}$	$n_{0i} - d_{0i}$	$n_i - d_i$
At Risk	n_{1i}	n_{0i}	n_i

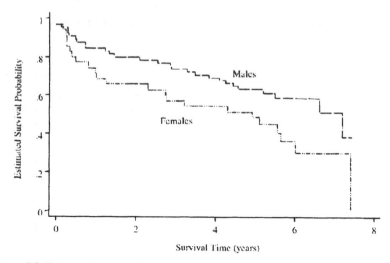

Figure 2.9 Estimated survival functions for males and females in the WHAS100 study.

of deaths is denoted by d_i. The contribution to the test statistic at each time is obtained by calculating the expected number of deaths in group 1 or 0, assuming that the survival function is the same in each of the two groups. This yields the usual "*row total times column total divided by grand total*" estimator. For example, using group 1, the estimator is

$$\hat{e}_{1i} = \frac{n_{1i}d_i}{n_i}.$$ (2.19)

Most software packages base their estimator of the variance of d_{1i} on the hypergeometric distribution, defined as follows

$$\hat{v}_{1i} = \frac{n_{1i}n_{0i}d_i(n_i - d_i)}{n_i^2(n_i - 1)}.$$ (2.20)

The contribution to the test statistic depends on which of the various tests is used, but each may be expressed in the form of a ratio of weighted sums over the observed survival times. These tests may be defined in general as follows:

$$Q = \frac{\left[\sum_{i=1}^{m} w_i (d_{1i} - \hat{e}_{1i}) \right]^2}{\sum_{i=1}^{m} w_i^2 \hat{v}_{1i}}, \tag{2.21}$$

where the w_i are weights whose values depend on the specific test. Under the null hypothesis that the two survival functions are the same, and assuming that the censoring experience is independent of group, and that the total number of observed events and the sum of the expected number of events is large, then the p-value for Q may be obtained using the chi-square distribution with one degree of freedom (i.e., $p = \Pr(\chi^2(1) \geq Q)$). Exact methods of inference for use with small samples have been implemented in the software package StatXact 7 but will not be discussed in this text.

The most frequently used test is based on weights equal to one, $w_i = 1$. In this case, the test mimics the Mantel-Haenszel test of the hypothesis that the stratum-specific odds-ratio is equal to one (see Mantel (1966) for further details). However, this test is most often called the "log-rank test," due to Peto and Peto (1972). The test is related to a test proposed by Savage (1956).

Gehan (1965) and Breslow (1970) generalized the Wilcoxon rank sum test to allow for censored data. This test uses weights equal to the number of subjects at risk at each survival time, $w_i = n_i$, and is called the "Wilcoxon" or "generalized Wilcoxon test" by most software packages.

SAS's lifetest procedure provides two ways of obtaining the same test, but different variance estimators are used. In SAS, if we define the grouping variable to be a stratification variable, the variance estimator $\hat{v}_{1i}$ is used. If we use SAS's test option, then the variance estimator

$$\hat{v}_{1i}^* = \frac{n_{1i} n_{0i}}{n_i^2}$$

is used, which assumes that $d_i = 1$ (i.e., there are no tied failure times). Thus, in any one example, we may obtain test statistics of similar magnitude but with slightly different values. Because survival time is often recorded in discrete units that may lead to ties, we recommend that the variance estimator $\hat{v}_{1i}$ be used.

The choice of weight influences the type of differences in the survival function the test is most apt to detect. The generalized Wilcoxon test, because it uses weights equal to the number at risk, will put relatively more weight on differences between the survival functions at smaller values of time. The log-rank test, because it uses weights equal to one, will place more emphasis than does the generalized Wilcoxon test on differences between the functions at larger values of time. Other tests have been proposed that use weight functions intermediate between these (e.g., Tarone and Ware (1977) suggested using $w_i = \sqrt{n_i}$).

Peto and Peto (1972) and Prentice (1978) suggested using a weight function that depends more explicitly on the observed survival experience of the combined sample. The weight function is a modification of the Kaplan-Meier estimator and is defined in such a way that its value is known just prior to the observed failure time. The value of any estimated survival function at a particular observed failure time is known only after the observation is made. The property of having the value known in advance of the actual observed failure is referred to as *predictable* in counting process terminology. This theory is needed to prove results concerning the distribution of the test statistics. The modified estimator of the survival function is

$$\tilde{S}(t) = \prod_{t_{(j)} \le t} \left(\frac{n_j + 1 - d_j}{n_j + 1} \right) \tag{2.22}$$

and the weight used is

$$w_i = \tilde{S}(t_{(i)}) . \tag{2.23}$$

A modified Peto-Prentice test uses weight

$$w_i = \tilde{S}(t_{(i-1)}) \times \frac{n_i}{n_i + 1} ,$$

that is equal to the unmodified weight when $d_j = 1$ in (2.22). Hence in the absence of ties, the two Peto-Prentice tests are identical. Most packages use the weight defined in (2.23), though SAS offers the test based on the modified weight.

Harrington and Fleming (1982) suggested a class of tests that incorporates features of both the log-rank and the Peto and Prentice tests. They suggest using weights

$$w_i = \left[\hat{S}(t_{(i-1)}) \right]^p \times \left[1 - \hat{S}(t_{(i-1)}) \right]^q . \tag{2.24}$$

If the powers are $p = q = 0$, then $w_i = 1$ and the test is the log-rank test. If the powers are $p = 1$ and $q = 0$, then the weight is the Kaplan-Meier estimator at the previous survival time, a weight similar to that of the Peto and Prentice test. If the powers are such that $p > q$, then the test puts relatively more weight on shorter survival times, while the reverse is true when $p < q$. This test has been implemented in STATA.

The principal advantage of the Peto-Prentice and Harrington-Fleming tests over the generalized Wilcoxon test is that they weight relative to the overall survival experience. The generalized Wilcoxon test uses the size of the risk set; weights depend both on the censoring as well as the survival experience. If the pattern of censoring is markedly different in each group, then this test may either reject or fail to reject, not on the basis of similarity or differences in the survival functions, but on the pattern of censoring. For this reason, most software packages will provide information as to the pattern of censoring in each of the two groups. This information should be checked for comparability, especially when the results of several of these tests are provided and yield markedly different significance levels.

A problem can occur if the estimated survival functions cross one another. This means that, in some time intervals, one group will have a more favorable survival experience, while in other time intervals, the other group will have the more favorable experience. This situation is analogous to having interaction present when applying Mantel-Haenszel methods to a stratified contingency table. Unfortunately, tests for the homogeneity across strata may not be used in most survival time applications because data in tables like Table 2.8 will be too thin to satisfy the necessary large sample criteria. Fleming, Harrington and O'Sullivan (1987) proposed a method that addresses the problem by using, as a test statistic, the maximum observed difference between the two survival functions. This test has not been implemented in any software package. We consider methods based on regression modeling to address this issue in Chapter 7. For the time being, our only check is via a visual examination of the plot of the Kaplan-Meier estimator for the groups being compared. If we see that the curves cross, then this "interaction" may be present.

When comparing the various tests for group differences it is not possible to say that one will always be more conservative than another one. In other words, it is not possible to provide a categorical rank ordering of the values of the various test statistics. The actual calculated values will depend on the observed survival and censoring times.

To illustrate the computation of each test, we have chosen a small subset of males and females from the WHAS100 study and modified their data slightly for purposes of illustration only. These data are listed in Table 2.9. Column 1 of Table 2.10 lists the eight distinct survival times. Columns 2 through 5 present the quantities defined by the notation shown in Table 2.8, and columns 6 and 7 present quantities defined in equations (2.19) and (2.20). Columns 8 through 11 present

Table 2.9 Listing of Males and Females Selected from the WHAS100 Study and Used to Illustrate the Tests for the Comparison of Two Survival Functions

Gender	Ordered Observed Survival Times
Male (0)	6, 44*, 98, 114
Female (1)	14, 44, 89*, 98, 104

* Denotes a censored observation.

values for the weight functions for the four tests, where "L" stands for log-rank test weights, "W" stands for generalized Wilcoxon test weights, "T" stands for Tarone-Ware weights, and "P" stands for the unmodified Peto-Prentice weights. The calculated values of the test statistics and their respective p-values are shown in Table 2.11, where the significance is provided only for the purpose of illustrating the calculations because, with only 7 total events and an expected number of events of 1.31 in group 1, the assumption that the sample sizes are large is clearly violated.

The Kaplan-Meier estimates of the survival functions for males and females in WHAS100 study shown in Figure 2.7 do not cross at any point, indicating that the previously described problem of "interaction" may not be present. An inspection of the proportion of values censored and the pattern of censoring (not shown) indicates that the censoring experience of the two groups is similar. Thus it would appear that the assumptions necessary for using the tests for equality of the survival functions seem to hold. The tests and their p-values are show in Table 2.12. All the tests have p-values of about 0.05, which support the impression seen in Figure 2.7 that females have a less favorable survival experience than do males. In practice, one could provide additional support for this conclusion by presenting the estimates of the within-gender median survival times with confidence interval estimates.

Each of the tests used to compare the survival experience in two groups may be extended to compare more than two groups. In the WHAS100 study, it was

Table 2.10 Listing of Quantities Needed to Calculate the Tests for the Equality of Two Survival Functions

Time	d_{1i}	n_{1i}	d_i	n_i	$\hat{e}_{1i}$	$\hat{v}_{1i}$	L	W	T	P
6	0	5	1	9	0.556	0.247	1	9	3.000	0.900
14	1	5	1	8	0.625	0.234	1	8	2.828	0.800
44	1	4	1	7	0.571	0.245	1	7	2.646	0.700
98	1	2	2	4	1.000	0.333	1	4	2.000	0.420
104	1	1	1	2	0.500	0.250	1	2	1.414	0.280
114	0	0	1	1	0.000	0.000	1	1	1.000	0.140

Table 2.11 Listing of the Test Statistics and p-values for the Equality of Two Survival Functions Computed from Table 2.10

Statistic	Value	p-value
Log-rank	0.427	0.513
Wilcoxon	0.075	0.784
Tarone-Ware	0.200	0.655
Peto-Prentice	0.105	0.746

hypothesized that age might be related to survival. Because age is a continuous variable, one approach to assessing a potential relationship is to use regression modeling. This is discussed in detail in Chapter 3. An approach used in practice, for preliminary analyses that can yield easily understood summary measures, is to break a continuous variable into several clinically relevant groups and use methods for grouped data on the categorized variable. We use this approach with groups based on the following intervals for age: $\{[32–59], [60–69], [70–79], [80–92]\}$. Table 2.13 presents the number of subjects, the number of deaths, the median survival time and associated Brookmeyer-Cowley 95 percent confidence interval for each age group.

The median survival time cannot be estimated for the first age group in Table 2.13 because the minimum value of the Kaplan-Meier estimate of the survival function for this group is larger than 0.5 (i.e., 0.68). The estimated median survival time decreases from 7.2 years to 2.3 years for the oldest three groups suggesting, not surprisingly, that age is negatively related to survival time. The goal in the four-group comparison will be to evaluate whether trends seen in the medians persist when the entire survival experience of the groups is compared. Before presenting the graphs of the Kaplan-Meier estimates of the survival functions for the four age groups, we present the details of the extension of the two-group tests to the multiple-group situation.

If we assume that there are K groups, then the calculations of the test statistics are based on a two (observed versus expected) by K table for each observed survival time. The general form of this table is presented in Table 2.13. In a manner similar to the two-group case, we estimate the expected number of events for each

Table 2.12 Test Statistics and p-values for the Equality of the Survival Functions for Males and Females in the WHAS100 Study

Statistic	Value	p-value
Log-rank	3.971	0.046
Wilcoxon	3.462	0.063
Tarone-Ware	3.686	0.055
Peto-Prentice	3.851	0.050

Table 2.13 The Number of Subjects, Events, Estimated Median Survival Time, and 95% Confidence Interval Estimates in Four Age Groups in the WHAS100 Study

Age Group	Freq	Deaths	Median	95 % CIE
< 60	25	8	*	*
60 - 69	23	7	7.18	(7.18, .)
70 -79	22	14	4.95	(0.75, 5.85)
≥ 80	30	22	2.30	(0.99, 5.51)

* Median not estimable.

group under an assumption of equal survival functions as

$$\hat{e}_{ki} = \frac{d_i n_{ki}}{n_i}, \ k = 1, 2, \ldots, K.$$ (2.25)

We compare the observed and expected number of events for $K-1$ of the K groups. The reason for this will be explained shortly. The easiest way to denote the $K-1$ comparisons is to use vector notation to represent both observed and estimated expected number of events as follows:

$$\mathbf{d}'_i = (d_{1i}, d_{2i}, \ldots, d_{K-1i}),$$

and

$$\hat{\mathbf{e}}'_i = (\hat{e}_{1i}, \hat{e}_{2i}, \ldots, \hat{e}_{K-1i}).$$

The difference between these two vectors is

$$(\mathbf{d}_i - \hat{\mathbf{e}}_i)' = (d_{1i} - \hat{e}_{1i}, d_{2i} - \hat{e}_{2i}, \ldots, d_{K-1i} - \hat{e}_{K-1i}).$$ (2.26)

For convenience, we have used the first $K-1$ of the K groups, but any collection of $K-1$ groups could be used.

To obtain a test statistic, we need an estimator of the covariance matrix of $\mathbf{d}_i$. The elements of this matrix are obtained assuming that the observed number of events follows a multivariate central hypergeometric distribution (see Johnson and

Table 2.14 Table Used for the Test for the Equality of the Survival Function in K Groups at Observed Survival Time $t_{(i)}$

Event/ Group	1	2	$\cdots$	k	$\cdots$	K	Total
Die	d_{1i}	d_{2i}	$\cdots$	d_{ki}	$\cdots$	d_{Ki}	d_i
Not Die	$n_{1i} - d_{1i}$	$n_{2i} - d_{2i}$	$\cdots$	$n_{ki} - d_{ki}$	$\cdots$	$n_{Ki} - d_{Ki}$	$n_i - d_i$
At Risk	n_{1i}	n_{2i}	$\cdots$	n_{ki}	$\cdots$	n_{Ki}	n_i

Kotz (1997)). The diagonal elements of the $K-1$ by $K-1$ covariance matrix of, $\mathbf{d}_i$ denoted $\hat{\mathbf{V}}_i$, are

$$\hat{v}_{kki} = \frac{n_{ki}(n_i - n_{ki})d_i(n_i - d_i)}{n_i^2(n_i - 1)}, \ k = 1, 2, \ldots, K-1 \tag{2.27}$$

and the off diagonal elements are

$$\hat{v}_{kli} = -\frac{n_{ki}n_{li}d_i(n_i - d_i)}{n_i^2(n_i - 1)}, \ k, l = 1, 2, \ldots, K-1, k \neq l. \tag{2.28}$$

The various multiple-group versions of the two-group test statistics are obtained by computing a weighted difference between the observed and expected number of events. The weights used at each distinct survival time can be any of the weights used in the two-group test, denoted in general at time $t_{(i)}$ by w_i. To obtain a formula similar to (2.21) for the general test statistic, we define a $K-1$ by $K-1$ diagonal matrix denoted $\mathbf{W}_i = \mathrm{diag}(w_i)$. This matrix has the value of the weight, w_i, at time $t_{(i)}$ in all $K-1$ positions along the diagonal of the matrix. The test statistic to compare the survival experience of the K groups is

$$Q = \left[\sum_{i=1}^{m} \mathbf{W}_i\left(\mathbf{d}_i - \hat{\mathbf{e}}_i\right)\right]' \left[\sum_{i=1}^{m} \mathbf{W}_i \hat{\mathbf{V}}_i \mathbf{W}_i\right]^{-1} \left[\sum_{i=1}^{m} \mathbf{W}_i\left(\mathbf{d}_i - \hat{\mathbf{e}}_i\right)\right]. \tag{2.29}$$

We use only $K-1$ of the K possible observed to expected comparisons to prevent the matrix in the center of the right hand side of (2.29) from being singular. If you are not familiar with matrix algebra, you can think of the problem of a singular matrix being similar to dividing by zero. The value of the test statistic in (2.29) is the same, regardless of which collection of $K-1$ groups are used.

The expression on the right hand side of (2.29) may look intimidating to those not familiar with matrix algebra calculations, but when $K=2$, it simplifies to the more easily understood statistic defined in (2.21). Software packages provide statistics for the same weights used for the case when $K=2$. These packages typically provide only the test statistic and a p-value. One exception is SAS's lifetest procedure, which provides the individual elements in (2.26) - (2.28) when the group variable is defined as a stratum variable. Under the hypothesis of equal survival functions, and if the summed estimated expected number of events is large, then Q will be approximately distributed as chi-square with $K-1$ degrees of freedom, and the p-value is $p = \Pr(\chi^2(K-1) \geq Q)$. The remarks made earlier about how the choice of weights in the two-group case can affect the ability of the test to detect differences apply to the multiple-group case as well.

The estimated survival functions for the four age groups are shown in Figure 2.10. The figure confirms our preliminary observations, based on estimates of median survival times, that overall survival worsens as age increases. In the first three months, the curves for the oldest three groups are similar. Over the remainder of the follow up period, these three curves become distinctly different, though the curves for the oldest two groups approach each other after about 5.75 years of follow up. The survival curves for the youngest two age groups demonstrate a possible interaction as they cross once at about 3.75 years. In the interval from time zero to 3.75, years the youngest age group has the more favorable survival experience. However, in the time interval beyond 3.75, years the age group 60-69 has the more favorable experience. Note that the number of events in both age groups is rather small beyond 3.75 years with only two events in each group. We begin by performing the overall test of equality of survival curves. This test will be followed by tests of more specific hypotheses.

The values of the four test statistics using their respective weights in (2.29) are given in Table 2.15. Because each statistic is significant at the 1% level, we reject the hypothesis that the survival functions for the four age groups are the same. We then test for overall group differences in survival experience with contrasts to describe more precisely the source(s) of the significance of the overall test. STATA offers this option by allowing the user to specify a trend test and to input a set of coefficients to test for trend when the groups are not equally spaced. The SAS package lifetest procedure has a test option that provides a trend test for a numeric covariate. The test does not yield the same numeric value as the trend test in STATA. We describe the test used in STATA, as it follows directly from the multiple group test in (2.29). The null hypothesis is that the survival functions are equal; the alternative is that they are rank-ordered and follow the trend specified by the coefficients denoted by the vector $\mathbf{c}' = (c_1, c_2, \ldots, c_{K-1}, c_K)$. If the groups are equally spaced, we may use $c_k = k$. The age groups we used in the WHAS100 study are not equally spaced, so we will use a vector of coefficients, whose values are the midpoints of the four groups, i.e., $\mathbf{c}' = (46, 65, 75, 86)$. Any linear transformation of these coefficients would yield the same value of the test statistic. The statistic to test for trend, with one degree-of-freedom, is

$$Q_{trend} = \frac{\mathbf{c}'\left[\sum_{i=1}^{m} \mathbf{W}_i\left(\mathbf{d}_i - \hat{\mathbf{e}}_i\right)\right]\mathbf{c}}{\mathbf{c}'\left[\sum_{i=1}^{m} \mathbf{W}_i\hat{\mathbf{V}}_i\mathbf{W}_i\right]\mathbf{c}}, \tag{2.30}$$

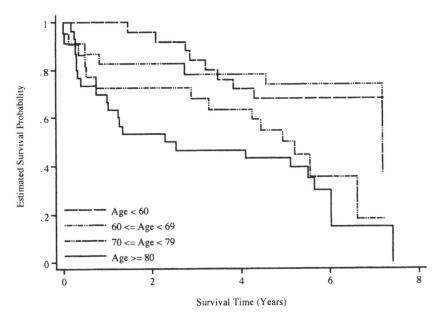

Figure 2.10 Estimated Survival Functions for the Four Age Groups in Table 2.13 (the WHAS100 Study).

where the p-value is computed using the chi-square distribution with one degree of freedom, i.e., $p = \Pr(\chi^2(1) \geq Q_{trend})$. Note that the vectors used in the test for trend in (2.30) have K components as opposed to $K - 1$ components for the tests for differences between groups. Table 2.16 presents the statistics and their p-values for the test of trend among the four age groups in the WHAS100 study. These values are each slightly smaller than the values in Table 2.15, providing strong evidence for a trend in survival experience that is inversely related to age. We explore this relationship in detail when we consider regression modeling in the next chapter.

As a follow up to our comments on a possible interaction with time in the two youngest age groups, we performed the log rank test, which was not significant, $p > 0.99$. This could mean that the two curves are within sampling variation of each other or that the differences between the groups prior to 3.75 years are "cancelled out" by the differences beyond 3.75 years. However, it could also mean that the better survival experience of the youngest group in the first 3.75 years is cancelled out in the sum of observed minus expected events used in the tests in the follow up exceeding 3.75 years, where this group has the poorer survival. One possible approach is to use a modification of the log rank test proposed by Lin and

**Table 2.15 Test Statistics, Degrees-of-Freedom and
p-values for the Equality of the Survival Functions
for the Four Age Groups in the WHAS100 Study**

Statistic	Value	df	*p*-value
Log-rank	15.57	3	0.001
Wilcoxon	12.30	3	0.006
Tarone-Ware	13.52	3	0.004
Peto-Prentice	14.54	3	0.002

Wang (2004). The test is based on the statistic $\hat{\Delta} = \sum_{i=1}^{m} \left(d_{1i} - \hat{e}_{1i} \right)^2$. While the estimator of the mean of $\hat{\Delta}$ is not especially complicated, the computations required to obtain the estimator of its standard error are. Lin and Wang show via simulations that their test has considerably more power than tests based on (2.21). However they do not compare its power to regression modeling based tests of time by covariate interactions discussed in Chapter 7. Also Lin and Wang do not provide the details of a multi-group extension. As yet this test has not been included in any software packages. Hence, we defer further discussion of this type of interaction until Chapter 7.

In the examples we have used from the WHAS100 study to illustrate the comparison of the survival functions over groups, the magnitude of the test statistics has not varied too dramatically with the choice of weight, and the significance or non-significance of all test statistics has mostly been consistent. However, this is not always the case and to illustrate this we use some data provided to us by our colleagues Drs. Carol Bigelow and Penny Pekow (at the University of Massachusetts) and Dr. Kathy Meyer (at Baystate Medical Center in Springfield, Massachusetts). These data were used as part of Ms. Shiaw-Shyuan Yuan's Masters degree project (Yuan (1993)). The purpose of the study was to determine factors that predict the length of time very low birth weight infants (<1500 grams) with bronchopulmonary dysplasia (BPD) were treated with oxygen. The data were collected retrospectively for the period December 1987 to March 1991. Beginning in August 1989, the treatment of BPD changed to include the use of surfactant replacement therapy. This was done with parental permission because this therapy was then considered experimental. A total of 78 infants met the study criteria, with 35 receiving surfactant replacement therapy and 43 not receiving this therapy. Five babies were still on oxygen at their last follow-up visit and are censored observations. We refer to this study as the BPD study and the data are available on the ftp site given in the Preface.

The outcome variable is the total number of days the baby required supplemental oxygen therapy. Figure 2.11 presents the Kaplan-Meier estimates of the survival functions for two groups defined by use of surfactant replacement therapy.

Table 2.16 Trend Test Statistics, Degrees of Freedom and *p*-values for the Equality of the Survival Functions among the Four Age Groups in the WHAS100 Study

Statistic	Value	df	*p*-value
Log-rank	12.44	1	<0.001
Wilcoxon	9.99	1	0.002
Tarone-Ware	10.70	1	0.001
Peto-Prentice	12.08	1	<0.001

The estimated median number of days of therapy for those babies who did not have surfactant replacement therapy is 107 {95% Brookmeyer-Crowley CIE: (71, 217)}, and the estimated median number of days for those who had the therapy is 71 {95% Brookmeyer-Crowley CIE: (56, 110)}. The median number of days of therapy for the babies not on surfactant is about 1.5 times longer than for those using the therapy, but there is considerable overlap in the confidence intervals. The plots of the survival functions in Figure 2.11 indicate a progressively larger difference in the survival curves between the two groups over time. Table 2.17 presents test statistics and associated *p*-values for the equality of the survival functions. The Wilcoxon test is not significant at the 5% level, but the log-rank test is significant. The difference in the magnitude of the test statistics is due to the difference in the weights used. The Wilcoxon test uses a weight equal to the size of the risk set and thus is more likely to detect early differences. The log-rank test uses a weight equal to one and is more likely to detect later differences in the survival functions.

In any statistical analysis where more than one test can be used, we need to make a decision about which results we will report. The log-rank test is the most frequently used and reported test for the comparison of survival functions. For most analyses, at least when each test has roughly the same level of significance, reporting only the results of the log-rank test is appropriate. When the tests give different results, then more than one result should be reported. This will provide the reader with a clearer picture as to where the survival functions may be different. The current example demonstrates the importance of computing several of the tests. Most packages have both the log-rank and Wilcoxon tests and we recommend that both be computed. The pattern of censoring can influence the magnitude of the tests, but the values of the Tarone-Ware and Peto-Prentice tests tend to be intermediate between the log-rank and Wilcoxon tests. It is vital that authors not choose to present the test that best agrees with their preconceived or preferred result. Instead, identifying the types of differences that should be detected, a priori, should determine which statistical test should be used.

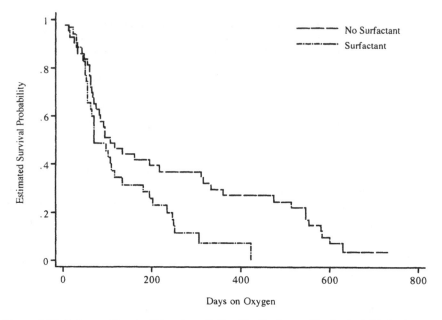

Figure 2.11 Estimated Survival Functions Defined by Surfactant Use in the BPD Study.

We conclude our presentation of the tests for comparison of survival functions with a brief discussion of the assumptions underlying the tests and the types of alternative hypotheses the tests are likely to have power to detect. Recall that the Kaplan-Meier estimator assumes that censoring is independent of survival time. In addition, the tests assume that the censoring is independent of the groups. Problems in study design and data collection can lead to differential effects due to censoring, and the best protection is a carefully designed study. However, it is good practice to examine the censoring pattern in the data.

In general, we cannot over-emphasize the importance of a careful study of the plot of the Kaplan-Meier estimates of the survival functions. Any tests comparing these functions, and within-group point estimates of quantiles, should support what

Table 2.17 Test Statistics and p-values for the Equality of the Survival Functions for Two Groups Defined by Surfactant Use in the BPD Study

Statistic	Value	df	p-value
Log-rank	5.618	1	0.018
Wilcoxon	2.490	1	0.115
Tarone-Ware	3.698	1	0.055
Peto-Prentice	2.534	1	0.111

is seen in the plot. The plot is also the basic diagnostic tool to determine whether the tests described previously should be used or, if used, have any chance of detecting a difference.

The alternative hypothesis that the tests are most likely to detect is a monotonic ordering of the survival functions (e.g., they lie one above another). The tests have little to no power to detect differences when the survival functions cross one another in a manner seen in Figure 2.10 for the two youngest age groups. None of the tests described in this section are able to detect this kind of difference.

2.5 OTHER FUNCTIONS OF SURVIVAL TIME AND THEIR ESTIMATORS

The Kaplan–Meier estimator of the survival function has been, and continues to be, the most frequently used estimator, largely due to the fact that it is routinely calculated by most software packages. To motivate the discussion of another estimator, we begin by providing a different representation of the survival function. If we assume that the underlying time random variable is absolutely continuous, then we may express the survival function as

$$S(t) = e^{-H(t)} \tag{2.31}$$

where $H(t)$ is the cumulative hazard function that will be discussed in more detail below and which can be written as $H(t) = -\ln(S(t))$. The expression in (2.31) suggests that estimators of the survival function could be based on an estimator of $H(t)$ instead of an estimator based on $S(t)$ (e.g., the Kaplan–Meier estimator). Aalen (1975, 1978), Nelson (1969, 1972) and Altshuler (1970) have proposed an easily computed estimator of $H(t)$, which we refer to as the Nelson-Aalen estimator.

The work by Aalen is considered to be one of the landmark contributions to the field, as virtually all recent statistical developments for the analysis of survival time data have been based on the counting process approach he used to derive his version of the estimator of $H(t)$. The statistical theory and use of this estimator in various applied settings are discussed in detail in Andersen, Borgan, Gill and Keiding (1993) and in Fleming and Harrington (1984, 1991). We use results derived from the counting process theory to justify various techniques discussed in this text. We do not present the counting process approach in any detail because fully appreciating and understanding it requires having had calculus-based courses in mathematical statistics and probability theory. For a brief introduction see Appendix 2.

Without providing any details as to its derivation the Nelson–Aalen estimator of $H(t)$ is

$$\tilde{H}(t) = \sum_{t_{(i)} \le t} \frac{d_i}{n_i}. \tag{2.32}$$

The estimator of the variance of the Nelson-Aalen estimator is

$$\hat{\text{Var}}\left[\tilde{H}(t)\right] = \sum_{t_{(i)} \le t} \frac{d_i}{n_i^2}, \tag{2.33}$$

and it follows that the endpoints of the confidence interval estimator are

$$\tilde{H}(t) \pm z_{1-\alpha/2} \times \hat{\text{SE}}\left[\tilde{H}(t)\right], \tag{2.34}$$

where $\hat{\text{SE}}\left[\tilde{H}(t)\right] = \sqrt{\hat{\text{Var}}\left[\tilde{H}(t)\right]}$. Thus the Nelson-Aalen estimator of the survival function is

$$\tilde{S}(t) = e^{-\tilde{H}(t)}. \tag{2.35}$$

and the associated confidence interval is obtained by exponentiating the negative of the endpoints in (2.34), e.g.,

$$\exp\left\{-\tilde{H}(t) \pm z_{1-\alpha/2} \times \hat{\text{SE}}\left[\tilde{H}(t)\right]\right\}. \tag{2.36}$$

One theoretical problem is that the expression in (2.31) is valid for continuous time, but the estimator in (2.35) is discrete. However, the estimator in (2.35) provides the basis for the estimator of the survival function used with the proportional hazards regression model discussed in Chapter 3. For this reason, we consider it in some detail.

Many packages now provide either the Nelson–Aalen estimator of the survival function or the estimator $\tilde{H}(t)$. One may show, by using a Taylor series expansion (see Appendix 1), that $d_i/n_i \le -\ln(1 - d_i/n_i)$ for each survival time. Thus, the Nelson–Aalen estimator of the survival function will always be greater than or equal to the Kaplan–Meier estimator. If the size of the risk sets relative to the number of events is large, then $d_i/n_i \cong -\ln(1 - d_i/n_i)$ and there will be little practical difference between the Nelson-Aalen and the Kaplan-Meier estimators of the survival function.

The WHAS100 study provides a good illustration of a situation in which there is no practical difference between the Kaplan-Meier and Nelson-Aalen estimators or their confidence limits. All were computed in STATA and are shown in Figure 2.12. We see that the two estimators of the survival function are nearly identical even though $\tilde{S}(t) \geq \hat{S}(t)$ at every observed value of time. Also, there is essentially no difference in the confidence limits.

The function $H(t)$ is an important analytic tool for the analysis of survival time data. In much of the survival analysis literature it is called the *cumulative hazard function*, but in the counting process literature, it is related to a function called the *cumulative* or *integrated intensity process*. The plot of the Nelson-Aalen estimator from (2.32) for the WHAS100 data is shown in Figure 2.13. Note that the curvature in the plot is similar to that seen the estimate of the survival function but in the reverse direction, as $H(t)$ increases, $S(t)$ decreases. Thus a sharp rise in the cumulative hazard is associated with a sharp decrease in the survival function. In Figure 2.13, we see that, except for the first and last half year, the increase in $\tilde{H}(t)$ is nearly constant. Because the scale of the cumulative hazard is not con-

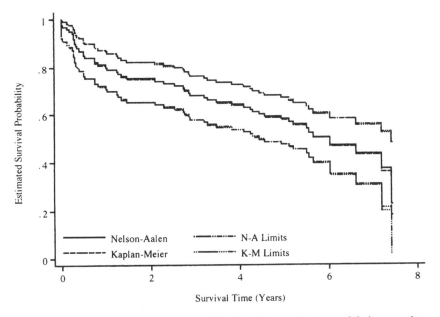

Figure 2.12 Graphs of the Nelson-Aalen and Kaplan-Meier estimators and their respective pointwise 95% confidence limits of the survival function from the WHAS100 study.

strained to be less than 1, it is sometimes preferred for plotting, especially when graphically assessing model assumptions, a point we return to in Chapter 6.

The term "hazard" is used to describe the concept of the risk of "failure" in an interval after time t, conditional on the subject having survived to time t. The word "cumulative" is used to describe the fact that its value is the "sum total" of the hazard up to time t. In mathematical terms, the cumulative hazard is the integral of the hazard from time 0 to time t namely

$$H(t) = \int_0^t h(u)du .$$

At this point, we focus on the hazard function itself, as it plays a central role in regression modeling of survival data.

Consider a subject in the WHAS100 study whose survival time is 5 years. For this subject to have died at 5 years, he/she had to be alive during their fourth year of follow up. The hazard at 5 years is the failure rate "per year," conditional on the

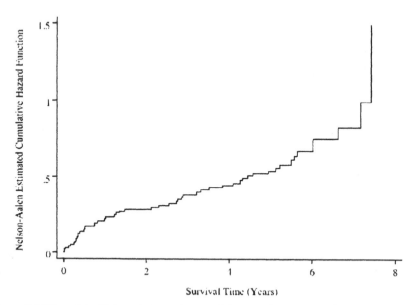

Figure 2.13 Plot of the Nelson-Aalen estimator of the cumulative hazard from the WHAS100 study.

fact that the subject has lived 4 years[2]. This is not the same as the unconditional failure rate "per year" at 5 years. The unconditional rate applies to subjects at time zero and, as such, does not use the information available as the study progresses about the survival experience in the sample. This accumulation of knowledge, over time, is generally referred to as *aging*. For example, of 100 subjects who enroll in a study, what fraction is expected to die at exactly 5 years? The conditional failure rate applies only to that subset of the sample that has survived to a particular time, thus it accounts for the aging that has taken place in the sample. The mathematical definition of the hazard function is

$$h(t) = \frac{f(t)}{S(t)}, \qquad (2.37)$$

where $S(t)$ is the survival function and $f(t)$ is the probability density function of the time variable. In more practical terms, the numerator of (2.37) is the unconditional probability of experiencing the event at time t, which is then scaled by the fraction alive at time t. The Nelson-Aalen estimator of the hazard function at observed survival time t_i is

$$\tilde{h}(t_i) = \tilde{H}(t_{i+1}) - \tilde{H}(t_i) = \frac{d_i}{n_i}. \qquad (2.38)$$

However, the estimator in (2.38) requires a large number of failures at each time point to be useful. Otherwise there is so much variability in the values that we are unable to draw any substantive conclusions as to its basic shape. Also the estimator is undefined at points where there are no observed events. One method of smoothing out some of the variability in the values is to use an elaborate method of averaging called kernel smoothing. This technique is available in STATA and is shown, along with 95 percent point-wise confidence limits, for the WHAS100 data in Figure 2.14. We refer the reader to Klein and Moeschberger (2003) for a detailed discussion of kernel smoothing methods applied to estimators of the hazard function. One problem with the kernel smoothed estimator is that it is estimating a smoothed hazard function, not the hazard function itself. However, the goal in plotting the smoothed estimate is to obtain a visual impression as opposed to providing precise point-wise estimates. We also note that the kernel smoothed estima-

---

[2] In this discussion we could use any unit of time, days, months or years. We have chosen years because all tables and graphs are based on years of follow up as the time variable for the WHAS100 data.

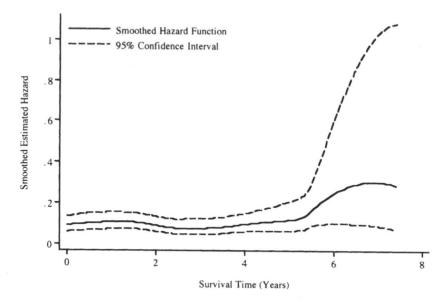

Figure 2.14 Plot of the kernel smoothed Nelson-Aalen estimator and 95 percent confidence limits of the hazard function for the WHAS100 data.

tors of the hazard function, and especially their confidence intervals, are not reliable in the right tail where the number of subjects still being followed is quite small. With these limitations in mind, the plot in Figure 2.14 seems to support our earlier impression that the hazard function is relatively constant over the first 5 ½ years of follow up and then increases.

Our interest in the hazard function stems from the fact that it is one of the functions that describes the underlying survival process being studied. In essence, if one is able to specify the hazard function, then the cumulative hazard, and hence, the survival function are also specified. The graphical non-parametric description of the survival experience of discrete groups of subjects, gender, age groups, etc., used in Section 2.4 is an effective analysis tool but is limited to univariable analysis of discrete covariates having only a few levels. Now we ask the question: How can we study the effect of a number of covariates on the survival experience in a manner similar to other regression models? Is it possible to characterize the hazard function, not only as a function of time but also as a function of subject and other study covariates, in such a way that resulting estimated parameters may be used to estimate covariate effects in a form that is easily understood by subject matter scientists? Stated in modeling terms, can the hazard function play the role of the systematic component in a regression analysis of survival time? The answer is, of course, yes, and we begin this task in the next Chapter.

Other texts presenting descriptive as well as other methods for survival data include: Collett (2003), Cox and Oakes (1984), Klein and Moeschberger (2003), Kleinbaum and Klein (2005), Le (1997), Lee and Wang (2003), Marubini and Valsecchi (1995) and Parmar and Machin (1995).

EXERCISES

1. Listed below are values of survival time in years for 6 males and 6 females from the WHAS100 study. Right-censored times are denoted by a "+" as a superscript.

   Males: $1.2, 3.4, 5.0^+, 5.1, 6.1, 7.1$
   Females: $0.4, 1.2, 4.3, 4.9, 5.0, 5.1^+$

   Using these data, compute the following by hand (and verify hand calculations when possible with a software package):
   (a) The Kaplan-Meier estimate of the survival function for each gender.
   (b) Pointwise 95 percent confidence intervals for the survival functions estimated in problem 1(a).
   (c) Point and 95 percent confidence interval estimates of the 25th, 50th and 75th percentiles of the survival time distribution for each gender.
   (d) The estimated mean survival time for each gender using all available times.
   (e) A graph of the estimated survival functions for each gender computed in problem 1(a) along with the pointwise and overall 95 percent limits computed in problem 1(b).

2. Repeat problem 1 using WHAS500 data. All calculations for this problem should be done using a software package.

3. Repeat problem 1 using the WHAS500 data with four groups defined by the age intervals: [40-59], [60, 69], [70, 79] and [80,90].

4. Compute by hand, and verify hand calculations with a software package, the log-rank, generalized Wilcoxon, and Peto–Prentice tests for the equality of the two survival functions estimated in problem 1(a).

5. Repeat problem 4 using data from the WHAS500 data in problem 2.

6. Repeat problem 4 using the WHAS500 data with four groups defined by the four age intervals in problem 3. Using the midpoints of the four age intervals, test for trend using the test statistic defined in (2.30). In addition, test whether the survival experience for the middle two age groups is the same or different from the youngest and oldest age groups.

7. Repeat problem 1 using the data from the ACTG 320 Study described in Table 1.5 with two groups defined by the dichotomized treatment indicator variable "tx."

8. Repeat problem 3 using the data from the ACTG 320 Study described in Table 1.5 and four age groups defined by the quartiles of age.

9. Because the minimum value of the Kaplan-Meier estimators in problem 7 is 0.869, any treatment differences in the plotted estimated survival functions are difficult to see. Explore plots of the Nelson-Aalen estimator of the cumulative hazard. Are treatment differences more easily seen? Interpret the plots in the context of the current study.

10. Repeat problem 1 using the data from the German Breast Cancer Study described in Table 1.4 using recurrence time with two groups defined by the use of hormone therapy.

11. Repeat problem 3 using the data from the German Breast Cancer Study described in Table 1.4 using recurrence time with groups defined by tumor grade.

12. Even if time-to-event is a normally distributed random variable, in most cases it would still be inappropriate to use a t-test to test for differences between groups. Why?

CHAPTER 3

Regression Models for Survival Data

3.1 INTRODUCTION

As we noted at the end of Chapter 2, our first question when considering regression modeling of survival data is: What are we going to model? Specifically, what will play the role of the systematic component in a regression model? The inherent aging process that is present when subjects are followed over time is what distinguishes survival time from other dependent variables. The presence of censoring in the data makes the study of survival time more interesting from a statistical research perspective, but from a practical point of view, it is an annoying technical detail that must be dealt with when we fit models. Of the functions describing the distribution of survival time discussed in Chapter 2, the hazard function best and most directly captures the essence of the aging process. Thus, a natural place to begin is to explore how to incorporate a regression model-like structure into the hazard function.

The simplest possible hazard function is one that is constant at all values of time. We saw in figure 2.14 that the kernel-smoothed hazard function from the WHAS100 data was nearly constant for the first 5½ years of follow-up, with a value approximately equal to 0.1. Thus for the WHAS100 data we might begin with the following model for the hazard function

$$h(t) = 0.1$$

or more generally

$$h(t) = \theta_0 . \tag{3.1}$$

Because the hazard function is a rate, it must be strictly positive. A desirable property for a statistical model to have is to be parameterized in such a way that the allowable range of parameter values is infinite. Parameter estimation is easier when this property holds. Hence, one difficulty with the form of (3.1) is that θ is constrained to be greater than zero. One approach to handle both issues is to parameterize the hazard function as

$$h(t) = e^{\beta_0} , \qquad (3.2)$$

where $\beta_0 = \ln(\theta_0)$ and is thus unconstrained. Given the form of (3.2), a natural way to include covariates is to have them be additive on the log scale. Specifically, for a covariate x the log-hazard function is

$$\ln[h(t,x)] = \beta_0 + \beta_1 x \qquad (3.3)$$

and the hazard function is

$$h(t,x) = e^{\beta_0 + \beta_1 x} . \qquad (3.4)$$

The hazard functions in (3.2) and (3.4) may be used to determine the cumulative hazard and hence the associated survival function. In this case, the resulting distribution is the exponential distribution, which is considered in detail in Chapter 8. The fact that the hazard function in (3.4) does not depend on time (i.e., it is constant over time) may be plausible in some settings but not so in others. For example the annual rate of death among healthy men in the US is more or less constant from age 20 to 40, while it increases after age 40 and dramatically so after age 70. In fact the hazard function for human life is often described as being "bathtub shaped." The model in (3.4) can be modified to include a function of time by using, for example, the Weibull model (see Chapter 8). It is possible (and indeed it is the aim of a fully parametric survival model) to characterize the hazard as an explicit function of time as well as study covariates. Every statistical distribution has an associated hazard function as determined from (2.37).

In essence, a fully parametric hazard function accomplishes two goals simultaneously: (1) It describes the basic underlying distribution of survival time (error component), and (2) It characterizes how that distribution changes as a function of the covariates (systematic component). In some applied settings it is important to use a model that accomplishes both goals, but in other settings, a model that addresses only the latter one is all that is necessary.

For example, if we want a model to predict the life-length of a particular brand of computer hard disk as a function of temperature and relative humidity, we need it to address both goals. The desired end product of the statistical modeling is an equation that may be used to predict survival time of the hard disk for specific operating conditions. In this case fully parametric models may be required. Lawless (2003) and Nelson (2004) provide a comprehensive study of parametric models. We consider several of these models in Chapter 8.

On the other hand, we are often in a setting where we may wish to see if survival is more favorable under a "new" treatment when compared with the "standard." For example, the goal of the ACTG 320 study, described briefly in Section 1.6, was to compare survival under a three-drug regimen to survival under a two-drug regimen. A complete description of survival time is of secondary importance to a description of how the new three-drug therapy modifies the survival experience relative to the two-drug therapy. We need a model whose parameters can be used to compare the relative survival experience of the two treatment groups, and this model may need to include/adjust for other patient characteristics. Fully parametric models can certainly be used to accomplish this goal. However, the assumptions required for their error components may be unnecessarily stringent or unrealistic, especially when we consider that we are going to base our inferences solely on the parameters in the systematic portion of the model. Survival time models that have a fully parametric regression structure but leave their dependence on time unspecified are called *semiparametric regression models* and these models are the major focus of this text.

3.2 SEMIPARAMETRIC REGRESSION MODELS

Suppose we wish to compare the survival experience of cancer patients on two different therapies. We noted in the previous section that a semiparametric rather than a fully parametric hazard function might be best suited for this problem. One form of a regression model for the hazard function that addresses the study goal is

$$h(t, x, \beta) = h_0(t)r(x, \beta). \tag{3.5}$$

The hazard function, as expressed in (3.5), is the product of two functions. The function, $h_0(t)$, characterizes how the hazard function changes as a function of survival time. The other function, $r(x, \beta)$, characterizes how the hazard function changes as a function of subject covariates. The functions must be chosen such that $h(t, x, \beta) > 0$. We note that $h_0(t)$ is the hazard function when $r(x, \beta) = 1$. When the function $r(x, \beta)$ is parameterized such that $r(x = 0, \beta) = 1$, $h_0(t)$ is frequently referred to as the *baseline hazard function*. Thus the baseline hazard function is, in some sense, a generalization of the intercept or constant term found in parametric regression models, a point we return to in Chapter 4. Under the model in (3.5) the ratio of the hazard functions for two subjects with covariate values denoted x_1 and x_0 is

$$\text{HR}(t, x_1, x_0) = \frac{h(t, x_1, \beta)}{h(t, x_0, \beta)} \ ,$$

so

$$\begin{aligned}
\text{HR}(t, x_1, x_0) &= \frac{h_0(t)\, r(x_1, \beta)}{h_0(t)\, r(x_0, \beta)} \\
&= \frac{r(x_1, \beta)}{r(x_0, \beta)} \ .
\end{aligned} \qquad (3.6)$$

The hazard ratio (HR) depends only on the function $r(x, \beta)$. If the ratio function $\text{HR}(t, x_1, x_0)$ has a clear clinical interpretation then, the actual form of the baseline hazard function is of little importance.

Cox (1972) was the first to propose the model in (3.6) when he suggested using $r(x, \beta) = \exp(x\beta)$. With this parameterization the hazard function is

$$h(t, x, \beta) = h_0(t)\, e^{x\beta} \qquad (3.7)$$

and the hazard ratio is

$$\text{HR}(t, x_1, x_0) = e^{\beta(x_1 - x_0)} \ . \qquad (3.8)$$

This model is referred to in the literature by a variety of terms, such as the *Cox model*, the *Cox proportional hazards model* or simply the *proportional hazards model*. Part of the appeal of the Cox model is the interpretation of (3.8) as a "relative risk"-type ratio. For example, when a covariate is dichotomous, such as gender, with a value of $x_1 = 1$ for males and $x_0 = 0$ for females, the hazard ratio in (3.8) becomes

$$\text{HR}(t, x_1, x_0) = e^{\beta} \ .$$

If the value of the coefficient is $\beta = \ln(2)$, then the interpretation is that males are "dying" at twice ($e^{\beta} = 2$) the rate of females. We defer further discussion of the interpretation of the ratio in (3.8) as a function of the coefficients to Chapter 4.

The Cox model in (3.7) is the most frequently used form of the hazard function . The term *proportional hazards* refers to the fact that, in expression (3.7), the hazard functions are multiplicatively related (i.e., their ratio is constant over survival time). This is an important assumption and methods for assessing its validity are presented in Chapter 6. Other parameterizations have been considered, most notably additive models. One example of an additive model is the *additive relative hazard model* whose hazard function is

$$h(t,x,\beta) = h_0(t)(1 + x\beta) . \tag{3.9}$$

This model is not commonly available in software packages. We discuss additive models in more detail in Chapter 9. Other more generally parameterized positive functions have been suggested [see Andersen, Borgan, Gill and Keiding (1993, Chapter VII)], but none are in wide practical use. We focus primarily on (3.7), the proportional hazards model, as it is the most frequently used model in applied settings.

Recall that the distribution of survival time can be specified through the hazard function. Thus, a natural question is: What is the survival function for a model with hazard function (3.5)? If we use the relationship shown in (2.31), then the survival function is

$$S(t,x,\beta) = e^{-H(t,x,\beta)} , \tag{3.10}$$

where $H(t,x,\beta)$ is the cumulative hazard function at time t for a subject with covariate x. We assume that survival time is absolutely continuous, in which case the value of the cumulative hazard function may be expressed, using methods of calculus, as

$$\begin{aligned} H(t,x,\beta) &= \int_0^t h(u,x,\beta)\, du \\ &= r(x,\beta)\int_0^t h_0(u)\, du \\ &= r(x,\beta)H_0(t). \end{aligned} \tag{3.11}$$

For those not comfortable with the methods of calculus, the expression in (3.11) may be considered as a measure of the cumulative baseline risk, $H_0(t)$, which is modified by the function, $r(x,\beta)$, for a subject with covariate x. Substituting the result (3.11) into (3.10), the survival function for the general semiparametric hazard function is

$$S(t,x,\beta) = e^{-r(x,\beta)H_0(t)} .$$

Thus, it follows that

$$\begin{aligned} S(t,x,\beta) &= \left[e^{-H_0(t)}\right]^{r(x,\beta)} \\ &= \left[S_0(t)\right]^{r(x,\beta)} , \end{aligned} \tag{3.12}$$

where $S_0(t) = e^{-H_0(t)}$ is the baseline survival function.

Under the Cox model, the survival function is

$$S(t,x,\beta) = \left[S_0(t)\right]^{\exp(x\beta)}. \tag{3.13}$$

The form of the expression for the survival function in (3.13) is a consequence of the multiplicative relationship between the baseline hazard function and the exponential function that describes the effect of the covariates. The value of the baseline survival function is always between zero and one (true of any survival function). Suppose the covariate is age, denoted a, which we model using $x = a - \bar{a}$. Then the baseline survival function corresponds to a subject whose age is equal to the mean age, $\bar{a}$, of the data. Assuming that the risk associated with age is positive (as is usually the case), then $\beta > 0$, and for $a > \bar{a}$ it follows that for $x > 0$, $\exp(x\beta) > 1$ and $S(t,x,\beta) < S_0(t)$. The interpretation is that the survival experience is less favorable for age a ($a > \bar{a}$) than at the mean age. In other words, at any point in time, the proportion of subjects alive at age a is smaller than the proportion alive at age $\bar{a}$. Similarly, if age is $a < \bar{a}$, then $x < 0$, $\exp(x\beta) < 1$ and $S(t,x,\beta) > S_0(t)$, implying that the survival experience is more favorable at age a than at the mean age.

In the next section, we consider estimation of the parameters in the proportional hazards model.

3.3   FITTING THE PROPORTIONAL HAZARDS REGRESSION MODEL

A natural place to begin studying the problem of estimating parameters is by seeing if we can apply the method of maximum likelihood to the proportional hazards model in (3.7).

Assume we have n independent observations, each containing information on the length of time a subject was observed, whether the observation was a survival time or was right censored and a single covariate whose value is determined at the time observation begins and remains at that value throughout the follow-up of the subject. Covariates whose values are fixed at the value measured at the beginning of follow-up are most commonly encountered in practice. However, covariates whose values change over time, generally referred to as *time varying covariates*, can be easily accommodated and are discussed in some detail in Chapter 7. For simplicity, as well as for basic applicability, we restrict consideration in this and the next few chapters to covariates whose values are fixed. Denote the triplet of observed time, covariate and censoring variable as (t_i, x_i, c_i), $i = 1, 2, ..., n$.

The first step in maximum likelihood estimation is to create the specific likelihood function to be maximized. In simplest terms, the likelihood function is an expression that yields a quantity similar to the probability of the observed data under the model. Suppose that the distribution of survival time for a subject with a single covariate can be described by the cumulative distribution function $F(t,\beta,x)$. For example, in the WHAS100 study, the value of the function $F(5,\beta,65)$ gives the proportion of 65-year-old subjects expected to die in less than or equal to 5 years. The survival function is obtained from the cumulative distribution function and is defined as $S(t,\beta,x) = 1 - F(t,\beta,x)$. The value of the function $S(5,\beta,65)$ gives the proportion of 65 year olds expected to live at least 5 years. To create the likelihood function, we also need a function that we think of, for the moment, as giving the "probability" that the survival time is exactly t. This function is derived mathematically from the distribution function and is called the density function. We denote the density function corresponding to $F(t,\beta,x)$ as $f(t,\beta,x)$. For example, the value of the function $f(5,\beta,65)$ gives the "probability" that a subject 65 years old survives exactly 5 years.[1]

We construct the actual likelihood function by considering the contribution of the triplets $(t,1,x)$ and $(t,0,x)$ separately. In the case of the triplet $(t,1,x)$ we know that the survival time was exactly t. Thus the contribution to the likelihood for this triplet is the "probability" that a subject with covariate value x dies from the disease of interest at time t units. This is given by the value of the density function $f(t,\beta,x)$. For the triplet $(t,0,x)$ we know that the survival time was at least t. Thus, the contribution to the likelihood function of this triplet is the *probability* that a subject with covariate value x survives at least t time units. This probability is given by the survival function $S(t,\beta,x)$. Under the assumption of independent observations, the full likelihood function is obtained by multiplying the respective contributions of the observed triplets, a value of $f(t,\beta,x)$ for a non-censored observation and a value of $S(t,\beta,x)$ for censored observations. In general, a concise way to denote the contribution of each triplet to the likelihood is the expression

$$\left[f(t,\beta,x) \right]^c \times \left[S(t,\beta,x) \right]^{1-c}, \tag{3.14}$$

where $c = 0$ or 1.

---

[1] Readers who have had some mathematical statistics know that the density function does not yield a probability but a probability per-unit of time over a small interval of time:
$f(t,\beta,x) = \lim_{\Delta t \to 0} \left\{ F(t + \Delta t, \beta, x) - F(t,\beta,x)/\Delta t \right\}.$

Because the observations are assumed to be independent, the likelihood function is the product of the expression in (3.14) over the entire sample and is

$$l(\beta) = \prod_{i=1}^{n} \left\{ \left[f(t_i,\beta,x_i) \right]^{c_i} \times \left[S(t_i,\beta,x_i) \right]^{1-c_i} \right\}. \tag{3.15}$$

To obtain the maximized likelihood with respect to the parameter of interest, β, we maximize the log-likelihood function

$$L(\beta) = \sum_{i=1}^{n} \left\{ c_i \ln \left[f(t_i,\beta,x_i) \right] + (1 - c_i) \ln \left[S(t_i,\beta,x_i) \right] \right\}. \tag{3.16}$$

Because the log function is monotone, the maximum of (3.15) and (3.16) occur at the same value of β; however, maximizing (3.16) is computationally simpler than maximizing (3.15). The procedure to obtain the values of the MLE involves taking the derivative of $L(\beta)$ with respect to β, the unknown parameter, setting these equations equal to zero, and solving for β. An application of methods from calculus shows that the density function is the product of the hazard function and the survival function, yielding the expression

$$f(t,x,\beta) = h(t,x,\beta) \times S(t,x,\beta). \tag{3.17}$$

Substituting (3.17) into the log-likelihood equation in (3.16) and simplifying using the form of the proportional hazards model in (3.13) yields

$$L(\beta) = \sum_{i=1}^{n} \left\{ c_i \ln \left[h_0(t_i) \right] + c_i x_i \beta + e^{x_i \beta} \ln \left[S_0(t_i) \right] \right\}. \tag{3.18}$$

Full maximum likelihood requires that we maximize (3.18) with respect to the unknown parameter of interest, β, and the unspecified baseline hazard and survival functions. As discussed in some detail in Kalbfleisch and Prentice (2002) it is not possible to use the log-likelihood function in (3.18). Therefore, the proportional hazards model in (3.18) is chosen to avoid having to specify explicitly the error component of the model.

Cox (1972) proposed using an expression he called a "partial likelihood function" that depends only on the parameter of interest. He speculated that the resulting parameter estimators from the partial likelihood function would have the same distributional properties as full maximum likelihood estimators. Rigorous mathematical proofs of this conjecture came later, and the counting process approach based on martingales simplified earlier work (see Andersen, Borgan, Gill and Keiding (1993, Chapter VII) and Fleming and Harrington (1991, Chapter 4). At this point, it is not vital that one understands the details of the mathematics. An intermediate level of presentation of the construction of the partial likelihood is provided in Collett (2003). The essential idea is similar to the one used to generate the conditional logistic regression model for matched case-control studies or other stratified designs that introduce a large number of nuisance parameters into the model [see Hosmer and Lemeshow (2000, Chapter 7)]. In the present setting, the partial likelihood is given by the expression

$$l_p(\beta) = \prod_{i=1}^{n} \left[\frac{e^{x_i\beta}}{\sum_{j \in R(t_i)} e^{x_j\beta}} \right]^{c_i}, \tag{3.19}$$

where the summation in the denominator is over all subjects in the risk set at time t_i, denoted by $R(t_i)$. Recall that the risk set consists of all subjects with survival or censored times greater than or equal to the specified time.

The expression in (3.19) assumes that there are no tied times, and it is often modified to exclude terms when $c_i = 0$, yielding

$$l_p(\beta) = \prod_{i=1}^{m} \frac{e^{x_{(i)}\beta}}{\sum_{j \in R(t_{(i)})} e^{x_j\beta}}, \tag{3.20}$$

where the product is over the m distinct ordered survival times and $x_{(i)}$ denotes the value of the covariate for the subject with ordered survival time $t_{(i)}$. The log partial likelihood function is

$$L_p(\beta) = \sum_{i=1}^{m} \left\{ x_{(i)}\beta - \ln \left[\sum_{j \in R(t_{(i)})} e^{x_j\beta} \right] \right\}. \tag{3.21}$$

We obtain the maximum partial likelihood estimator by differentiating the right hand side of (3.21) with respect to β, setting the derivative equal to zero and solving for the unknown parameter. The derivative of (3.21) with respect to β is

$$\frac{\partial L_p(\beta)}{\partial \beta} = \sum_{i=1}^{m} \left\{ x_{(i)} - \frac{\sum\limits_{j \in R(t_{(i)})} x_j e^{x_j \beta}}{\sum\limits_{j \in R(t_{(i)})} e^{x_j \beta}} \right\}$$

$$= \sum_{i=1}^{m} \left\{ x_{(i)} - \sum_{j \in R(t_{(i)})} w_{ij}(\beta) x_j \right\}$$

$$= \sum_{i=1}^{m} \left\{ x_{(i)} - \bar{x}_{w_i} \right\},$$

(3.22)

where

$$w_{ij}(\beta) = \frac{e^{x_j \beta}}{\sum\limits_{l \in R(t_{(i)})} e^{x_l \beta}}$$

and

$$\bar{x}_{w_i} = \sum_{j \in R(t_{(i)})} w_{ij}(\beta) x_j .$$

All software packages provide the maximum partial likelihood estimator, which we denote as $\hat{\beta}$.

The estimator of the variance of the estimator of the coefficient is obtained in the same manner as variance estimators are obtained in most maximum likelihood estimation applications. The estimator is the inverse of the negative of the second derivative of the log partial likelihood at the value of the estimator. In particular, taking the derivative of (3.22) we obtain the following expression

$$\frac{\partial^2 L_p(\beta)}{\partial \beta^2} = -\sum_{i=1}^{m} \left\{ \frac{\left[\sum\limits_{j \in R(t_{(i)})} e^{x_j \beta} \right] \left[\sum\limits_{j \in R(t_{(i)})} x_j^2 e^{x_j \beta} \right] - \left[\sum\limits_{j \in R(t_{(i)})} x_j e^{x_j \beta} \right]^2}{\left[\sum\limits_{j \in R(t_{(i)})} e^{x_j \beta} \right]^2} \right\}.$$

(3.23)

The form of this expression may be simplified by using the definition of $w_{ij}(\beta)$. The simplified expression is

$$\frac{\partial^2 L_p(\beta)}{\partial \beta^2} = -\sum_{i=1}^{m} \sum_{j \in R(t_{(i)})} w_{ij}(\beta) \left(x_j - \bar{x}_{w_i} \right)^2 .$$

(3.24)

The negative of the second derivative of the log partial likelihood in (3.23) or (3.24) is called the *observed information*, and we will denote it as

$$\mathbf{I}(\beta) = -\frac{\partial^2 L_p(\beta)}{\partial \beta^2} \, . \tag{3.25}$$

Later in this chapter we will consider models containing more than one covariate and the result in (3.25) will be called the *observed information matrix*. The estimator of the variance of the estimated coefficient is the inverse of (3.25) evaluated at $\hat{\beta}$ and is

$$\hat{\mathrm{Var}}(\hat{\beta}) = \mathbf{I}(\hat{\beta})^{-1} \, . \tag{3.26}$$

The estimator of the standard error, denoted $\hat{\mathrm{SE}}(\hat{\beta})$, is the positive square root of the variance estimator in (3.26).

As an example, we return to the ACTG320 study described in Section 1.3 (see Table 1.5) and studied in more detail in exercises at the end of Chapter 2. The goal of this study is to examine the effectiveness of a new three drug treatment regimen when compared to the standard two drug regimen in improving survival among HIV infected patients. We begin by fitting a model containing the treatment indicator variable, tx. The results are shown in Table 3.1 where the value of the estimated coefficient is $\hat{\beta} = -0.684$, and the estimated standard error of the estimated coefficient is $\hat{\mathrm{SE}}(\hat{\beta}) = 0.2149$. We defer discussing the interpretation of the estimated coefficient to Chapter 4.

Typically, the first steps following the fit of a regression model are the assessment of the significance of the model and the formation of a confidence interval for key estimated parameters. We discuss methods that can be used for each of these tasks.

Three related tests to assess the significance of the coefficient are: the partial likelihood ratio test, the Wald test and the score test.

The partial likelihood ratio test, denoted G, is calculated as twice the difference between the log partial likelihood of the model containing the covariate and the log partial likelihood for the model not containing the covariate. Specifically

$$G = 2\left\{ L_p(\hat{\beta}) - L_p(0) \right\}, \tag{3.27}$$

where the log partial likelihood evaluated at $\beta = 0$ is

$$L_p(0) = -\sum_{i=1}^{m} \ln(n_i) \tag{3.28}$$

Table 3.1 Estimated Coefficient, Standard Error, z-Score, Two-Tailed p-value, and 95% Confidence Interval Estimate for the Proportional Hazards Model Containing Treatment (tx)

Variable	Coeff.	Std. Err.	z	p>|z|	95% CIE
tx	–0.684	0.2149	–3.18	0.001	–1.105, –0.263

and n_i denotes the number of subjects in the risk set at observed survival time $t_{(i)}$.

Under the null hypothesis that the coefficient is equal to zero (along with other mathematical assumptions), this statistic will follow a chi-square distribution with 1 degree of freedom and thus can be used to obtain p-values to test the significance of the coefficient. The mathematical details using a counting process approach to the partial likelihood may be found in Andersen, Borgan, Gill and Keiding (1993) and Fleming and Harrington (1991). In practice, the assumption of a "sufficiently" large sample size cited for likelihood ratio tests translates in this case into having the number of observed non-censored survival times be large relative to the number of parameters. There are 96 deaths in the ACTG320 data, which would be judged large enough for a model containing one covariate, by even the most conservative "rule of thumb." For a categorical covariate, such as tx, there must be a large enough number of events at each level of the covariate. The minimum cell frequency in the four-fold table cross-classifying censor and tx is 33, again a reasonably large number. We will consider this point in more detail when we discuss numerical fitting problems at the end of Chapter 5.

Software packages fitting the proportional hazards model typically provide the value of the log partial likelihood for the fitted model and the value of G. For the example in Table 3.1, these values are $L_p(\hat{\beta}) = -653.118$ and $G = 10.70$. We can use (3.27) to obtain the log partial likelihood of model zero[2] as

$$L_p(0) = L_p(\hat{\beta}) - G/2 = (-653.118) - (10.70/2) = -658.468.$$

The p-value for the test is $\Pr(\chi^2(1) \geq 10.70) = 0.001$, so we reject the null hypothesis and conclude that the new three-drug treatment regimen is significantly related to survival time.

Another test for significance of the coefficient is the ratio of the estimated coefficient to its estimated standard error. This ratio is commonly referred to as a *Wald statistic*. Under the same mathematical assumptions required for the log partial likelihood ratio test, the Wald statistic follows a standard normal distribu-

---

[2] This will be useful later when we extend the partial likelihood ratio test to the mutivariable regression setting.

tion. The Wald statistic and its p-value are typically reported by software packages. However, some statistical packages (e.g., SAS) report the square of the Wald statistic, which follows a chi-square distribution with one degree-of-freedom under the null hypothesis. Unlike normal errors linear regression where the square of the t-statistic for the coefficient in a univariable model is equal to the F-test for significance, the Wald and log partial likelihood ratio test are not numerically related, but are usually of quite similar magnitude. The equation for the Wald statistic is

$$z = \frac{\hat{\beta}}{\widehat{SE}(\hat{\beta})}. \qquad (3.29)$$

The value shown in Table 3.1 is

$$z = \frac{-0.684}{0.2149} = -3.18$$

and its two-tailed p-value is $\Pr(|z| > -3.18) = 0.001$.

The score test is a third test we are likely to encounter. The test statistic is the ratio of the derivative of the log partial likelihood, equation (3.22), to the square root of the observed information (equation (3.25)) all evaluated at $\beta = 0$. Thus the equation for the score test is

$$z^* = \frac{\partial L_p / \partial \beta}{\sqrt{I(\beta)}}\bigg|_{\beta=0}. \qquad (3.30)$$

Under the hypothesis that the coefficient is equal to zero and the same mathematical conditions required for the Wald and partial likelihood ratio tests, this statistic also follows the standard normal distribution. The value of the score test for the example in Table 3.1 is $z^* = 3.25$, and the two-tailed p-value is $\Pr(|z^*| > 3.25) = 0.001$. The score test, when computed by a software package such as SAS or SPSS, may be reported as the square of the value of (3.30) which, under the null hypothesis, follows a chi-square distribution with one degree of freedom.

In practice, the numeric values of the three tests $(\sqrt{G}, z \text{ and } z^*)$ are usually quite similar and thus lead one to draw the same conclusion about the significance of the coefficient. In situations where there is disagreement, making it necessary to choose one test, the partial likelihood ratio test is the preferred test.

A clear advantage of the score test is that it may be computed without evaluating the maximum partial likelihood estimator of the coefficient. For this reason, the score test has gained some favor as a test to use in model building applications in which evaluation of the estimator is computationally intensive. We consider this point further when we discuss statistical methods for variable selection in Chapter 5.

The confidence interval for the coefficient shown in Table 3.1 is called the Wald-statistic-based interval. Its endpoints are based on the same assumptions as the Wald test for significance, i.e., that the estimator is distributed normally with standard error estimated by the square root of (3.26). The endpoints of a $100(1-\alpha)$ percent confidence interval for the coefficient are

$$\hat{\beta} \pm z_{1-\alpha/2}\widehat{\text{SE}}(\hat{\beta}).$$

The endpoints of the 95 percent confidence interval shown in Table 3.1 are computed as

$$-0.684 \pm 1.96 \times 0.2149,$$

yielding the interval reported in Table 3.1, $-1.105 \le \beta \le -0.263$. The fact that this interval does not include zero suggests, as did each of the three tests, that the three-drug treatment is associated with survival time.

Up to this point, we have considered models in which only one covariate is of interest. One advantage of using regression modeling in any statistical analysis is the ability to include multiple covariates in the model simultaneously. We now focus on the extension of the proportional hazards model to include a collection of p covariates whose values are measured on each individual at the time follow-up begins and remain fixed over time.

Let the p covariates for subject i be denoted by the vector $\mathbf{x}_i' = (x_{i1}, x_{i2}, \ldots, x_{ip})$. (Note that we use a bold non-italicized font for vectors and matrices.) This vector can include any collection of covariates: continuous covariates, design variables for nominal scale covariates, products of covariates (interactions) and other higher-order terms. Denote the triplet of observed time, covariates and censoring variable as $(t_i, \mathbf{x}_i, c_i)$, $i = 1, 2, \ldots, n$. The partial likelihood for the multivariable model is obtained by replacing the single covariate, x, in (3.19) with the vector of covariates, $\mathbf{x}$. Its expression is so similar to (3.19) that it is not repeated.

There are p equations, one for each covariate, similar to (3.22) which, when set equal to zero and solved, yield the maximum partial likelihood estimators. We denote the vector of coefficients as $\boldsymbol{\beta}' = (\beta_1, \beta_2, \ldots, \beta_p)$. The equation for the k-th covariate is

$$\frac{\partial L_p(\boldsymbol{\beta})}{\partial \beta_k} = \sum_{i=1}^{m} \left\{ x_{(ik)} - \frac{\displaystyle\sum_{j \in R(t_{(i)})} x_{jk} e^{\mathbf{x}_j'\boldsymbol{\beta}}}{\displaystyle\sum_{j \in R(t_{(i)})} e^{\mathbf{x}_j'\boldsymbol{\beta}}} \right\} \tag{3.31}$$

$$= \sum_{i=1}^{m} \left\{ x_{(ik)} - \overline{x}_{w_ik} \right\},$$

$$\overline{x}_{w_ik} = \sum_{j \in R(t_{(i)})} w_{ij}(\boldsymbol{\beta}) x_{jk}$$

and

$$w_{ij}(\boldsymbol{\beta}) = \frac{e^{\mathbf{x}_j'\boldsymbol{\beta}}}{\displaystyle\sum_{l \in R(t_{(i)})} e^{\mathbf{x}_l'\boldsymbol{\beta}}}.$$

We use $x_{(ik)}$ to denote the value of covariate x_k for the subject with observed ordered survival time $t_{(i)}$. We denote the maximum partial likelihood estimator as $\hat{\boldsymbol{\beta}}' = (\hat{\beta}_1, \hat{\beta}_2, \ldots, \hat{\beta}_p)$.

The elements of the p by p information matrix are obtained by extending the definition in (3.25) to include all second-order partial derivatives, namely

$$\mathbf{I}(\boldsymbol{\beta}) = -\frac{\partial^2 L(\boldsymbol{\beta})}{\partial \boldsymbol{\beta}^2}.$$

The general form of the elements in this matrix is obtained from (3.24). The diagonal elements are

$$\frac{\partial^2 L_p(\boldsymbol{\beta})}{\partial \beta_k^2} = -\sum_{i=1}^{m} \sum_{j \in R(t_{(i)})} w_{ij} \left(x_{jk} - \overline{x}_{w_ik} \right)^2 \tag{3.32}$$

and the off-diagonal elements are

$$\frac{\partial^2 L_p(\boldsymbol{\beta})}{\partial \beta_k \partial \beta_l} = -\sum_{i=1}^{m} \sum_{j \in R(t_{(i)})} w_{ij} \left(x_{jk} - \overline{x}_{w_ik} \right)\left(x_{jl} - \overline{x}_{w_il} \right). \tag{3.33}$$

The estimator of the covariance matrix of the maximum partial likelihood estimator is obtained by extending (3.26) and is the inverse of the observed information matrix evaluated at the maximum partial likelihood estimator

$$\hat{\text{Var}}(\hat{\boldsymbol{\beta}}) = \mathbf{I}(\hat{\boldsymbol{\beta}})^{-1}. \tag{3.34}$$

Software packages typically provide the value of the estimated standard error for all estimated coefficients in the model. Most packages provide the user with the option of obtaining the full estimated covariance matrix for the estimated parameters.

As an example, we return to the ACTG320 data used to illustrate fitting a model containing a single covariate in Table 3.1. There we saw that the sample size is 1151 but there are only 96 events, which limits the size of a multivariable model that can be fit to these data. Again, the goal of the study is to examine the effectiveness of the new three-drug treatment regimen, but due to the limited number of events, we are only going to be able to control for a few variables, hence model parsimony is vital. We begin by fitting a five-variable model containing: treatment (tx), age, sex, CD4 count, and prior months use of ZDV (priorzdv). We show the results of the fit in Table 3.2.

As is the case when fitting any regression model, we first test for the overall significance of the model. The log partial likelihood ratio test is shown in (3.27). From testing the significance of the univariable model containing treatment (tx), we found that the log partial likelihood for model 0 is $L_p(0) = -658.468$. The log partial likelihood for the fitted multivariable model in Table 3.2 is $L_p(\hat{\beta}) = -618.826$, and the value of the log partial likelihood ratio test is

$$G = 2\big[(-618.826)-(-658.468)\big] = 79.28 .$$

Under the null hypothesis that all five coefficients are simultaneously equal to zero and, under the mathematical regularity and large sample conditions referred to above, G will follow a chi-square distribution with five degrees of freedom (one for each coefficient). The p-value for the test in this example is $\Pr\left(\chi^2(5) \geq 79.28\right) \leq 0.001$, providing evidence that at least one of the coefficients in the model is significantly associated with survival time.

The multivariable score and Wald tests for the multiple proportional hazards regression model are most easily defined using matrix notation. Specifically, we denote the vector of first partial derivatives whose elements are given in (3.31) as $\mathbf{u}(\boldsymbol{\beta})$. Under the hypothesis that all coefficients are equal to zero, and under the mathematical conditions needed for the partial likelihood ratio test, the vector of scores $\mathbf{u}(\mathbf{0}) = \mathbf{u}(\boldsymbol{\beta})|_{\boldsymbol{\beta}=\mathbf{0}}$ will be distributed as multivariate normal with mean vector

Table 3.2 Estimated Coefficients, Standard Errors, z-Scores, Two-Tailed p-values, and 95% Confidence Interval Estimates for the Proportional Hazards Model Containing Treatment (tx), Age, Sex, CD4 Count (cd4), and Prior Months Use of ZD (priorzdv)

Variable	Coeff.	Std. Err.	z	$p > \lvert z \rvert$	95% CIE
tx	−0.659	0.2153	−3.06	0.002	−1.081, −0.237
age	0.028	0.0300	2.52	0.012	0.006, 0.050
sex	0.097	0.2841	0.34	0.732	−0.460, 0.654
cd4	−0.017	0.0025	−6.51	<0.001	−0.022, −0.012
priorzdv	−0.003	0.0037	−0.08	0.937	−0.008, 0.007

equal to zero and covariance matrix given by the information matrix evaluated at the coefficient vector equal to zero, $I(0) = I(\beta)\big|_{\beta=0}$. The elements in this matrix are obtained by evaluating the expressions in (3.32) and (3.33) with the coefficient vector equal to zero. The score test statistic is

$$ u'(0)\big[I(0)\big]^{-1} u(0), $$

which is distributed asymptotically as chi-square with p degrees-of-freedom, $p = 5$ in our example. Under the same assumptions, the estimator of the coefficient, $\hat{\beta}$, will be asymptotically normally distributed with mean vector equal to zero and a covariance matrix estimated by the expression in (3.34). The multiple variable Wald test statistic is

$$ \hat{\beta}'I(\hat{\beta})\hat{\beta}, $$

which is also distributed asymptotically as chi-square with p degrees of freedom. Both the score and Wald test require matrix calculations that, while not difficult from a purely technical perspective, are not as easy to perform in most packages as the partial likelihood ratio test. For this reason, we do not often use the multiple variable score and Wald tests in this text. The values for the multiple variable score and Wald tests for the model in Table 3.2 are 63.15 ($p < 0.001$) and 55.71 ($p < 0.001$), respectively.

During the model building process, the univariate Wald tests based on individual estimated coefficients can provide guidance to possible variables that might be eliminated from the model without compromising model performance. The individual p-values in Table 3.2 suggest that the coefficients for sex and priorzdv may not be significant. To explore this further, we fit a reduced model that excludes these two covariates. The results are shown in Table 3.3. The output from

Table 3.3 Estimated Coefficients, Standard Errors, z-Scores, Two-Tailed p-values, and 95% Confidence Intervals for the Proportional Hazards Model Containing Treatment (tx), Age, and CD4 count (cd4)

Variable	Coeff.	Std. Err.	z	$p>|z|$	95% CIE
tx	−0.659	0.2150	−3.06	0.002	−1.080, −0.370
age	0.028	0.0111	2.49	0.013	0.006, 0.050
cd4	−0.017	0.0025	−6.52	<0.001	−0.021, −0.012

the fit of the model shows that the partial likelihood ratio test for the model has $p <$ 0.001. Each of the three variables remaining in the model have a significant p-value for their Wald statistic, indicating that at least from a statistical point of view, none should removed from the model.

Next we calculate the partial likelihood ratio test for exclusion of sex and priorzdv, keeping tx, age and cd4 in the model, by comparing the values of the logpartial likelihood function for the models in Tables 3.2 and 3.3. This test is analogous to the partial F-test in linear regression, in that two models having a common set of covariates are being compared. As in any multivariable analysis, we must make sure that both models have been fit to the same set of data. Because the ACTG320 data we are using has no missing values, this is not an issue. The value of the log partial likelihood function for the reduced model in Table 3.3 is $L(3) = -618.885$ which, when compared with that of the larger model in Table 3.2, yields a test statistic whose value is

$$G = 2\left[(-618.826) - (-618.885)\right] = 0.118.$$

Under the null hypothesis that the coefficients for sex and priorzdv have co-effcients equal to zero, given that the main effects for tx, age and cd4 are in the model, this statistic will follow a chi-square distribution with two degrees of freedom. The p-value for the test statistic is $\Pr(\chi^2(2) \geq 0.118) = 0.942$, indicating that the two variables do not contribute to a model containing tx, age, and cd4. As noted above, we defer discussion of interpretation of coefficients from the fitted models until Chapter 4.

In summary, the basic techniques for fitting the proportional hazards model are identical to those used in other modeling scenarios, such as the logistic and Poisson regression models. Maximum likelihood methods are used to obtain estimators of the coefficients and their standard errors. We use log-likelihood functions in a standard manner to obtain test statistics used with the chi-square distribution to assess the overall significance of the model and to compare nested models. The only difference between the analysis of the proportional hazards model and other models is that the likelihood function is a partial, rather than a full, likelihood function.

3.4 FITTING THE PROPORTIONAL HAZARDS MODEL WITH TIED SURVIVAL TIMES

The partial likelihood function methods described in the previous section are based on the assumption that there were no tied values among the observed survival times. Because most, if not all, applied settings are likely to have some tied observations, modifications to handle ties are needed. A number of approaches have been suggested and, of these, three are used by software packages: an exact expression that is derived in Kalbfleisch and Prentice (2002) and approximations due to Breslow (1974) and to Efron (1977). The analyses presented in the previous section used the Breslow approximation described below. We give a general description of each method. Therneau and Grambsch (2000) discuss them in greater detail.

We will not present the mathematical expression for the exact partial likelihood. The basis for its construction assumes that the d ties at a particular survival time are due to lack of precision in measuring survival time. Thus the tied values could actually have been observed in any one of the possible d factorial arrangements of their values. The exact partial likelihood is obtained by modifying the denominator of (3.19) to include each of these arrangements at each risk set. The SAS and STATA software packages include the option of using the exact partial likelihood.

The approximations derived by Breslow (1974) and Efron (1977) are designed to provide expressions more easily computed than the exact partial likelihood, yet that still account for the fact that ties are present among the observed values of survival time. For ease of notation, we present the approximations to the exact partial likelihood for the case when the model contains a single covariate. The Breslow approximation uses as the partial likelihood

$$l_{p1}(\beta) = \prod_{i=1}^{m} \frac{e^{x_{(i)+}\beta}}{\left[\sum_{j \in R(t_{(i)})} e^{x_j\beta} \right]^{d_i}} , \qquad (3.35)$$

where d_i denotes the number of subjects with survival time $t_{(i)}$ and $x_{(i)+}$ is equal to the sum of the covariate values over the d_i subjects. That is,

$x_{(i)+} = \sum_{j \in D(t_{(i)})} x_j$, where $D(t_{(i)})$ represents the subjects with survival times equal to $t_{(i)}$. The Efron approximation is a bit more complicated and yields a slightly better approximation to the exact partial likelihood than the Breslow approximation. It uses the approximation

$$l_{p2}(\beta) = \prod_{i=1}^{m} \frac{e^{x_{(i)+}\beta}}{\prod_{k=1}^{d_i} \left[\sum_{j \in R(t_{(i)})} e^{x_j\beta} - \frac{k-1}{d_i} \sum_{j \in D(t_{(i)})} e^{x_j\beta} \right]} . \tag{3.36}$$

Note that when $d_i = 1$, the terms in the numerators and denominators of (3.20), (3.35), and (3.36) are identical.

The maximum partial likelihood estimator for β in the presence of ties is obtained in the same manner as in the non-tied data case, with the exception that derivatives are taken with respect to the unknown parameter in the log of either the Breslow (1974) or Efron (1977) approximation to the partial likelihood. These equations are similar in form to (3.22). The estimator of the variance of the estimated coefficient is obtained from the second partial derivative evaluated at the value of the estimator, and results are similar to (3.23) - (3.25).

There are few ties in any of the data sets described in Section 1.3. To provide a good example of tied data, we use the WHAS100 data and first convert follow up time in days to months, then round months to the nearest quarter year, replacing values rounded to zero to 1.5 months. This yields 27 distinct survival times among the 100 subjects, with the number of deaths at a particular time ranging from 1 to 14. If there are major differences in the estimators obtained from the three versions of the partial likelihood with ties, it should be apparent in this example. The values of the estimator using each of the three methods are shown in Table 3.4 for the model containing bmi and gender.

The results shown in Table 3.4 support the fact that the Efron (1977) method of correcting for tied survival times yields estimates closer to those obtained from the exact partial likelihood than estimates obtained from the Breslow (1974) approximation. While this is true in a strict numeric sense, all three point estimates are close to one another. The Breslow estimates differ from the exact estimates by about 4 percent, and the Efron estimates differ by 0.4 to 1 percent. The estimated standard errors differ by 1-2 percent. Hence, we would reach the same scientific conclusion using the estimates from the Breslow partial likelihood as we would with the estimates from the other two partial likelihoods. Thus, given a choice, we prefer to use the Efron approximation, but in this example, the Breslow approximation yields acceptably close estimates.

Table 3.4 Estimated Coefficients and Standard Errors for Age and IV Drug Use Obtained from the Exact Partial Likelihood, Breslow and Efron Approximations for tied observations for modified WHAS100 data

Method	bmi		gender	
	Coeff.	Std. Err.	Coeff.	Std. Err.
Exact	−0.0921	0.03378	0.5391	0.28755
Breslow	−0.0885	0.03299	0.5181	0.28302
Efron	−0.0925	0.03343	0.5332	0.28278

The Breslow (1974) approximation is available in many software packages. The Efron (1977) approximation is available in the SAS and STATA. In many, if not most, applied settings there will be little or no practical difference between the estimators obtained from the two approximations. Because of this, and because the Breslow approximation is more commonly available, unless stated otherwise, analyses presented in this text will be based on Breslow.

3.5 ESTIMATING THE SURVIVAL FUNCTION OF THE PROPORTIONAL HAZARDS REGRESSION MODEL

An estimator of the baseline survival function, $S_0(t)$, of the proportional hazards model is available as an output option in most software packages. This estimator may be used, when combined with the estimated coefficients and specific covariate values, to estimate the survival experience of subgroups of subjects of particular interest and is discussed in detail in Chapter 4. In this section we present how the estimator itself is obtained.

The expression for the proportional hazards survival function in (3.13) allowing for more than one covariate is repeated here for convenience

$$S(t,\mathbf{x},\boldsymbol{\beta}) = \left[S_0(t)\right]^{\exp(\mathbf{x}'\boldsymbol{\beta})}. \tag{3.37}$$

This indicates that, once we have an estimator of the regression coefficients, all we need is an estimator of the baseline survival function. A likelihood-based approach, which assumes that the hazard is constant between observed survival times, is the foundation of the method. Lawless (2003) provides details that we sketch here. Fleming and Harrington (1991) and Andersen, Borgan, Gill and Keiding (1993) use the counting process approach to derive the estimator.

The essential idea of the likelihood approach is to mimic the arguments that lead to the Kaplan–Meier estimator of the survival function described in Chapter

2, equation (2.1). The key point in that development is the use of the quantity $\hat{\alpha}_i = 1 - d_i/n_i$ as an estimator of the conditional survival probability at observed ordered survival time $t_{(i)}$. The Kaplan–Meier estimator of the survival function is the product of estimators of the individual conditional survival probabilities. The expression for the conditional survival probability that leads to this estimator is $\alpha_i = S(t_{(i)})/S(t_{(i-1)})$. To extend this argument to the proportional hazards model, we define the conditional baseline survival probability as $\alpha_{0i} = S_0(t_{(i)})/S_0(t_{(i-1)})$, and it follows that the survival probability is

$$\frac{S(t_{(i)},\mathbf{x},\boldsymbol{\beta})}{S(t_{(i-1)},\mathbf{x},\boldsymbol{\beta})} = \left\{ \frac{\left[S_0(t_{(i)})\right]^{\exp(\mathbf{x}'\boldsymbol{\beta})}}{\left[S_0(t_{(i-1)})\right]^{\exp(\mathbf{x}'\boldsymbol{\beta})}} \right\} = \left\{ \frac{S_0(t_{(i)})}{S_0(t_{(i-1)})} \right\}^{\exp(\mathbf{x}'\boldsymbol{\beta})} = \alpha_{0i}^{\exp(\mathbf{x}'\boldsymbol{\beta})}.$$

Maximum likelihood methods are employed, conditional on the partial likelihood estimator of the regression coefficients, $\hat{\boldsymbol{\beta}}$, in the model. To simplify the notation, we let $\hat{\theta}_l = \exp(\mathbf{x}_l'\boldsymbol{\beta})$, and the estimator of the conditional baseline survival probability is obtained by solving the equation

$$\sum_{l \in D_i} \frac{\hat{\theta}_l}{1 - \alpha_{0i}^{\hat{\theta}_l}} = \sum_{l \in R_i} \hat{\theta}_l , \qquad (3.38)$$

where R_i denotes the subjects in the risk set at ordered observed survival time $t_{(i)}$ and D_i denotes the subjects in the risk set with survival times equal to $t_{(i)}$.

If there are no tied survival times, D_i contains one subject and the solution to (3.38) is

$$\hat{\alpha}_{0i} = \left[1 - \frac{\hat{\theta}_i}{\sum_{l \in R_i} \hat{\theta}_l} \right]^{\hat{\theta}_i^{-1}}. \qquad (3.39)$$

If there are tied survival times, then (3.38) is solved by iterative methods. The estimator of the baseline survival function is the product of the individual estimators of the conditional baseline survival probabilities

$$\hat{S}_0(t) = \prod_{t_{(i)} \leq t} \hat{\alpha}_{0i} , \qquad (3.40)$$

where $\hat{\alpha}_{0i}$ is the solution to (3.38). This estimator is used in some software packages, for example, SAS and STATA. Other packages may use an approximation to the solution for (3.38) from Breslow (1974). To obtain this solution, one replaces $\alpha_{0i}^{\hat{\theta}_l}$ on the left-hand side of (3.38) with the approximation $\alpha_{0i}^{\hat{\theta}_l} \approx 1 + \hat{\theta}_l \ln(\alpha_{0i})$. The solution is

$$\tilde{\alpha}_{0i} = \exp\left[-d_i \Big/ \sum_{l \in R_i} \hat{\theta}_l \right],\tag{3.41}$$

and the estimator of the baseline survival function is again the product of the individual conditional survival probabilities. We use (3.40) with the estimator in (3.41). The two solutions, iterative and approximate, yield estimators equivalent, respectively, to the Kaplan-Meier and Nelson-Aalen estimators. This is easily seen by noting that the above expressions simplify to these estimators. When $\beta = 0$ it follows that $\hat{\theta}_i = 1$ and $\sum_{l \in R_i} \hat{\theta}_l = n_i$.

The estimator of the survival function in (3.37) is obtained by substituting the estimators of the baseline survival function and the estimator of the coefficients using covariate values of interest. Software packages typically provide the value of the estimator of the survival function using the observed time and covariates for all (non-censored as well as censored) subjects.

Some software packages provide an estimator of the baseline hazard function, which is a simple function of the estimator of the conditional survival probabilities, namely

$$\hat{h}_0(t_{(i)}) = 1 - \hat{\alpha}_{0i}.$$

The individual pointwise estimators of the baseline hazard function will typically be very "noisy" or unstable. The estimator of the cumulative baseline hazard function is more practical to use because it is less noisy than the estimator of the baseline hazard function. Its estimator is obtained using the expression for the survival function shown in (2.31), namely

$$\hat{S}_0(t) = e^{-\hat{H}_0(t)}.$$

Thus the estimator of the cumulative baseline hazard function is

$$\hat{H}_0(t) = -\ln\left[\hat{S}_0(t) \right].$$

The estimator of the cumulative hazard function for a specific value of the covariates is

$$\hat{H}(t, \mathbf{x}, \hat{\boldsymbol{\beta}}) = -\ln\left[\hat{S}(t, \mathbf{x}, \hat{\boldsymbol{\beta}})\right]$$
$$= -e^{\mathbf{x}\hat{\boldsymbol{\beta}}} \ln\left[\hat{S}_0(t)\right],$$

(3.42)

which, when plotted as a function of time, provides a useful graphical descriptor of the "risk" experience.

We do not present an application of the estimators of the cumulative hazard function or survival function in this chapter. Instead we defer it to Chapter 4, where we discuss the interpretation of the estimated regression coefficients as well as a fitted proportional hazards model.

EXERCISES

1. Using the data from the German Breast Cancer Study with recurrence time as the survival time variable and recurrence status as the censoring variable, do the following:

   (a) Fit the proportional hazards model containing age, menopause status, hormone therapy, tumor size, number of nodes, number of progesterone receptors, and number of estrogen receptors.

   (b) Assess the significance of the model using the partial log likelihood ratio test. If it is possible in the software package, assess for the significance of the model using the multivariable score and Wald tests. Is the statistical decision the same for the three tests?

   (c) Using the univariate Wald tests, which variables do not appear to contribute to the model? Fit a reduced model and test for the significance of the variables removed using the partial log likelihood ratio test.

   (d) Estimate the baseline survival function for the model fit in problem 1(c). Plot the estimated baseline survival function as a step function versus recurrence time. What covariate pattern is the "baseline" subject for the fitted model?

   (e) Repeat problem 1(d) fitting the model in 1(c) centering all continuous covariates at their median. Explain why the range of the estimated baseline survival functions in problems 1(d) and 1(e) are different.

   (f) Using the model fit in problem 1(c) estimate the value of the survival function for each subject at her respective observed value of recurrence time. Graph the values of the estimated survival function versus recurrence time.

Why is there scatter in this plot that was not present in the plots in problems 1(d) and 1(e)?

2. For this problem, using the German Breast Cancer Study, convert recurrence time (days) into months by dividing by (365.25/12). Round months to quarter years, replacing any values rounded to zero to 1.5 months (midway between 0 and 3). Using rounded month as the survival time variable, fit the reduced model in problem 1(c) using the Breslow, Efron, and exact methods for tied survival times. Compare the estimates of the coefficients and standard errors obtained from the three methods for handling tied survival times and with the results from 1(c), the fitted model before recurrence time was rounded. Are the results similar or different?

3. Repeat problem 1 using the WHAS500 data using as covariates: Age, Gender, Initial Heart Rate, Initial Systolic Blood Pressure, Initial Diastolic Blood Pressure, Body Mass Index, History of Cardiovascular Disease, MI Order, and MI Type.

4. Repeat problem 2 using the reduced model from problem 3.

CHAPTER 4

Interpretation of a Fitted Proportional Hazards Regression Model

4.1 INTRODUCTION

The interpretation of a fitted proportional hazards model requires that we be able to draw practical inferences from the estimated coefficients in the model. We begin by discussing the interpretation of the coefficients for nominal (Section 4.2) and continuous (Section 4.3) scale covariates. In Section 4.4 we discuss the issues of statistical adjustment and the interpretation of estimated coefficients in the presence of statistical interaction. The chapter concludes with a discussion of the interpretation of fitted values from the model and covariate adjusted survivorship functions.

In any regression model, the estimated coefficient for a covariate represents the rate of change of a function of the dependent variable per-unit change in the covariate. Thus, to provide a correct interpretation of the coefficients, we must determine the functional relationship between the independent and dependent variables and we must define the unit change in the covariate likely to be of interest.

In Chapters 2 and 3 we recommended that the hazard function be used in regression analysis to study the effect of one or more covariates on survival time. We must first determine what transformation of the hazard function is linear in the coefficients. In the family of generalized linear models (i.e., linear, logistic, Poisson, and other regression models) this linearizing transformation is known as the *link function* (see McCullagh and Nelder (1989)). This same terminology can be applied to proportional hazards regression models.

The proportional hazards model can be used when the primary goal of the analysis is to estimate the effect of study variables on survival time. Suppose that we have a regression model containing a single covariate. Because the hazard function for the proportional hazards regression model is:

$$h(t, x, \beta) = h_0(t) e^{x\beta},$$

it follows that the link function is the natural log transformation. We denote the log of a hazard function as $g(t,x,\beta) = \ln[h(t,x,\beta)]$. Thus, in the case of the proportional hazards regression model, the log-hazard function is

$$g(t,x,\beta) = \ln[h_0(t)] + x\beta. \tag{4.1}$$

The difference in the log-hazard function for a change from $x = a$ to $x = b$ is

$$
\begin{aligned}
\left[g(t, x = a, \beta) - g(t, x = b, \beta) \right] &= \left\{ \ln[h_0(t)] + a\beta \right\} - \left\{ \ln[h_0(t)] + b\beta \right\} \\
&= a\beta - b\beta \\
&= (a - b)\beta. \tag{4.2}
\end{aligned}
$$

Note that because the baseline hazard function, $h_0(t)$, is a component of the log hazard when $x = a$ as well as when $x = b$, it disappears when we compute the difference in the log hazards. We also note that the difference in the log hazards does not depend on time. This is the *proportional hazards* assumption and it is examined in detail in Chapter 6, when we discuss methods for assessing model adequacy and assumptions.

The log hazard is the correct function to assess the effect of change in a co-variate. However, it is not as easily interpreted as the expression we obtain when we exponentiate (4.2), namely

$$
\begin{aligned}
\mathrm{HR}(t, x = a \text{ versus } x = b, \beta) &= \mathrm{HR}(t, a, b, \beta) \\
&= \exp\left[g(t, x = a, \beta) - g(t, x = b, \beta) \right] \\
&= \frac{h(t, a, \beta)}{h(t, b, \beta)} \\
&= e^{(a-b)\beta}. \tag{4.3}
\end{aligned}
$$

The quantity defined in (4.3) is the *hazard ratio*, and it plays the same role in interpreting and explaining the results of proportional hazards regression that the odds ratio plays in a logistic regression.[1] We will return to this point in the next section.

The results in (4.2) and (4.3) are important because they provide the method that must be followed to correctly interpret the coefficients in any proportional hazards regression model. The presence of censored observations of survival time

---

[1] See Hosmer and Lemeshow (2000) Chapter 3 for a detailed discussion of the interpretation of the coefficients in a logistic regression model.

in the data does not alter the interpretation of the coefficients. Censoring in the observations of time is an estimation issue dealt with when we constructed the partial likelihood function (see (3.17)) and, once we have accounted for the censoring, we can ignore it.

4.2 NOMINAL SCALE COVARIATE

We begin by considering the interpretation of the coefficient for a dichotomous covariate. Dichotomous or binary covariates occur regularly in applied settings. They may be truly dichotomous (e.g., gender) or they may be derived from continuous covariates (e.g., age greater than 65 years).

Assume that we have a model containing a single dichotomous covariate, denoted X, coded 0 or 1. The first step in interpreting the coefficient for X is to calculate the difference in the log hazard corresponding to a one-unit change in the covariate. This difference, from (4.2) yields:

$$g(t,1,\beta) - g(t,0,\beta) = (1-0)\beta = \beta .$$

Thus, in the special case when the dichotomous covariate is coded zero and one, the coefficient is equal to the change of interest in the log hazard. We can exponentiate, following (4.3), the difference in log hazards to obtain the hazard ratio:

$$\mathrm{HR}(t,1,0,\beta) = e^{\beta} . \qquad (4.4)$$

The form of the hazard ratio in (4.4) is identical to the form of the odds ratio from a logistic regression model for a dichotomous covariate. However, in the context of a proportional hazards model, it is a ratio of rates rather than of odds. To expand on this difference, suppose that we followed a large cohort of males and females for 60 months (5 years) and record if a subject "died" during this period. Subjects alive after 60 months of follow up are considered censored. In this hypothetical setting, we might be tempted to analyze the end-of-study binary variable, death during follow-up (yes = 1), using a logistic regression model. We should note that this binary variable is the censoring variable for the observation of time to death. Suppose the value of the odds ratio for gender (1 = female) is 2.0. This is interpreted to mean, under conditions where the odds ratio approximates the relative risk, that the probability of death by the end of the study is 2 times higher for females than for males. A hazard ratio of 2 obtained from (4.4) means that, at any time during the study, the per-month rate of death among males is twice that of females. Thus, the hazard ratio is a comparative measure of survival experience over the entire time period, whereas the odds ratio is a comparative measure of event occurrence at the study endpoint. They are two different measures, and the fact that they may, under certain circumstances, be of similar magnitude in an applied setting is irrelevant. Note that, if one is able to observe the survival time for all subjects, then the censoring variable is equal to one for all subjects and logistic regression cannot be used because the outcome is constant.

To expand on the interpretation of the hazard ratio for a dichotomous covariate, survival times were created for a hypothetical cohort of 5,000 females (sex = k = 1) and 5,000 males (sex = k = 0) with a theoretical hazard ratio of 2.0. Subjects whose survival time exceeded 60 months were considered censored at 60 months. At each month of follow up the number at risk, the number of deaths, the estimated hazard rates, $h_k(t) = d_k(t)/n_k(t)$, $k = 0,1$ and the hazard ratio $\hat{HR}(t) = h_1(t)/h_0(t)$, were computed. These quantities are listed in Table 4.1 for the first 12 months and the last 12 months of this study. The hazard ratio is graphed for the 60–month study period in Figure 4.1. The average estimated hazard ratio, $2.007 = (1/60) \times \sum_{t=1}^{60} \hat{HR}(t)$, is included in Figure 4.1 for reference. The hazard rates and their ratios indicate that, during each of the 60 months of follow up, the death rate for females is approximately twice that of males. The scatter about 2.0 is due to the randomness in the number of deaths observed at each month.

The increase in the scatter over time in Figure 4.1 is due to the fact that the number in the risk sets decreases over time. By design of the example, all values of time greater than or equal to 60 months are censored, so hazards and their ratio are not estimable after this point.

In most applied settings, there will be too much variability in the point-wise estimators of the hazard ratios, $\hat{HR}(t)$, for a figure like Figure 4.1 to be particularly informative about the value of the hazard ratio or to determine if it is constant over time.

Table 4.2 presents the results of fitting the proportional hazards model containing the dichotomous variable gender in the WHAS100 data. The point estimate of the coefficient is $\hat{\beta} = 0.555$. Because gender was coded as 1 = female and 0 = male, we know from (4.3) that we can obtain the point estimator of the hazard ratio by exponentiating the estimator of the coefficient. In this example the estimate is:

$$\hat{HR} = e^{0.555} = 1.74.$$

Like the odds–ratio estimator in logistic regression, the sampling distribution of the estimator of the hazard ratio is skewed to the right, so confidence interval estimators based on the Wald statistic (for the hazard ratio) and its assumption of normality may not have good coverage properties unless the sample size is quite large. Comparatively speaking, the sampling distribution of the estimator of the coefficient is better approximated by the normal distribution than the sampling distribution of the estimated hazard ratio. As a result, its Wald statistic–based confidence interval (for the coefficient) will have better coverage properties. In

Table 4.1 Partial Listing of the Number of Deaths, the Number at Risk, the Estimated Hazard Rate in Two Hypothetical Groups, and the Estimated Hazard Ratio at Time t

t	$d_0(t)$	$n_0(t)$	$h_0(t)$	$d_1(t)$	$n_1(t)$	$h_1(t)$	$\widehat{HR}(t)$
1	190	5000	0.038	361	5000	0.072	1.895
2	114	4810	0.024	272	4639	0.059	2.458
3	119	4696	0.025	219	4367	0.05	2.00
4	112	4577	0.024	191	4148	0.046	1.917
5	107	4465	0.024	190	3957	0.048	2.000
6	97	4358	0.022	183	3767	0.049	2.227
7	100	4261	0.023	190	3584	0.053	2.304
8	117	4161	0.028	174	3394	0.051	1.821
9	101	4044	0.025	170	3220	0.053	2.12
10	94	3943	0.024	131	3050	0.043	1.792
11	95	3849	0.025	129	2919	0.044	1.760
12	93	3754	0.025	141	2790	0.051	2.040
⋮	⋮	⋮	⋮	⋮	⋮	⋮	⋮
49	43	1465	0.029	21	447	0.047	1.621
50	34	1422	0.024	31	426	0.073	3.042
51	26	1388	0.019	15	395	0.038	2.000
52	32	1362	0.023	20	380	0.053	2.304
53	31	1330	0.023	18	360	0.05	2.174
54	49	1299	0.038	18	342	0.053	1.395
55	25	1250	0.02	19	324	0.059	2.950
56	32	1225	0.026	18	305	0.059	2.269
57	32	1193	0.027	13	287	0.045	1.667
58	21	1161	0.018	11	274	0.04	2.222
59	17	1140	0.015	13	263	0.049	3.267
60	14	1123	0.012	4	250	0.016	1.333

this case, we obtain the end-points of a 95 percent confidence interval for the hazard ratio by exponentiating the endpoints of the confidence interval for the coefficient. In the current example these are:

$$\exp\left[\hat{\beta} \pm 1.96 \times \widehat{SE}\left(\hat{\beta}\right)\right] = \exp\left[0.555 \pm 1.96 \times 0.2824\right] = 1.002, 3.031 \,.$$

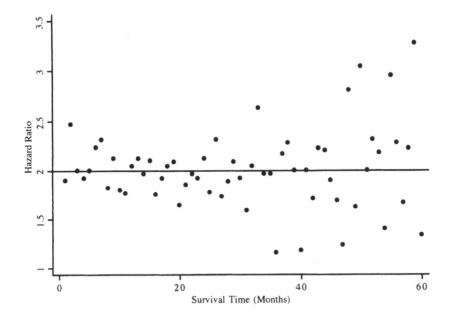

Figure 4.1 Graph of the estimated hazard ratios and the mean hazard ratio ($\overline{HR} = 2.0$) for the hypothetical data from Table 4.1.

Alternative confidence interval estimators have been studied, one of which is based on the partial likelihood. To date, this method has not been implemented in most software packages.

The interpretation of the estimated hazard ratio of 1.74 is that females die at about 1.74 times the rate of males, throughout the study period. The confidence interval suggests that ratios as low as 1.002 or as high as 3.031 are consistent with the observed data at the 95 percent level of confidence. Another way of expressing the hazard ratio that can be more meaningful to subject matter scientists is to describe it as a percentage increase over the null value of 1. In this example, one would say that the death rate among females is 74 percent larger than among males throughout the study period, and it could be as little as 0.2 percent larger or as much as 203 percent larger with 95 percent confidence.

Table 4.2 Estimated Coefficient, Standard Error, z-Score, Two-Tailed p-value, and 95% Confidence Interval Estimate for Gender for the WHAS100 Study

Variable	Coeff.	Std. Err.	z	$p>|z|$	95% CIE
Gender	0.555	0.2824	1.97	0.049	0.002, 1.109

As discussed in Chapter 3, the partial likelihood ratio test, the Wald test and the score test can be used to assess the significance of a coefficient. In the current example, the value of the partial likelihood ratio test is $G = 3.75$, with a p–value equal to 0.053. The Wald test statistic is $z = 1.97$, with a p–value equal to 0.049. Here one test is significant at the 5 percent level and the other just barely not so. The confidence interval for the hazard ratio does not include 1.0, a result consistent with the Wald test. In such cases, we believe that the best approach is to report all the results. The reader then has the option to evaluate the differing significance levels within the context of his/her own research objectives.

In the WHAS100 example in Table 4.2, the covariate value "1," female, is associated with poorer survival experience. In many settings, the treatment of interest may result in improved survival experience. In these cases, the estimate of the coefficient is negative and the estimated hazard ratio is less than one. Our experience is that subject matter scientists seem to have more trouble interpreting the effect when it is protective. Hence we consider an example of this type, the three-drug versus two-drug regimens in the ACTG320 study. The results of fitting a proportional hazards model containing the indicator variable for the three-drug treatment are shown in Table 4.3.

The Wald test of the coefficient for treatment in Table 4.3 is highly significant. The partial likelihood ratio test (results not shown) is also significant with $p < 0.01$. The estimated hazard ratio and 95 percent confidence interval based on the results in Table 4.3 are, respectively, $\hat{\text{HR}} = 0.505$ and $(0.33, 0.77)$. The interpretation of the estimated hazard ratio is that the rate of progression to AIDS or death among patients on the three-drug regimen is 0.505 times that of patients on the two-drug regimen; this could be as little as 0.77 times or as much as 0.33 times with 95 percent confidence. The percentage change interpretation is that the rate of progression of AIDS or death of patients on the three-drug regimen is 49.5 percent less than the rate of progression of AIDS or death of patients on the two-drug regimen; this decrease could be as little as 23 percent or as much as 67 percent with 95 percent confidence. Both forms of the interpretation are found in the subject matter literature. Which form is used in an applied setting should be based on which is thought to be more easily understood by the target audience for the research.

We also point out that, if one changes the 0–1 coding using the equation $new = 1 - old$, then the numeric output is the same but with the signs of the estimated coefficient and its confidence interval reversed. For example, if we coded

Table 4.3 Estimated Coefficient, Standard Error, z-Score, Two-Tailed p-value, and 95% Confidence Interval Estimate for Gender from the ACTG320 Study

Variable	Coeff.	Std. Err.	z	$p>|z|$	95% CIE
tx	−0.684	0.2149	−3.18	0.001	−1.106, −0.263

the two-drug treatment as 1, then the estimated coefficient would be 0.684 with an estimated hazard ratio of 1.982. If one uses enough decimal places in the calculations then the results are exact, $HR_{new} = 1/HR_{old}$. This fact is useful because it often explains why an estimated coefficient has a sign opposite of what was expected (i.e., the coding has been reversed).

Note that Table 4.2 and Table 4.3 do not contain an intercept term. This is the price we pay for choosing the semiparametric proportional hazards model. The intercept, were one present in Table 4.2, would correspond to the log baseline hazard function, in this case for females. The implication of this in practice is that we cannot, from the regression output of a proportional hazards model, reconstruct group–specific hazard rates. Only hazard ratios can be estimated. If it is critical to have individual estimates of group–specific hazard rates, then we would use one of the fully parametric models discussed in Chapter 8.

Occasionally, the coded values for a dichotomous variable are not 0 and 1 (e.g., +1 and −1 may be used instead). In this case, it may not be possible to obtain the estimator of the hazard ratio by simply exponentiating the estimator of the coefficient. One can always obtain the correct estimator by explicitly evaluating (4.2) and (4.3). If, as shown in (4.2) and (4.3), the two values are denoted as a and b, then the estimator of the hazard ratio is:

$$\widehat{HR}(t,a,b,\beta) = e^{(a-b)\hat{\beta}}. \tag{4.5}$$

The end-points of a $100(1-\alpha)$ percent confidence interval estimator for the hazard ratio can be obtained by exponentiating the end-points of the confidence interval estimator for $(a-b)\beta$,

$$\exp\left[(a-b)\hat{\beta} \pm |a-b| z_{1-\alpha/2}\widehat{SE}(\hat{\beta})\right], \tag{4.6}$$

where $|a-b|$ denotes the absolute value of $(a-b)$.

If a nominal scale covariate has more than two levels, denoted in general by K, we must model the variable using a collection of $K-1$ "design" (also known as "dummy" or "indicator") variables. The most frequent method of coding these

Table 4.4   Coding of the Three Design Variables for the Age Groups in the WHAS100 Study

Age Group	AGE_2	AGE_3	AGE_4
< 60	0	0	0
[60 – 69]	1	0	0
[70 – 79]	0	1	0
≥ 80	0	0	1

design variables is to use *reference cell coding*. With this method, we choose one level of the variable to be the reference level, against which all other levels are compared. The resulting hazard ratios compare the hazard rate of each group to that of the referent group. Note that different software packages use different groups as the default referent group and options might need to be specified or adjusted if the default referent group is not the preferred referent group.

In Chapter 2, we considered an example in which age of subjects in the WHAS100 study was categorized into four groups < 60, $[60 - 69]$, $[70 - 79]$ and ≥ 80. Our goal was to describe, qualitatively, how survival experience in the cohort changes with age, through plots of estimated survivorship functions and a log–rank test. We can continue along these same lines by fitting a proportional hazards model to these data. The estimated hazard ratios provide a convenient and easily interpreted summary measure of the comparative survival experience of the four groups.

The methods discussed in this example may be applied to any covariate with multiple groups. The coding for the three design variables based on the four age groups, using the youngest age group as the referent group, is shown in Table 4.4. The results of fitting a proportional hazards model using these three design variables are presented in Table 4.5.

The value of the partial likelihood ratio test for the overall significance of the coefficients is $G = 15.32$ and the p–value, computed using a chi–square distribution with three degree of freedom, is 0.002. This suggests that at least one of the three older age groups has a hazard rate significantly different from the youngest age group. The p–values of the individual Wald statistics indicate that the hazard rate in each of the two oldest groups is significantly different from that in the youngest (the referent) age group.

Before we can use (4.2) and (4.3) to obtain estimators of the hazard ratios, we need the equation for the log–hazard function. The log–hazard function, ignoring the log baseline hazard function, $h_0(t)$, for the model fit in Table 4.5 is:

$$g(t, \text{four Age groups}, \boldsymbol{\beta}) = \beta_1 \text{AGE}\_2 + \beta_2 \text{AGE}\_3 + \beta_3 \text{AGE}\_4 .$$

The estimator of the hazard ratio comparing Age group 2 to Age group 1 is obtained by first calculating the difference in the estimators of the log–hazard functions, (4.2),

$$\left[g(t, \text{Age group 2}, \hat{\boldsymbol{\beta}}) - g(t, \text{Age group 1}, \hat{\boldsymbol{\beta}}) \right]$$
$$= (\hat{\beta}_1 1 + \hat{\beta}_2 0 + \hat{\beta}_3 0) - (\hat{\beta}_1 0 + \hat{\beta}_2 0 + \hat{\beta}_3 0) = \hat{\beta}_1 .$$

Exponentiating the result, we obtain:

$$\hat{HR}(\text{Age group 2 versus 1}) = e^{\hat{\beta}_1}.$$

We obtain the estimators of the other two hazard ratios by proceeding in a similar manner, and these are:

$$\hat{HR}(\text{Age group 3 versus 1}) = e^{\hat{\beta}_2}$$

and

$$\hat{HR}(\text{Age group 4 versus 1}) = e^{\hat{\beta}_3}.$$

We calculate the value of the estimates in the example, shown in the second column of Table 4.6, by exponentiating the values of the coefficients, from Table 4.5.

When reference cell coding is used to create the design variables, the estimators of the hazard ratios comparing each group to the referent group are obtained by exponentiating the respective estimators of the coefficients.

We construct confidence interval estimators of the hazard ratios by exponentiating the endpoints of the confidence intervals for the individual coefficients. For example, the endpoints of the 95 percent confidence interval estimate for $HR(\text{Age group 3 versus 1})$ shown in Table 4.6 are:

$$\exp\left[\hat{\beta}_2 \pm 1.96 \times \hat{SE}(\hat{\beta}_2)\right] = \exp\left[0.986 \pm 1.96 \times 0.4454\right] = 1.12, 6.42.$$

Similar calculations yield the endpoints for the other two confidence interval estimates shown in Table 4.6.

The hazard ratios in Table 4.6 suggest: (1) subjects in their sixties are dying at a rate that is about the same as subjects younger than 60, (2) subjects in their 70's are dying at a rate that is about 2.7 times greater than subjects younger than 60 and (3) subjects 80 or older have a mortality rate that is approximately 3.5 times greater than subjects younger than 60.

Given the similarity of the hazard ratios comparing each of the two older age groups to the referent group, it would make sense to test whether the survival experience in these two groups differs. We can estimate their hazard ratio and determine whether it is different from 1.0. We do this by using the general approach

Table 4.5 Estimated Coefficients using Referent Cell Coding, Standard Errors, z-Scores, Two-Tailed p-values, and 95% Confidence Intervals Estimates for Age Categorized into Four Groups from the WHAS100 Study

Variable	Coeff.	Std. Err.	z	p>|z|	95% CIE
AGE_2	0.047	0.5186	0.09	0.928	−0.970, 1.063
AGE_3	0.986	0.4454	2.21	0.027	0.113, 1.859
AGE_4	1.263	0.4155	3.04	0.002	0.449, 2.077

Table 4.6 Estimated Hazard Ratios (HR) and 95% Confidence
Intervals Estimates for Age Categorized into Four Groups from
the WHAS100

Age Group	HR	95% CIE
< 60	1.00	
$[60 - 69]$	1.05	0.38, 2.90
$[70 - 79]$	2.68	1.12, 6.42
≥ 80	3.54	1.57, 7.98

in (4.2) and (4.3). The specific difference in the hazard functions for the two
groups is:

$$\left[g\left(t, \text{Age group } 4, \hat{\boldsymbol{\beta}} \right) - g\left(t, \text{Age group } 3, \hat{\boldsymbol{\beta}} \right) \right]$$
$$= \left(\hat{\beta}_1 0 + \hat{\beta}_2 0 + \hat{\beta}_3 1 \right) - \left(\hat{\beta}_1 0 + \hat{\beta}_2 1 + \hat{\beta}_3 0 \right)$$
$$= \hat{\beta}_3 - \hat{\beta}_2 \ .$$

The estimator of the hazard ratio is:

$$\widehat{\text{HR}} \left(\text{Age group } 4 \text{ versus } 3 \right) = e^{\left(\hat{\beta}_3 - \hat{\beta}_2 \right)}$$

and is equal to $\exp(1.263 - 0.986) = 1.319$. To obtain a confidence interval, we
need an estimator for the variance of the difference between the two coefficients.
Specifically:

$$\widehat{\text{Var}}(\hat{\beta}_3 - \hat{\beta}_2) = \widehat{\text{Var}}(\hat{\beta}_3) + \widehat{\text{Var}}\left(\hat{\beta}_2 \right) - 2\widehat{\text{Cov}}\left(\hat{\beta}_2, \hat{\beta}_3 \right),$$

where $\widehat{\text{Var}}$ denotes the estimator of the variance of the estimator in the parentheses and $\widehat{\text{Cov}}$ denotes the estimator of the covariance of the two estimators in the
parentheses. These estimates may be obtained from most software packages by
requesting the estimated covariance matrix of the estimated coefficients. Table 4.7

Table 4.7 Estimated Variances and Covariances for the Three
Estimated Coefficients in Table 4.5

Variable (Coeff.)	AGE_2	AGE_3	AGE_4
AGE_2	0.2690	0. 1260	0. 1251
AGE_3	0.1260	0.1984	0.1260
AGE_4	0.1251	0.1260	0.1727

presents the covariance matrix for the estimated coefficients for the three age groups.

The estimated variances and covariance needed are $\hat{\mathrm{Var}}\left(\hat{\beta}_2\right) = 0.1984$, $\hat{\mathrm{Var}}\left(\hat{\beta}_3\right) = 0.1727$, and $\hat{\mathrm{Cov}}\left(\hat{\beta}_2, \hat{\beta}_3\right) = 0.1260$. The estimate of the variance of the difference in the two coefficients is:

$$\hat{\mathrm{Var}}\left(\hat{\beta}_3 - \hat{\beta}_2\right) = 0.1727 + 0.1984 - 2 \times 0.1260 = 0.1191$$

and the estimated standard error is:

$$\hat{\mathrm{SE}}\left(\hat{\beta}_3 - \hat{\beta}_2\right) = \sqrt{0.1191} = 0.3451.$$

The end-points of the 95 percent confidence interval estimate are:

$$\exp\left[\left(\hat{\beta}_3 - \hat{\beta}_2\right) \pm 1.96 \times \hat{\mathrm{SE}}\left(\hat{\beta}_3 - \hat{\beta}_2\right)\right]$$
$$= \exp\left[(1.263 - 0.986) \pm 1.96 \times 0.3451\right]$$
$$= 0.67, 2.59.$$

The confidence interval includes 1.0, suggesting that the hazard rates for the two older age groups may, in fact, be the same.

Instead of using the confidence interval, we could test the hypothesis of the equality of two coefficients via a Wald test. Many software packages allow the user to test whether specified contrasts of model coefficients are equal to zero. This is a convenient feature, especially when contrasts of interest are more complicated than simple differences. The Wald test for the contrast $\hat{\beta}_3 - \hat{\beta}_2$ is:

$$z = \frac{\hat{\beta}_3 - \hat{\beta}_2}{\hat{\mathrm{SE}}\left(\hat{\beta}_3 - \hat{\beta}_2\right)} = \frac{1.263 - 0.986}{0.3451} = 0.803,$$

and the two–tailed p-value computed from the standard normal distribution is 0.42. Because the p-value is greater than 0.05, we fail to reject the hypothesis that the two coefficients are equal and conclude that there is no evidence that the death rates in the two age groups differ.

The test for a general contrast among the $K - 1$ coefficients for a nominal scaled covariate with K levels is described as follows. Let the vector of estimators of the coefficients be denoted:

$$\hat{\boldsymbol{\beta}}' = \left(\hat{\beta}_1, \hat{\beta}_2, \ldots, \hat{\beta}_{K-1} \right)$$

and the estimator of the covariance matrix be denoted $\hat{\mathbf{V}}\left(\hat{\boldsymbol{\beta}}\right)$. Let the vector of constants specifying the contrast be denoted:

$$\mathbf{c}' = \left(c_1, c_2, \ldots, c_{K-1} \right),$$

where the sum of the constants is zero. The single degree of freedom Wald test for the contrast is:

$$Q = \frac{\mathbf{c}'\hat{\boldsymbol{\beta}}}{\sqrt{\mathbf{c}'\hat{\mathbf{V}}\left(\hat{\boldsymbol{\beta}}\right)\mathbf{c}}} \qquad (4.7)$$

and the two–tailed p–value is obtained using the standard normal distribution. Most software packages will report the square of the Wald test and use the chi-square distribution to calculate the p–value. The equivalence of these two approaches follows from the fact that the distribution of the square of a $N(0,1)$ random variable follows a χ^2 distribution with one degree of freedom.

In the WHAS100 study, it may be of interest to determine whether the log hazard ratio of the second age group is equal to the average of the log hazard ratios of two oldest age groups. The vector of constants for this contrast is $\mathbf{c}' = (1.0, -0.5, -0.5)$, the vector of estimated coefficients is given in Table 4.5, and the covariance matrix is shown in Table 4.7. We used STATA to perform the calculations, but other software packages (e.g., SAS) could have been used. The value of the test statistic is $Q = 6.69$ with a p–value equal to 0.01. We conclude that the oldest two age groups have an average hazard rate significantly greater than the average hazard rate of the younger two age groups.

The method of using a contrast to compare coefficients can be especially useful when trying to pool categories of a nominal scale covariate recorded with more levels than the data can support (e.g., categories with few events). Considerations regarding meaningful interpretations are of primary importance in deciding which categories to combine, but contrasts may be used to judge whether the hazard rates of clinically similar groups are statistically similar.

Referent cell coding as used above is the most frequently applied scheme for coding design variables; however, it is just one of many possible methods. An alternative is *deviation from means coding*. This type of design variable coding may be used when one simply needs an overall assessment of differences in hazard rates. To illustrate the method, we apply it to the four age groups in the WHAS100 study. This coding is obtained by replacing the first row of zeros in Table 4.4 with a row in which each value is equal to -1. The resulting estimated coefficient for an age group estimates the difference between the log hazard of the group and the arithmetic mean of the log hazards of all K groups. The exponentiated estimated coefficient provides the ratio of the hazard rate of the particular group to the geometric mean of the hazard rates of all K groups.

The results of fitting a proportional hazards model using the deviation from means coding are shown in Table 4.8. The value of the partial likelihood ratio test for the overall significance of the coefficients is identical to that obtained using reference cell coding and is $G = 15.32$ with a p-value, computed using a chi-square distribution with three degree of freedom, of 0.002. The value of -0.527 for the estimated coefficient of design variable AGE_2 is equal to the estimate of the difference between the log–hazard rate for age group 2, [60, 69], and the estimate of the mean log–hazard rate over all four groups (including group 2). The Wald statistic has a p-value of 0.089, indicating that the difference between the log–hazard rate for this age group and the average log–hazard rate is significant at between the 5 and 10 percent level. The coefficient for group 4 is 0.689 and its Wald statistic has $p = 0.002$. Thus, the log–hazard rate for this age group is significantly larger than the average log–hazard rate.

The estimated difference between the log hazard for the first age group and the average log–hazard rate is the negative of the sum of the coefficients in Table 4.8 and is -0.574. The easiest way to obtain an estimate of its standard error, Wald statistic, etc., is to make a small change in the coding of the design variables and refit the model. We merely switch the row coded -1 with any other row. We do not recommend that hazard ratios be reported when using deviation from means coding, because the ratio cannot be interpreted in the same manner as the ratio from referent cell coding. The comparison is not a comparison of two distinct groups, but rather of one group to the geometric mean hazard rate of all groups combined.

Many other methods for coding design variables are possible. For example, coding that compares each group to the next largest group or each group to the average of the higher groups. These methods tend to be appropriate in special circumstances and will not be discussed further in this text. In our experience, the method of referent cell coding, perhaps followed by contrasts, has provided a useful and informative analysis in most circumstances.

Table 4.8   Estimated Coefficients Using the Deviation from Means Coding, Standard Errors, z-Scores, Two-Tailed p-values, and 95% Confidence Intervals Estimates for Age Categorized into Four Groups from the WHAS100 Study

Variable	Coeff.	Std. Err.	z	$p>|z|$	95% CIE
AGE_2	−0.527	0.3100	−1.70	0.089	−1.135, 0.081
AGE_3	0.412	0.2456	1.68	0.094	−0.070, 0.893
AGE_4	0.689	0.2189	3.15	0.002	0.260, 1.118

4.3 CONTINUOUS SCALE COVARIATE

At first glance it might seem that interpreting the coefficient for a continuous co-variate would be easier than that of a nominal scale variable because indicator variables and coding schemes need not be introduced. Looking more deeply reveals that this is not necessarily true. Before we can use (4.2) and (4.3) to obtain an estimator of a hazard ratio for a continuous covariate, we must address two issues. First and foremost, we must verify that we have included the variable in its correct scale in the model. In this section, we will assume that the log hazard is linear in the covariate of interest. Methods to assess the scale are presented in Chapter 5. Second, we must decide what a clinically meaningful unit of change in the covariate is. Once these two steps are accomplished we may apply (4.2) and (4.3).

We illustrate the method using the WHAS100 study and age as the covariate. The results of fitting a proportional hazards model containing age are shown in Table 4.9. The estimated coefficient in Table 4.9 gives the change in the log hazard corresponding to a 1-year change in age. Often a 1-year change in age is not of clinical interest. The investigators conducting the study may, for example, be more interested in a 5-year change in age.

We obtain the correct change in the log-hazard function for a change of c units in a continuous covariate by using (4.2) and (4.3) with $a = x + c$ and $b = x$. This yields the following change in the log hazard

$$
\begin{aligned}
\left[g(t, x+c, \beta) - g(t, x, \beta) \right] &= \left\{ \ln\left[h_0(t) \right] + (x+c)\beta \right\} - \left\{ \ln\left[h_0(t) \right] + x\beta \right\} \\
&= (x+c)\beta - x\beta \\
&= c\beta.
\end{aligned}
\tag{4.8}
$$

The change is simply equal to the value of the change of interest times the coefficient. The estimator of the hazard ratio is

$$
\hat{HR}(c) = e^{c\hat{\beta}}
\tag{4.9}
$$

and the end-points of a $100(1-\alpha)$ percent confidence interval estimator of the hazard ratio are

$$
\exp\left[c\hat{\beta} \pm z_{1-\alpha/2} |c| \hat{SE}(\hat{\beta}) \right].
\tag{4.10}
$$

Applying (4.9) and (4.10) for a 5-year change in age in the WHAS100 study, we obtain an estimated hazard ratio of

$$
\hat{HR}(5 \text{ year increase in age}) = e^{5 \times 0.046} = 1.26
$$

Table 4.9 Estimated Coefficient, Standard Error, z-Score, Two-Tailed p-value, and 95% Confidence Interval for Age in the WHAS100 Study

Variable	Coeff.	Std. Err.	z	$p>|z|$	95% Conf. Int.
AGE	0.046	0.0120	3.82	<0.001	0.022, 0.069

and the endpoints of a 95 percent confidence interval are

$$\exp\left[5 \times 0.046 \pm 1.96 \times 5 \times 0.0120\right] = 1.12, 1.42 .$$

Alternatively, we could have calculated the endpoints of the 95 percent confidence interval by multiplying the endpoints in Table 4.9 by 5 and then exponentiating. We suggest, for continuous covariates, that the hazard ratio for the clinically interesting unit of change, along with its confidence interval, be reported in any table of results. The unit of change should be indicated in the table heading or in a footnote.

The interpretation of an estimated hazard ratio of 1.26 is that the hazard rate increases by 26 percent for every 5-year increase in age and is independent of the age at which the increase is calculated. The independence of the increase in age is due to the fact that the log hazard was assumed to be linear in age and subtracts itself from the calculation in (4.8). The confidence interval estimate suggests that an increase in the hazard rate of between 12 and 42 percent is consistent with the data at the 95 percent level of confidence.

As is the case with a nominal scaled covariate, our experience is that subject matter investigators are more comfortable interpreting the effect of a continuous, linearly modeled covariate when increasing values are associated with poorer survival experience (i.e., positive coefficients and estimated hazard ratios that exceed one). The covariate CD4 count in the ACTG320 study provides an example of a protective effect. The results of fitting this model are shown in Table 4.10.

The coefficient in Table 4.10 estimates the decrease in the log hazard rate for every increase of one unit in the CD4 count. With a range in CD4 count from 0 to 392, a change of one is not clinically meaningful. The three quartiles are, respectively, 23, 75 and 136.5. The estimated standard deviation is approximately 70. In settings where 2, 5, or 10 do not provide a meaningful change, one might consider alternative, choices such as one-half the inter quartile range or the standard deviation. As an example, the estimated hazard ratio for a one standard deviation in-

Table 4.10 Estimated Coefficient, Standard Error, z-Score, Two-Tailed p-value, and 95% Confidence Interval Estimates for CD4 Count in the ACTG320 Study

Variable	Coeff.	Std. Err.	z	$p>|z|$	95% CIE
CD4	−0.016	0.0025	−6.47	<0.001	−0.021, −0.011

crease in CD4 count is

$$\hat{\text{HR}} = e^{-0.016 \times 70} = 0.326 \,.$$

The end-points of a 95 percent confidence interval estimate are

$$\exp\left(-0.016 \times 70 \pm 1.96 \times 70 \times 0.0025\right) = \left(0.232, 0.459\right).$$

The interpretation is that the rate of AIDS-defining diagnosis or death is estimated to decrease by 67.4 percent for every increase of 70 in the CD4 count and a decrease of between 54.1 and 76.8 percent is consistent with the data at the 95 percent level of confidence.

In summary, it is important to remember that the interpretation of the estimated hazard ratio for a continuous covariate depends on having included it in the model in the correct scale (linear in the examples in this section) and adhering to the basic premise of a proportional hazards model. Methods for checking these assumptions are considered in detail in Chapters 5 and 6, respectively.

4.4 MULTIPLE-COVARIATE MODELS

One of the primary reasons for using a regression model is to include multiple covariates to adjust statistically for possible imbalances in the observed data before making statistical inferences. This process of adjustment has been given different names in various fields of study. In traditional statistical applications, it is called *analysis of covariance*, while in clinical and epidemiological investigations it is often called *control of confounding*. A statistically related issue is the inclusion of higher-order terms in a model representing interactions between covariates. These are also called *effect modifiers*. In this section we discuss the strengths and limitations of statistical adjustment and inclusion of interactions and establish a set of basic guidelines that we employ when discussing model development in the next chapter.

Suppose for the moment we are in a setting where we have two variables: a primary risk factor or treatment variable, denoted as d, and another covariate, denoted x. To simplify things, assume that the covariate x is significantly associated with the outcome. In addition to being a contributor to the model itself, the covariate x could be: (1) a confounder of the association of the primary covariate of interest, d, with the outcome; (2) an effect modifier of the association and (3) neither a confounder of the association of the primary covariate of interest, d, with the outcome nor an effect modifier of the association. We use examples from various data sets to demonstrate each of these possibilities. As we show in the series of examples, determining the status of the covariate, x, involves fitting three models: (1) the model containing d but not containing x; (2) the model containing both d and x and (3) the model containing d, x and their interaction $x \times d$.

Before we consider the examples, we continue with the two-variable setting, as it is helpful conceptually to understand and graphically to describe confounding and interaction as they are manifested in a regression model.

Suppose that our primary risk factor, d, has two levels (coded 0 = absent and 1 = present) and that our primary analysis goal is to estimate the hazard ratio for d. The proportional hazards model that contains only d has log-hazard function

$$g(t,d,\theta_1) = \ln[h_0(t)] + d\theta_1 .$$

The difference in the log-hazard at the two levels of d is

$$[g(t,d=1,\theta_1) - g(t,d=0,\theta_1)] = \{\ln[h_0(t)] + 1\theta_1\} - \{\ln[h_0(t)] + 0\theta_1\}$$
$$= \theta_1 . \tag{4.11}$$

Suppose that we have a second model that contains both d and x. The log-hazard function for this model is

$$g(t,d,x,\boldsymbol{\beta}) = \ln[h_0(t)] + d\beta_1 + x\beta_2 . \tag{4.12}$$

The adjusted difference in the log-hazard from (4.12) is

$$[g(t,d=1,x,\boldsymbol{\beta}) - g(t,d=0,x,\boldsymbol{\beta})] = \{\ln[h_0(t)] + 1\beta_1 + x\beta_2\} - \{\ln[h_0(t)] + 0\beta_1 + x\beta_2\}$$
$$= \beta_1 + (x-x)\beta_2$$
$$= \beta_1 . \tag{4.13}$$

The results shown in (4.11) and (4.13) indicate that we have two estimators of the effect of our risk factor: (1) a so-called crude or unadjusted estimator $\hat{\theta}_1$, obtained from (4.11) by fitting the model that does not include x, and (2) an adjusted estimator $\hat{\beta}_1$ obtained from (4.13) by fitting a model that includes x. If the two estimators are similar, then x is not a confounder of the association of d and survival time, as measured by the difference in the log-hazard. If the estimators are different, then adjustment is needed and the variable x may be a confounder of the association. The extent of adjustment, or difference, between $\hat{\theta}_1$ and $\hat{\beta}_1$ is a function of the difference in the distribution of x within the two groups defined by d and the magnitude of $\hat{\beta}_2$, the association between x and survival time.

Suppose that the model containing d and x, (4.12), is the correct model, and denote the average value of x among subjects with $d=1$ as $\bar{x}_1$ and among those with $d=0$ as $\bar{x}_0$. An approximation of the average log-hazard functions [see

Fleming and Harrington (1991) page 134 for an exact expression] for the two groups defined by d is

$$g(t, d = 0, \boldsymbol{\beta}) = \ln\left[h_0(t)\right] + \bar{x}_0\beta_2$$

and

$$g(t, d = 1, \boldsymbol{\beta}) = \ln\left[h_0(t)\right] + \beta_1 + \bar{x}_1\beta_2 \, .$$

If we use the results from the fitted crude and adjusted models and take the difference between these two expressions, the crude or unadjusted log-hazard ratio is approximately

$$\hat{\theta}_1 \approx \hat{\beta}_1 + \hat{\beta}_2 \times \left(\bar{x}_1 - \bar{x}_0\right). \tag{4.14}$$

Thus, the crude estimator will be approximately equal to the adjusted estimator if the difference in the mean of x of the two groups defined by d is zero or if the coefficient for x is zero. The two estimators will differ if at least one of the two is large or both are moderate in size. The above two-variable model is based on a dichotomous and a continuous covariate. However, it may be generalized to covariates on other measurement scales, for example d continuous.

The magnitude of the confounding by x expressed in (4.14) is on the scale of the coefficients or difference in the log-hazard. Hence, we believe that any measure of difference in the two estimators of effect be defined using estimated coefficients. Others may prefer to use exponentiated coefficients, i.e., hazard ratios. The measure of difference in the two coefficients we prefer to use is the percentage change

$$\Delta\hat{\beta}\% = 100\frac{\hat{\theta} - \hat{\beta}}{\hat{\beta}} \, , \tag{4.15}$$

where $\hat{\theta}$ denotes the estimator from the model that does not contain the potential confounder (the smaller model) and $\hat{\beta}$ denotes the estimator from the model that does include the potential confounder (the larger model). This particular measure of confounding works well with our favorite approach to model building, discussed in Chapter 5.

If we assume that (4.14) is correct, then the percentage change in terms of the model is

$$\Delta\hat{\beta}_1\% = 100\frac{\hat{\theta}_1 - \hat{\beta}_1}{\hat{\beta}_1} \approx \frac{100\left(\bar{x}_1 - \bar{x}_0\right)\hat{\beta}_2}{\hat{\beta}_1} \, . \tag{4.16}$$

The right hand side of (4.16) expresses the amount of confounding as a percentage of the adjusted estimator. In practice, one would evaluate only (4.15). The expressions in (4.14) and (4.16) are provided as a tool to assist in explaining why the crude and adjusted estimators could be different. We explore this in more detail in the examples that follow our general discussion.

Under the model in (4.12), once we include the covariate x in the model, the adjusted estimate of effect for d is constant, i.e., does not depend on the value of x. Recall that the fact that it also does not depend on time is due to the assumption that the hazards are proportional. We say that the covariate x is an effect modifier if the effect of d does depend on the value of x. For example, suppose d represents a treatment and x represents age. If the effect of the treatment varies with age, then age is said to be an effect modifier. The simplest, and most frequently used, way to determine whether x is an effect modifier is to include the product term $x \times d$ in the model. Specifically

$$g(t, d, x, \boldsymbol{\beta}) = \ln\left[h_0(t)\right] + d\beta_1 + x\beta_2 + x \times d\beta_3 . \qquad (4.17)$$

Using the model in (4.17) the difference in the log hazard function at the two levels of d is

$$
\begin{aligned}
\left[g(t, d = 1, x, \boldsymbol{\beta}) - g(t, d = 0, x, \boldsymbol{\beta})\right] &= \left\{\ln\left[h_0(t)\right] + 1\beta_1 + x\beta_2 + 1x\beta_3\right\} \\
&\quad - \left\{\ln\left[h_0(t)\right] + 0\beta_1 + x\beta_2 + 0x\beta_3\right\} \qquad (4.18) \\
&= \beta_1 + x\beta_3,
\end{aligned}
$$

which clearly depends on the value of x through the coefficient β_3. Thus for the covariate x to be an effect modifier, the coefficient, β_3, must be different from zero. Hence, we see that, while confounding by x depends on two quantities [see (4.14)], its effect modification depends only on the magnitude of a single coefficient and thus is typically examined via the Wald test for the interaction coefficient or the partial likelihood ratio test comparing the model in (4.17) to the model in (4.12). It may be the case that prior research has clearly demonstrated that x is an effect modifier and, under these circumstances, empirical evidence is less important for justifying the inclusion of the product term $d \times x$ in the model.

Once we make the decision that there is evidence that a covariate is an effect modifier, discussion of its role as a confounder is no longer relevant. In particular, the estimator of β_1 in (4.13) provides an "x" adjusted estimator of the effect of d that holds for all values of x. However, the main effect coefficient for d, β_1, in (4.18) provides an estimator of effect only at a single specific covariate value (which, for a non-centered continuous covariate, is a value likely not to be clinically plausible), but not for other values of x. The point here is that a $\Delta\hat{\beta}\%$ calculation comparing estimated coefficients from the models in (4.12) and (4.17) is of no interest.

The estimator of the hazard ratio from (4.18) is

$$\widehat{HR}(d = 1, d = 0, x) = e^{\hat{\beta}_1 + x\hat{\beta}_3} . \tag{4.19}$$

End-points of its confidence interval estimator are first calculated on the log-hazard scale and then exponentiated. To obtain these we use the estimator of the standard error

$$\widehat{SE}(\hat{\beta}_1 + x\hat{\beta}_3) = \left[\widehat{Var}(\hat{\beta}_1) + x^2\widehat{Var}(\hat{\beta}_3) + 2x\widehat{Cov}(\hat{\beta}_1, \hat{\beta}_3)\right]^{1/2} . \tag{4.20}$$

The end-points of the $100(1-\alpha)$ percent confidence interval on the log hazard ratio scale are

$$(\hat{\beta}_1 + x\hat{\beta}_3) \pm z_{1-\alpha/2} \times \widehat{SE}(\hat{\beta}_1 + x\hat{\beta}_3) \tag{4.21}$$

and the end-points for the corresponding confidence interval for the estimated hazard ratio are

$$\exp\left\{(\hat{\beta}_1 + x\hat{\beta}_3) \pm z_{1-\alpha/2} \times \widehat{SE}(\hat{\beta}_1 + x\hat{\beta}_3)\right\} . \tag{4.22}$$

Now we consider examples to illustrate each of the confounder and effect modifier possibilities listed in the second paragraph. Because a covariate may or may not be a confounder, and may or may not be an effect modifier (but never both simultaneously), we present the results of three fitted models for each example: (1) a model containing only the risk factor of interest, referred to as the crude model; (2) a model containing the risk factor and the potential adjustment variable, referred to as the adjusted model and (3) a model containing main effect terms for both variables and one that is the arithmetic product of the two, referred to as the interaction model.

We begin with an example from the German Breast Cancer Study (see Section 1.3) where the risk factor of interest is hormone therapy and the potential confounder (or, perhaps, effect modifier) is the size of the tumor. The results of fitting the three models are shown in Table 4.11.

The results for the crude model indicate that hormone therapy significantly reduces the rate of cancer recurrence; the estimated coefficient is negative with $P = 0.004$. This effect could be influenced by imbalances in the distribution of another variable. The adjusted model in Table 4.11 adds tumor size to the model.

In this case, the calculated value of the amount of confounding due to differences in the distribution of size in the two hormone therapy groups is

$$\Delta\hat{\beta}\% = \frac{100 \times \left[-0.364 - (-0.373) \right]}{-0.373} = -2.41\%.$$

We see that the crude estimator is only 2.41% smaller than the adjusted estimator. The results in Table 4.11 show that size is a significant risk factor with $p < 0.001$, hence we conclude [based on (4.14)] that the mean size of the tumor in the two-hormone therapy groups must be quite similar. In fact they are, with values respectively of 29.6 mm and 28.8 mm. In this case, the estimated hazard ratios for both the crude and adjusted models are quite similar (approximately 0.7). Thus use of hormone therapy is estimated to reduce the rate of tumor recurrence by about 30 percent.

The results for the interaction model show that the p-value for the Wald test for the inclusion of the product variable is not significant, $p = 0.928$. Although we don't present the details here, the p-value for the likelihood ratio test comparing the adjusted and interaction models (results not shown) is also 0.928. Hence, there is no statistical evidence of tumor size modifying the effect of hormone therapy in these data. The fact that size is such a significant risk factor in its own right would lead us to prefer the adjusted model.

To provide an example of a covariate that is a confounder, we turn to the UIS data described in Section 1.3, whose variables are listed in Table 1.3. The reader who is not yet familiar with this study is encouraged to read the short description on pages 10-12. The outcome in this study is the time from randomization to treatment to self-reported return to drug use. The primary risk factor for this example is a dichotomous variable, drug, obtained by recoding the variable history of IV drug use, ivhx in Table 1.3, into none versus any use. The potential confounder (or, perhaps, effect modifier) is age of the subject at randomization to treatment. The results of fitting the three models are shown in Table 4.12.

Table 4.11 **Estimated Coefficients, Standard Errors, z-Scores, Two-Tailed p-values, and 95% Confidence Interval Estimates for Three Models Fit to the German Breast Cancer Study Data, $n = 686$**

Model	Variable	Coeff.	Std. Err.	z	$p>|z|$	95% CIE
Crude	hormone	−0.364	0.1250	−2.91	0.004	−0.609, −0.119
Adjusted	hormone	−0.373	0.1252	−2.98	0.003	−0.619, −0.128
	size	0.015	0.0036	4.28	<0.001	0.008, 0.022
Interaction	hormone	−0.394	0.2602	−1.51	0.130	−0.904, 0.116
	size	0.015	0.0047	3.18	0.001	0.006, 0.024
	hormone × size	0.0007	0.0072	0.09	0.928	−0.013, 0.015

The results for the crude model indicate that having any history of IV drug use significantly increases the rate of returning to drug use; the estimated coefficient is positive with $P = 0.001$. The adjusted model shows that increasing age at randomization significantly decreases the rate of returning to drug use; the estimated coefficient is negative with $P = 0.001$.

The calculated value of the amount of confounding due to differences in the distribution of age in the two drug use groups is

$$\Delta \hat{\beta}\% = \frac{100 \times [0.321 - 0.439]}{0.439} = -26.88\% .$$

We see that the crude estimator is 26.88 percent smaller than the adjusted estimator. At this point we need to consider a criterion for how much change in an estimated coefficient is important. This decision is more driven by research experience than statistical thresholds. In general, our preference is to use 20 percent as a cutoff value. As the reader will see in examples we will consider in later chapters, we do not adhere strictly to this value, varying it up and down as common sense dictates. However, for now we use 20 percent. Thus we say that age at randomization confounds the drug history effect. Age is quite significant, but there could also be a difference in the mean ages of the two drug history groups. In fact this is the case the mean age of those without a history is 29.64 whereas the mean age for those with a history is 34.05. To explore this further we evaluate (4.14) as follows

$$0.324 = 0.439 - 0.026 \times (34.05 - 29.64).$$

Here the approximation to the crude estimator from (4.14) is quite close. Thus, assuming the fitted model is correct, the confounding can be explained by the significance of age at randomization and the fact that subjects with a history of IV drug use are, on average, five years older than subjects without such history.

Table 4.12 **Estimated Coefficients, Standard Errors, z-Scores, Two-Tailed p-values, and 95% Confidence Interval Estimates for Three Models Fit to the UIS Data, $n = 605$**

Model	Variable	Coeff.	Std. Err.	z	$p>|z|$	95% CIE
Crude	drug	0.321	0.0948	3.39	0.001	0.135, 0.507
Adjusted	drug	0.439	0.1007	4.36	<0.001	0.242, 0.637
	age	−0.026	0.0078	−3.37	0.001	−0.042, −0.011
Interaction	drug	−0.012	0.5484	−0.02	0.982	−1.087, 1.063
	age	−0.037	0.0152	−2.44	0.015	−0.067, −0.007
	drug × age	0.015	0.0178	0.84	0.403	−0.020, 0.050

The results for the interaction model in Table 4.12 show that the p-value for the Wald test for the inclusion of the product variable is not significant, $p = 0.403$. The p-value for the likelihood ratio test comparing the adjusted and interaction models (results not shown) is 0.402. Hence, there is no statistical evidence that age at randomization modifies the effect of history of IV drug use in these data.

Because age is a strong confounder, we would use the estimated coefficient for drug in the adjusted model to estimate the effect of history of IV drug use. The estimated hazard ratio from this model is 1.55, suggesting that a history of IV drug use increases the rate of return to drug use by 55 percent.

To provide an example of a variable that is an effect modifier, we turn to the Worcester Heart Study data, WHAS500, where we consider gender as the risk factor of interest and age as the other covariate. The results of the three fitted models are shown in Table 4.13. The results for the crude model indicate that females, gender = 1, are dying, after hospitalization for a heart attack, at a rate that is significantly greater than males. The estimated coefficient is positive and $p < 0.001$. The results for the adjusted model show that, when age is added to the model, gender is no longer significant. When we calculate the percentage change in the coefficient for gender after adding age to the model, we obtain

$$\Delta \hat{\beta}\% = \frac{100 \times \left[0.381 - (-0.066) \right]}{-0.066} = -682\% .$$

This states that the crude estimate is approximately 682 percent larger than the adjusted estimate. This huge number is due to the fact that the adjusted estimate is almost zero. Regardless of the magnitude of the number, the effect of gender more or less disappears when we add age to the model. Why is this the case? The mean age of females is 74.72 versus 66.60 for males and, evaluating (4.14), we obtain

$$0.477 = -0.066 + 0.067 \times \left(74.72 - 66.60 \right) .$$

Hence, we see that a large portion of the crude effect is due to the fact that age is highly significant in the adjusted model and the difference in the means is large.

When we examine the interactions model in Table 4.13, we see that the Wald test for the product variable is significant with $p = 0.015$. The p-value for the likelihood ratio test comparing the interaction model to the adjusted model (details not presented) also has $p = 0.016$. Hence, age is a significant modifier of the effect of gender in these data. Because age is an effect modifier, we cannot interpret the estimated coefficient for gender in the interactions model in the same way as we do in the adjusted model. Namely, the value of –0.066 provides an age adjusted estimate of effect of female gender, but 2.329 is the estimate of the effect of female gender only for participants with age equal to zero years. Because the effect of female gender depends on age, it is completely inappropriate to use the adjusted model to provide an age adjusted estimate of effect and pretend that it applies to all ages. We must use the interaction model and the results in (4.18) – (4.22) to provide individual age specific estimates of the effect of female gender.

The relevant estimator of the log hazard in the presence of an interaction is shown in (4.17), and the log-hazard ratio in (4.18). Because the estimator depends on a continuous covariate, age in this example, we have a choice of using a plot and/or a table. We find that a plot of the log hazard as well as one of the relevant log-hazard ratio can be useful for understanding the source of the interaction, but often these plots are not specific enough to provide the kind of detailed information about the actual values of estimated hazard ratios that subject matter investigators are interested in knowing.[2] Hence, we typically use the plot to identify key values of the covariate and prepare a table for presentation to the investigators, that contains the point and confidence interval estimates of the hazard ratio at these values.

Following this suggested approach we present, in Figure 4.2, a plot of the estimated log hazard from the interaction model in Table 4.13. Under a model with no interaction, the lines for the log hazards for two genders are parallel and the vertical distance between them is the age adjusted log hazard ratio. The plot of the lines for the interaction model shows the departure from being parallel and the significance of the interaction coefficient in Table 4.13 tells us that the two lines are statistically significantly different. The two lines intersect at approximately 77 years. The fact that the line for females lies above that of males for ages less than 77 means that they are dying at a rate greater than that of males. The reverse is true for ages greater than 77. The estimated age-specific log hazard ratio is the vertical distance between the two lines at any specified age.

Table 4.13   Estimated Coefficients, Standard Errors, z-Scores, Two-Tailed p-values, and 95% Confidence Interval Estimate for Three Models Fit to the Worcester Heart Attack Data, $n = 500$

Model	Variable	Coeff.	Std. Err.	z	$p>|z|$	95% CIE	
Crude	gender	0.381	0.1376	2.77	0.006	0.112,	0.651
Adjusted	gender	−0.066	0.1406	−0.47	0.641	−0.341,	0.210
	age	0.067	0.0062	10.79	<0.001	0.055,	0.079
Interaction	gender	2.329	0.9923	2.35	0.019	0.384,	4.273
	age	0.078	0.0080	9.77	<0.001	0.063,	0.094
	gender × age	−0.030	0.0125	−2.43	0.015	−0.055,	−0.006

---

[2] For both plots, we ignore the contribution of the baseline hazard function to the log-hazard function because under the proportional hazards assumption, it does not depend on the covariates.

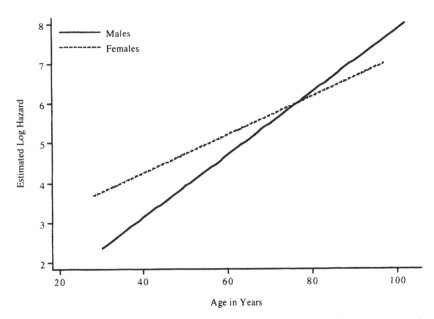

Figure 4.2 Plot of the estimated log hazard for males and females from the interaction model in Table 4.13 versus age.

In Figure 4.3 we plot the estimated log hazard ratio given by (4.18) and 95 percent pointwise confidence limits from (4.21) using estimated coefficients from the interaction model in Table 4.13. In addition, we have added a scale on the right that indicates the corresponding value of the estimated hazard ratio. We should note that the confidence bands in Figure 4.3 have the same hyperbolic shape as confidence bands for a fitted univariable linear regression model. This is a consequence of the parametric form of (4.18), which looks like a linear regression model and the fact that the confidence bands are narrowest at approximately the overall mean age, 68 years in these data.

In Figure 4.3 the horizontal line at log hazard equal to zero and hazard ratio equal to one corresponds to no gender effect. This line is contained within the confidence limits between the ages of 58 and 89. This tells us that the rate of death among females is not significantly different from males between the ages of 58 and 89. Females have a significantly higher rate of death for age less than 65 and the reverse is true for age greater than 85. Based on the above graph, Table 4.14 presents estimated hazard ratios and confidence intervals for ages 40, 50, 60, 65, 85 and 90. Obviously we have fit a simple model that ignores many other known risk factors for death following an MI. Keeping this in mind, the results in Table 4.14 show that the rate of death among 40–year-old women is estimated to

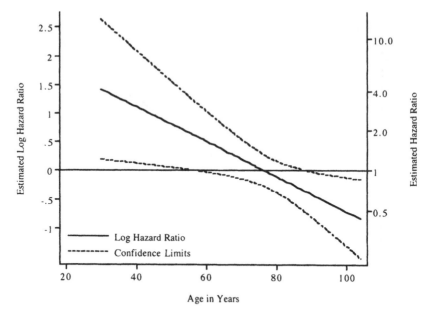

Figure 4.3 Plot of the age specific estimated log hazard ratio for female gender and 95 percent pointwise confidence limits versus age for the interaction model in Table 4.13

be three times that of males and drops to a 1.63-fold increase at age 60. Females over the age of 90 are dying at a rate estimated to be approximately 34% less than that of males. This interpretation must be tempered by the fact that only 16 men and 13 women of the 500 subjects are 90 or older.

We return to the German Breast Cancer Study data for our final example where, again, the covariate is an effect modifier. Again we use hormone therapy as the covariate of interest and the modifying covariate is the count of the number

Table 4.14   Age-Specific Estimated Hazard Ratios for Gender and 95% Confidence Interval Estimates from the Interactions Model in Table 4.13

Age	$\widehat{HR}$	95% CIE
40	3.04	1.139, 8.107
50	2.24	1.061, 4.736
60	1.65	0.977, 2.799
65	1.42	0.928, 2.174
85	0.77	0.564, 1.059
90	0.66	0.448, 0.983

of nodes involved. The results of fitting three models containing these two covariates are presented in Table 4.15.

The results for the crude model in Table 4.15 are the same as those for the crude model in Table 4.11, which indicate that use of hormone therapy significantly reduces the rate of recurrence. The results for the adjusted model in Table 4.15 show that increased nodal involvement significantly increases the rate of recurrence. The estimated coefficient for hormone therapy is only 2 percent different from the crude estimate. This is due to the fact that the mean number of nodes involved for the two treatment groups are nearly identical: 5.1 for those receiving therapy and 4.9 for those not receiving therapy. Hence, we conclude that nodal involvement does not confound the estimate of the effect of hormone therapy in these data.

The Wald test for the interaction coefficient in Table 4.15 is significant with $p = 0.011$. Although not shown, the likelihood ratio test is also significant ($p = 0.015$). For this example we show only the plot of the node specific estimated log hazard ratio with its 95 percent confidence bands in Figure 4.4.

As in Figure 4.3, the horizontal line in Figure 4.4 represents no effect. Furthermore, we see that the no effect line is contained within the confidence bands for 10 or more nodes involved. Hence use of hormone therapy significantly reduces the rate of recurrence only when 9 or fewer nodes are involved. While the number of nodes involved ranges from 1 to 51, 85 percent of the subjects had 9 or fewer nodes involved, with 43 percent having one or two. This suggests that we should focus our attention in the low end of the range, and to this end, we present node-specific estimated hazard ratios and confidence intervals for 1, 3, 5, 7 and 9 nodes in Table 4.16. The point estimates of the hazard ratios demonstrate that the benefit of hormone therapy ranges from a 43 percent reduction in the rate of recurrence among women with one node involved to a 23 percent reduction for women with 9 nodes involved.

Each of the examples in this section involved only two covariates. In subse-

Table 4.15 Estimated Coefficients, Standard Errors, z-Scores, Two-Tailed p-values, and 95% Confidence Interval Estimate for Three Models Fit to the German Breast Cancer Study Data, $n = 686$

Model	Variable	Coeff.	Std. Err.	z	$p > |z|$	95% CIE
Crude	hormone	−0.364	0.1250	−2.91	0.004	−0.609, −0.119
Adjusted	hormone	−0.357	0.1252	−2.85	0.004	−0.602, −0.112
	Nodes	0.058	0.0067	8.66	<0.001	0.045, 0.071
Interaction	hormone	−0.606	0.1635	−3.71	<0.001	−0.926, −0.286
	Nodes	0.049	0.0082	6.03	<0.001	0.033, 0.065
	hormone × nodes	0.038	0.0150	2.55	0.011	0.009, 0.068

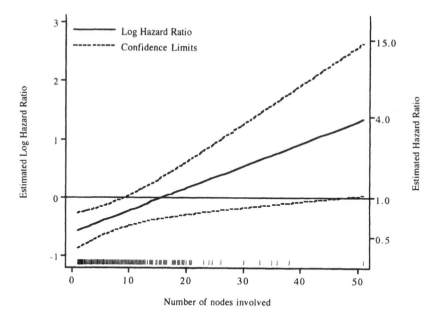

Figure 4.4 Plot of the node-specific estimated log-hazard ratio for hormone therapy and 95 percent pointwise confidence limits versus nodes for the interaction model in Table 4.15

quent chapters we consider more realistic, and thus more complicated, multi-variable models containing covariates that confound and/or interact with other model covariates. Regardless of how complicated a model might be, the simple examples in this section provide the basic paradigm for estimating and interpreting hazard ratios. We must remember that model-based inferences are only as good as the model upon which they are based. Hence, it is vital that one pays close attention to the all the model building and model assessment details discussed in Chapters 5 and 6 before using a fitted model to estimate hazard ratios.

Table 4.16 Node-Specific Estimated Hazard Ratios and 95% Confidence Interval Estimate from the Interactions Model in Table 4.15

Nodes	$\widehat{HR}$	95% CIE
1	0.57	0.419, 0.767
3	0.61	0.466, 0.803
5	0.66	0.513, 0.850
7	0.71	0.558, 0.911
9	0.77	0.598, 0.990

4.5 INTERPRETING AND USING THE ESTIMATED COVARIATE-ADJUSTED SURVIVAL FUNCTION

Methods for estimating the survival function following the fitting of a proportional hazards model were presented in Section 3.5. The key step presented in that section is the estimation of the baseline survival function, $\hat{S}_0(t)$, shown in (3.40). This estimator may be combined with the estimators of the coefficients in the model using (3.37) to obtain the estimator of the survival function, adjusting for the covariates, as follows

$$\hat{S}(t,\mathbf{x},\hat{\boldsymbol{\beta}}) = \left[\hat{S}_0(t)\right]^{\exp(\mathbf{x}'\hat{\boldsymbol{\beta}})}. \tag{4.23}$$

All software packages allow the user to request that the estimator of the baseline survival function be calculated and saved. This estimator may be used to derive other functions of survival time. For example, the estimator in (4.23) is essential for graphical description of the results of the analysis and for other analyses, such as model assessment. We discuss graphical methods and estimation of quantiles and their interpretation in this section and model assessment in Chapter 6.

We begin with an example from the German Breast Cancer Study fitting a model containing the dichotomous treatment variable, hormone therapy. The model containing only hormone therapy was fit as the crude model in two examples in the previous section, see Table 4.11 and Table 4.15. For convenience, we repeat the results of this fit in Table 4.17.

The estimator of the baseline survival function for this model is an estimator of the survival function for hormone = 0. If we request that the baseline survival function be computed as part of the analysis, then the software evaluates (3.40), denoted

$$\hat{S}_0(t_i), \quad i = 1, 2, \ldots, n \tag{4.24}$$

for each subject in the study, regardless of their survival status or hormone use. It follows from (3.40) that the estimator $\hat{S}_0(t)$ is constant between observed survival times. Thus, the estimated value for subjects who were censored is equal to the value at the largest observed survival time for which they were still at risk.

Table 4.17   Estimated Coefficients, Standard Errors, z-Scores, Two-Tailed p-values, and 95% Confidence Interval Estimate for a Model Fit to the German Breast Cancer Study Data, $n = 686$

Variable	Coeff.	Std. Err.	z	$p>|z|$	95% CIE
hormone	–0.364	0.1250	–2.91	0.004	–0.609, –0.119

We can compute an estimate of the survival function for hormone = 1 by using the previously calculated value of the baseline survival function and evaluating

$$\hat{S}\left(t_i, \text{hormone} = 1, \hat{\beta}_1 = -0.364\right) = \left[\hat{S}_0\left(t_i\right)\right]^{\exp(-0.364)}, \quad i = 1, 2, \ldots, 686 \qquad (4.25)$$

where the value of the coefficient for hormone is obtained from Table 4.17. The graphs of the two estimated survival functions, and (4.25), are shown in Figure 4.5. The plot has been drawn with steps connecting the points to emphasize the fact that the estimator is constant between observed survival times. It follows from and (4.25) that each function has been plotted at exactly the same $n = 686$ values of time. The shape of the two curves is a consequence of the proportional hazards assumption. The ratio of the hazards at each point in Figure 4.5 is forced to be equal to $0.69 = \exp(-0.364)$.

One of the treatment specific Kaplan-Meier estimators may have a plot similar in appearance to Figure 4.5. However, there is an important distinction, as the Kaplan-Meier estimators use only the data in each hormone use group and do not assume the hazards are proportional.

We can also think of the curves plotted in Figure 4.5 as being like "fitted" or "predicted" regression lines. Here the "prediction" is on the survival probability scale. The upper curve predicts or estimates the survival experience among those having hormone therapy if: (1) the estimate of the baseline survival function correctly describes the survival experience in the no-hormone therapy group (the lower curve), and (2) the proportional hazards model is correct.

In the GBCS data, the observed range of times is nearly identical for the two hormone groups. This may not always be the case. For example, consider a study where the survival experience is much poorer in an "exposed" group than an unexposed group. In this case, we might expect to see few long follow-up times in the exposed group and it is possible that the range of times would be less than that of the unexposed group. Yet a plot of the estimated survival function for the exposed group, using the estimated baseline survival function from the fitted proportional hazards model, would extrapolate this group's survival experience beyond their observed range. This extrapolation can be avoided by simply restricting the plot for each group to the observed times in the group. However, in reading someone else's analyses in the literature, it may be quite difficult to determine if there has been an inappropriate extrapolation in plots of proportional hazards covariate adjusted survival curves. We leave as an exercise plotting the two estimated survival functions in Figure 4.5 over their specific times, e.g., a plot with a total of 686 points.

If the observed range of survival times is comparable for each group, as it is in our example, we recommend a plot like Figure 4.5 because it uses all the data and best presents the fitted model and its assumptions. However, if there is a clinically important difference in the observed range of survival times, then we recommend plotting over each group's specific times. The best approach in practice is to pro-

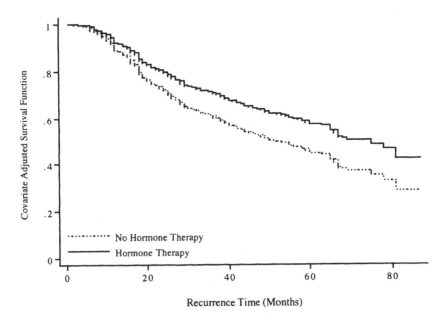

Figure 4.5 Graph of the estimated proportional hazards model survival functions for hormone use for the German Breast Cancer Study. Points are plotted at each of 686 observed values of time for both curves.

vide results from both a thorough univariate analysis of survival experience in subgroups of special interest, as well as results from any regression analyses.

As noted in the previous section, the principal reason for regression modeling is to adjust statistically for possible imbalances in the observed data. As an example of a more complicated model, suppose we fit the proportional hazards model containing hormone therapy and tumor size. If the goal is to present survival functions for the two hormone therapy groups, controlling for tumor size, then we must give some thought to what we mean by *controlling for tumor size*.

We would like the estimated survival function to use the covariates in the same way that covariates are controlled for in a linear regression. In linear regression, a point on the regression line (or plane for a multiple variable model) is the model-based estimate of the conditional mean of the dependent variable among subjects with values of the covariates defined by the point. The analogy to linear regression can help our thinking, but the situation is a bit more complicated in a proportional hazards regression analysis. Because the model does not contain an intercept, we do not have a fully parametric hazard function and thus the model cannot predict an individual point estimate of the conditional "mean" survival time. The estimated survival function in (4.23) is the proportional hazards model-based estimator of the conditional statistical distribution of survival time. In this case, the word "conditional" means restricting observation to a cohort with covariate values equal to values specified. Pursuing this notion further, suppose we were able to follow an extremely large cohort of subjects for 5 years. Furthermore, suppose that the cohort is large enough that we can perform a fully stratified analysis and compute the Kaplan–Meier estimator of the survival function for each possible set of values of the covariates, such as use of hormone therapy and tumor size 25mm. If the proportional hazards model is correct, then the estimator and the Kaplan–Meier estimator should be similar, within statistical variation. We can use the estimator to describe survival time graphically and to compute estimates of quantiles, such as the median, in the same way we used the Kaplan–Meier estimator in Chapter 2.

Estimated survivor functions are most frequently used in applied settings to provide curves, similar to those in Figure 4.5, to compare groups visually, controlling for other model covariates. If the model does not contain grouping variable by covariate interactions, then the resulting survival functions are in a sense "parallel" in a way similar to lines with the same slope in a linear regression. In practice, one would choose one set of "typical" values of the other covariates. For a continuous covariate like tumor size, we usually choose the mean, median or other central value. In the GBCS data, the median tumor size is 25mm and the mean is 29.3. Thus, 25 is a good value to use for tumor size in this example. If we fit the proportional hazards model containing hormone therapy and tumor size, then the baseline survival function estimates the survival experience for no hormone therapy and tumor size equal to 0 mm. To obtain the estimates of the two more realistically size-adjusted survival functions, we have to evaluate the expression in using the coefficients from the fitted model with $(\text{hormone} = 0, \text{size} = 25)$ and $(\text{hormone} = 1, \text{size} = 25)$. This approach, while algebraically correct, could cause unwanted round off and computational error in some situations due to exponentiating large positive or negative numbers, though we have rarely encountered this problem in our own work.

We can avoid this problem by centering continuous covariates. In the current example, we fit the model using $\text{size\_c} = \text{size} - 25$, and the results are shown in Table 4.18. These results are identical to those for the adjusted model in Table 4.11 obtained with size uncentered; the only difference is in the baseline survival function. When we center tumor size, the estimate of the baseline survival func-

Table 4.18 Estimated Coefficients, Standard Errors, z-Scores, Two-Tailed p-values, and 95% Confidence Interval Estimates for the Model Containing Hormone Therapy and Tumor Size Centered at 25mm in the German Breast Cancer Study

Variable	Coeff.	Std. Err.	z	$p>|z|$	95% CIE
hormone	−0.373	0.1252	−2.98	0.003	−0.619, −0.128
size_c	0.015	0.0036	4.28	<0.001	−0.008, 0.022

tion corresponds to no hormone therapy and tumor size 25mm, the zero value for the two covariates in the model. To obtain the second estimated survival function, specific for women receiving hormone therapy and having a tumor size of 25 mm, we compute

$$\hat{S}\left(t_i, \text{hormone} = 1, size\_c = 25, \hat{\beta}\right) = \left[\hat{S}_0\left(t_i\right)\right]^{\exp(-0.373)}, \quad i = 1, 2, \ldots, 686.$$

A graph of the two estimated survival functions, plotted at each of the 686 observed values of time, is shown in Figure 4.6. The curves in this graph provide proportional hazards estimates of the survival experience of two cohorts, each with a 25 mm tumor but differing in their hormone therapy use.

The shapes of the curves in Figure 4.6 are determined by the proportional hazards assumption, hormone therapy status, and size equal to 25 mm. If we centered size at a larger number, say 40 mm, then the resulting curves would look similar to those in Figure 4.6 but with poorer survival experience because the rate of recurrence increases with increasing tumor size. The reverse would be true if we centered at 15mm. In all three cases, the two plotted curves would be based on a hazard ratio of $0.69 = \exp(-0.373)$ at all time points.

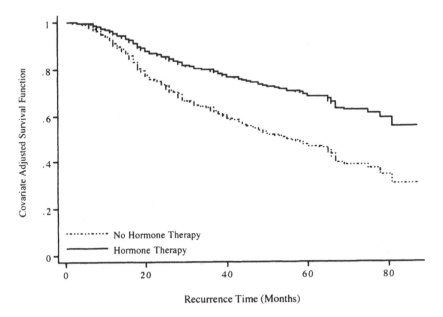

Figure 4.6 Graph of the tumor size adjusted estimated proportional hazards survival functions for hormone therapy in the German Breast Cancer Study. Functions are plotted at 686 values of time for each group.

When the fitted model is even moderately complex, it may be difficult to decide what combination of covariate values best represents the middle of the data. In these situations, plots based on values of the *risk score* are frequently used in practice. The risk score is the value of the linear portion of the proportional hazards model and its estimator for the ith subject from a model containing p covariates is

$$\hat{r}_i = \hat{r}\left(\mathbf{x}_i, \hat{\boldsymbol{\beta}}\right) = \sum_{k=1}^{p} \hat{\beta}_k x_{ik} . \tag{4.26}$$

Most software packages will calculate and save the values of (4.26). The baseline survival function corresponds to a risk score equal to zero, which may or may not be clinically relevant. We can provide a graphical description of survival experience by plotting the estimated survival function for various quantiles of the risk score, which we can easily get from the descriptive statistics. Typically, one might do this plot for the quartiles of the risk score or other quantiles. The estimator of the survival function for the qth quantile of the risk score, $\hat{r}_q$, is

$$\hat{S}\left(t_i, \hat{r}_q, \hat{\boldsymbol{\beta}}\right) = \left[\hat{S}_0\left(t_i\right)\right]^{\exp(\hat{r}_q)}, i = 1, 2, \ldots, n . \tag{4.27}$$

As an example of a typical multivariable survival model, we fit the proportional hazards model to the German Breast Cancer Study data containing hormone therapy, tumor grade with grade one as the referent value, tumor size and the natural logarithm of the number of progesterone receptors[3], denoted as ln_prg. The results for the fitted model are given in Table 4.19. As in the previously fit models use of hormone therapy significantly reduces the rate of tumor recurrence as does an increase in the number of progesterone receptors, while rate of tumor recurrence increases significantly for grade two and three tumors and the size of the tumor.

Table 4.19 Estimated Coefficients, Standard Errors, z-Scores, Two-Tailed p-values, and 95% Confidence Interval Estimates for the Model Containing Hormone Therapy, Tumor Grade, Tumor Size, and the Natural Logarithm of the Number of Progesterone Receptors from the German Breast Cancer Study

Variable	Coeff.	Std. Err.	z	p>|z|	95% CIE
hormone	−0.326	0.1262	−2.58	0.010	−0.573, −0.079
grade_2	0.624	0.2508	2.49	0.013	0.133, 1.116
grade_3	0.629	0.2758	2.28	0.023	0.088, 1.170
size	0.014	0.0036	3.70	<0.001	0.006, 0.021
ln_prg	−0.181	0.0315	−5.74	<0.001	−0.242, −0.119

---

[3] We discuss the rationale for using the natural logarithm of the number of progesterone receptors in Chapter 5.

To get a general feeling for time-to-tumor recurrence as a function of model covariates, we plot in Figure 4.7 the estimated survival function for the 10th, 25th, 50th, 75th, and 90th percentiles of the estimated risk score. These values are –0.487, –0.118, 0.239, 0.593, and 0.899, respectively. The basic "parallelism" seen in Figure 4.7 is a consequence of the proportional hazards assumption and the fact that each estimated survival function is plotted over all 686 values of recurrence time. As expected, as the risk score increases, the survival experience worsens. We can quantify the differences empirically in the estimated curves by reporting their respective estimated median time to cancer recurrence. Because the minimum value of the estimated survival function for the 10th percentile curve is 0.602, the estimator of the median does not have a finite value. The estimates for the remaining curves are 81, 65, 46, and 32 months, respectively, are obtained by applying (2.11) to each estimated survival function. Methods have not been developed to provide confidence interval estimates for these risk quantile survival curves, to test for their equality, or to provide confidence intervals for their respective median time to response. As a result, the type of presentation shown in Figure 4.7, while providing a useful description of survival experience as a function of risk, is not likely to be helpful for inferential purposes when the study has a key exposure or risk factor.

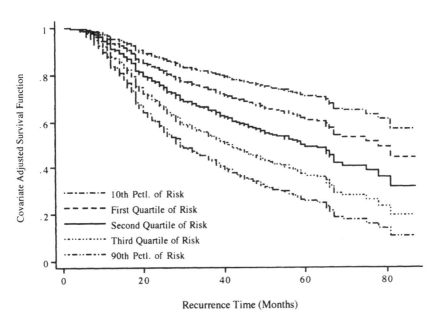

Figure 4.7 Graph of the estimated proportional hazards survival functions at the 10th, 25th, 50th, 75th, and 90th percentiles of the estimated risk score for fitted model in Table 4.19.

The risk score procedure may be modified when we wish to graph the estimated survival functions for any discrete grouping variable, controlling for a risk score based on the remaining covariates. Most often the grouping variable is the key treatment or exposure variable. To accomplish this, we subtract the contribution of the grouping variable to the risk score and calculate the median value that remains. We calculate covariate adjusted survival functions at the median risk with the effect of the grouping variable absent and then with its effect added to the median risk. Suppose the grouping variable is dichotomous and is the first of the p covariates in the model. The modified risk scores, obtained by removing the effect of the grouping variable, are

$$\hat{rm}_i = \hat{r}_i - \hat{\beta}_1 x_{i1}, \ i = 1, 2, \ldots, n.$$

If we denote the median of the modified risk scores as $\hat{rm}_{50}$, then the estimates of the survival functions for the two groups at this median are

$$\hat{S}\left(t_i, x_1 = 0, \hat{rm}_{50}, \hat{\boldsymbol{\beta}}\right) = \left[\hat{S}_0\left(t_i\right)\right]^{\exp\left(\hat{rm}_{50} + \hat{\beta}_1 \times 0\right)} \tag{4.28}$$

and

$$\hat{S}\left(t_i, x_1 = 1, \hat{rm}_{50}, \hat{\boldsymbol{\beta}}\right) = \left[\hat{S}_0\left(t_i\right)\right]^{\exp\left(\hat{rm}_{50} + \hat{\beta}_1 \times 1\right)} \tag{4.29}$$

for each of the $i = 1, 2, \ldots, n$ subjects.

As an example, we use the fitted model in Table 4.19 with hormone therapy as the dichotomous covariate of interest. As noted above, this model has been chosen for demonstration purposes only. The estimated hazard ratio for hormone use is $\hat{HR} = \exp(-.326) = 0.72$ with an associated 95 percent confidence interval of $(0.564, 0.924)$. The estimate indicates that use of hormone therapy reduces the rate of cancer recurrence by about 28 percent.

In this example, the equation for the estimated risk score from Table 4.19 for the ith subject is

$$\hat{r}_i = -0.326 \times \text{hormone} + 0.624 \times \text{grade\_2} + 0.629 \times \text{grade\_3} \\ + 0.014 \times \text{size} - 0.181 \times \text{ln\_prg},$$

and the modified estimated risk score is

$$\hat{rm}_i = \hat{r}_i - \left(-0.326 \times \text{hormone}_i\right).$$

The median value of the modified risk score is 0.35 and the equations for the estimators of the modified risk score-adjusted survival functions obtained from (4.28) and (4.29) are

$$\hat{S}\left(t_i, hormone = 0, \hat{rm}_{50}, \hat{\boldsymbol{\beta}}\right) = \left[\hat{S}_0\left(t_i\right)\right]^{\exp(0.35)} \tag{4.30}$$

and

$$\hat{S}\left(t_i, hormone = 1, \hat{rm}_{50}, \hat{\boldsymbol{\beta}}\right) = \left[\hat{S}_0\left(t_i\right)\right]^{\exp(0.35-0.326)}. \tag{4.31}$$

Because the observed range of survival times in the two treatment groups is comparable, we chose to use all 686 observed survival times to plot (4.30) and (4.31). These are shown in Figure 4.8.

The two curves in Figure 4.8 reflect the effect of the use of hormone therapy, adjustment of model covariates via the median modified risk score and the assumption of proportional hazards. We can use the adjusted estimated survival functions, as we did with those shown in Figure 4.7, to estimate the adjusted median time to recurrence. Rounded to whole months, the estimates are 55 months for no hormone therapy and 69 months for users of hormone therapy. Hence, the conclusion, based on this typical model, is that use of hormone therapy is estimated to delay the median time to recurrence by a little over one year.

As noted earlier in this section confidence interval estimators for the risk score covariate-adjusted estimator of the survival function and its median survival time have not been developed. However, if one is able to specify the values of all

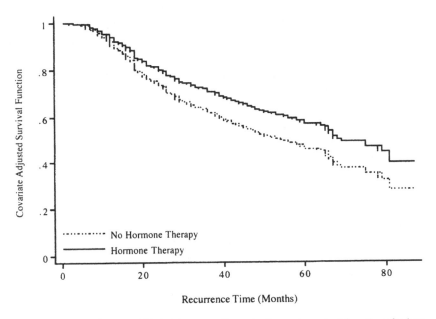

Figure 4.8 Graph of the modified risk score-adjusted estimated survival functions for hormone use based on the fitted model in Table 4.19.

model covariates then one may use an estimator presented by Andersen, Borgan, Gill and Keiding (1993), equation (7.2.33), page 506| of the variance of the log of the covariate-adjusted survival function to derive a confidence interval estimator. Their estimator is identical to one presented by Marubini and Valsecchi (1995, in the Appendix to Chapter 6). As noted in Chapter 2, better coverage properties are obtained if a confidence interval for the survival function is based on the log-log transformation of the function. An expression for a variance estimator for this further transformation is also given by Andersen, Borgan, Gill and Keiding (1993) following (7.2.33). We do not consider this method further because the compli-cated models encountered in practice make it almost impossible to specify a set of covariates that describes the "middle" of the data.

The estimated survival function and its variations discussed in this section are effective tools for describing the results of a regression analysis of survival time. We wish to reemphasize the importance of giving careful thought to the plotted range of the curve and estimates of survival probabilities. It is all too easy, with current statistical software, to present graphs and predictions that may inappropri-ately extrapolate the fitted model.

EXERCISES

1. For this problem, use the WHAS500 data with non-missing values for both gen-der and bmi. Use length of follow up as the survival time variable, status at last follow up as the censoring variable, and 10 percent as the level of signifi-cance.

(a) Fit the proportional hazards model containing gender and estimate the haz-ard ratio, pointwise and confidence interval. Interpret, in words, the point and interval estimates.

(b) Add bmi to the model fit in 1(a). Is bmi a confounder of the effect of gen-der? Explain the reasons for your answer.

(c) Estimate the bmi-adjusted hazard ratio, pointwise and confidence interval. Interpret, in words, the point and interval estimates.

(d) Estimate the gender adjusted hazard ratio, pointwise and confidence inter-val for a 5 kg/m^2 increase in bmi. Interpret, in words, the point and interval es-timates.

(e) Is there a significant interaction between bmi and gender?

(f) Explain why the main effect coefficients for gender in the models fit in 1(b) and 1(d) are different.

(g) Using the interaction model fit in 1(e), estimate and interpret the hazard ratio and associated confidence interval for gender, for bmi equal to 15, 20, 25, 30, and 35.

(h) Using the interaction model fit in 1(e), graph the estimate of the hazard ratio for gender with confidence bands as a function of bmi.

(i) Using the interaction model fit in 1(e), estimate the hazard ratio, pointwise, and confidence interval, for a 5 kg/m^2 increase in bmi for each gender.

(j) Using the interaction model fit in 1(e), compute and then graph the estimated survival functions for males and females with a bmi of 25 kg/m^2. Interpret the survival experience presented in this graph.

(k) Using the covariate adjusted survival functions from 1(j) estimate the median survival time for males and females with bmi = 25 kg/m^2.

2. Repeat problem 1 parts (a)-(c) and (e), using MI order as the risk factor of interest and MI type as the controlling covariate.

(f) Using the interactions model fit in 2(e), estimate the hazard ratio and associated confidence interval for MI type: recurrent, for Q-wave and non Q-wave MI's.

(g) Using the interaction model fit in 2(e), compute and then graph the four possible covariate adjusted-survival functions.

3. Using the data from the WHAS500 data with length of follow-up as the survival time variable and status at last follow up as the censoring variable, do the following:

(a) Fit the proportional hazards model containing gender, age (centered at 65 years), the gender by age interaction, MI type, MI order, the MI type by MI order interaction, heart rate (centered at 85 bpm), and congestive heart failure. Obtain the estimated baseline survival function and the risk score.

(b) Graph the baseline survival function and explain the cohort of subjects whose survival experience is being estimated.

(c) Graph the four risk-score adjusted survival functions at each of the quartiles of the risk score. How does increasing risk score influence time to death following hospital admission for an MI in this cohort?

(d) Using the modified risk score method graph the covariate adjusted survival functions at the two levels of congestive heart failure. Using the estimated survival functions, estimate the median survival time for each group as well as the one-year survival probability. Which of these two measures, median survival time or one-year probability, do you think might be most clinically useful?

CHAPTER 5

Model Development

5.1 INTRODUCTION

In any applied setting, performing a proportional hazards regression analysis of survival data requires a number of critical decisions. It is likely that we will have data on more covariates than we can reasonably expect to include in the model, so we must decide on a method to select a subset. We must consider such issues as clinical importance and adjustment for confounding, as well as statistical significance. Once we have selected the subset, we must determine whether the model is "linear" in the continuous covariates and, if not, what transformations are suggested by the data and clinical considerations. Which interactions, if any, should be included in the model is another important decision. In this chapter, we discuss these and other practical model development issues.

The end use of the estimated regression model will most often be a summary presentation and interpretation of the factors that have influenced survival. This summary may take the form of a table of estimated hazard ratios and confidence intervals and/or estimated covariate–adjusted survival functions. Before this step can be taken, we must critically examine the estimated model for adherence to key assumptions (e.g., proportional hazards) and determine whether any subjects have an undue influence on the fitted model. In addition, we may calculate summary measures of goodness-of-fit to support our efforts at model assessment. Methods for model assessment are discussed and illustrated in Chapter 6.

The methods available to select a subset of covariates to include in a proportional hazards regression model are essentially the same as those used in any other regression model. In this chapter, we present three methods for selecting a subset of covariates. Purposeful selection is a method completely controlled by the data analyst, while stepwise and best subsets selection of covariates are statistical methods. We also discuss an iterative method called "multivariable fractional polynomials" that makes statistical decisions regarding which covariates to include in the model as well as possible transformations of continuous covariates. These approaches to covariate selection have been chosen because use of one or more will yield, in the vast majority of model building applications, a subset of statistically and clinically significant covariates.

132

A word of caution: statistical software for fitting regression models to survival data is, for the most part, easy to use and provides a vast array of sophisticated statistical tools and techniques. One must be careful, therefore, not to lose sight of the problem and end up with the software prescribing the model to the analyst rather than the other way around.

Regardless of which method is used for covariate selection, any survival analysis should begin with a thorough univariable analysis of the association between survival time and each of the covariates under consideration. These methods are discussed in detail in Chapter 2. For categorical covariates, this should include Kaplan–Meier estimates of the group–specific survival functions, point and interval estimates of the median (and/or other quantiles of) survival time and use of one or more of the significance tests to compare survival experience across the groups defined by the covariate. For descriptive purposes, continuous covariates could be broken into quartiles, or other clinically meaningful groups, and the methods for categorical covariates could then be applied. Alternatively, point and interval estimates of the hazard ratio for a clinically relevant change in the covariate could be used in conjunction with the significance level of the partial likelihood ratio test. These results should be displayed using the tabular conventions of the scientific field.

5.2 PURPOSEFUL SELECTION OF COVARIATES

Modern statistical software is so powerful and easy to use that it is sometimes difficult to avoid shortcuts in analyses. The expression "cutting to the chase" is not appropriate to describe multivariable model building. We feel that one should approach multivariable model building with patience and a keen eye for the details that differentiate a good model from one that is merely adequate for the job. A good model is one that has been chosen by using a careful, well thought out, covariate selection process that gives thoughtful consideration to issues of adjustment and interaction (confounding and effect modification) and thoroughly evaluates the model for assumptions, influential observations, and tests for goodness-of-fit. We feel that the method described below comes as close to this ideal as any method.

Our purposeful selection method consists of the following seven steps:

Step 1: We begin by fitting a multivariable model containing all variables significant in the univariable analysis at the 20-25 percent level, as well as any other variables not selected with this criterion but judged to be of clinical importance. (If there are adequate data to fit a model containing all study covariates, this full model could be the beginning a multivariable model. We will provide further details regarding our perspective on what adequate data means toward the end of this section.) The rationale for choosing a relatively modest level of significance is based on recommendations for linear regression by Bendel and Afifi (1977), for discriminant analysis by Costanza and Afifi (1979), and for change in coefficient modeling in epidemiology by Mickey and Greenland (1989). Use of this level of significance should lead to the inclusion, in the preliminary multivariable model, of any statistically significant variable or one with the potential to be an important confounder.

Step 2: Following the fit of the initial multivariable model, we use the *p-values* from the Wald tests of the individual coefficients to identify covariates that might be deleted from the model. Some caution should be taken at this point not to reduce the size of the model by deleting too many seemingly non-significant variables at one time. The *p*-value of the partial likelihood ratio test should confirm that the deleted covariate is not significant. This is especially important when a nominal scale covariate with more than one design variable has been deleted, because we typically make a rough guess about overall significance based on the significance levels of the individual coefficients of the design variables.

Step 3: Following the fit of the reduced model, we assess whether removal of the covariate has produced an "important" change in the coefficients of the variables remaining in the model. In general, we use a value of about 20 percent as an indicator of an important change in a coefficient. If the variable excluded is an important confounder, it should be added back into the model. This process continues until no covariates can be deleted from the model.

Step 4: At this point, we add to the model, one at a time, all variables excluded from the initial multivariable model to confirm that they are neither statistically significant nor an important confounder. We have encountered situations in practice where a variable had a univariable test *p*-value that exceeded 0.8 but became highly significant when added to the multivariable model obtained at step (3). We refer to the model at the conclusion of this step as the *preliminary main effects model*.

Step 5: We now examine the scale of the continuous covariates in the preliminary main effects model. A number of techniques are available, all of which are designed to determine whether the data support the hypothesis that the effect of the covariate is linear in the log hazard and, if not, what transformation of the covariate is linear in the log hazard. Discussion of these methods is somewhat involved and would interfere with the flow of the presentation of purposeful selection, if done at this point. Hence, we discuss these methods in Section 5.2.1. We refer to the model at the end of step (5) as the *main effects model*.

Step 6: The final step in the variable selection process (but not the final step in the model building process) is to determine whether interactions are needed in the model. In this setting, an interaction term is a new variable that is the product of two covariates in the model. Special considerations may dictate that a particular interaction term or terms be included in the model, regardless of the statistical significance of the coefficient(s). If this is the case, these interaction terms and their component terms should be added to the main effects model and the larger model fit before proceeding with a statistical evaluation of other possible interactions. However, in most settings, there will be insufficient clinical theory to justify automatic inclusion of interactions.

The selection process begins by forming a set of plausible interaction terms from the main effects in the model. Each individual interaction is assessed by comparing the model with the interaction term to the main effects model via the partial likelihood ratio test. All interactions significant at the 5 percent, or other, level are then added jointly to the main effects model. Wald statistic p-values are used as a guide to selecting interactions that may be eliminated from the model, but significance should be checked by the partial likelihood ratio test. Often when an interaction term enters a model, the coefficient of one of its component main effects may have a non-significant Wald statistic. We firmly believe that all main effects of significant interactions should remain in the model because, as shown in Section 4.4, estimates of effect require both main effect and interaction coefficients.

Several points should be kept in mind when selecting interaction terms. Because interactions are included to improve inferences and obtain a more realistic model, we feel that all interaction terms should be statistically significant at usual levels of significance, such as 5 or 10 percent, and perhaps as low as 1 percent in some settings. Inclusion of any interaction term in a model makes interpretation more difficult, but often more informative. However, if the interaction term is not significant, then standard error estimates will needlessly increase, thus unnecessarily widening confidence interval estimates of hazard ratios.

Step 7: We refer to the model at the conclusion of step (6) as the *preliminary model*. It does not become the *final model* until we thoroughly evaluate it. Model evaluation should include: checking for adherence to key model assumptions using casewise diagnostic statistics to check for influential observations and testing for overall goodness-of-fit. This step is mandatory for any model building strategy, not just purposeful selection. We discuss evaluation methods in Chapter 6.

A modification that is sometimes used in a clinical trial setting where there is a clear "treatment" variable is to exclude the treatment variable from the variable selection process. After the preliminary main effects model containing all other variables associated with outcome, treatment is then added to the model. This approach provides an estimate of the additional effect of treatment, adjusting for other covariates, in contrast to modeling in epidemiological studies where "treatment" would be the risk factor of interest. In these settings, selection of variables may be based on the change in the coefficient (estimate of effect) of the risk factor variable. Thus, rather than being the last variable to enter, the risk factor enters the model first. This points out that one must have clear goals for the analysis and proceed thoughtfully, using a variety of statistical tools and methods. The variable selection methods discussed may be an integral part of this analysis.

We mentioned in the beginning of this section that it is likely that we will have data on more covariates than we can reasonably expect to include in a single model. This might mean that the number of covariates showing a statistically significant association with survival from the univariable analyses will be much larger than can be expected to be included as a beginning multivariable model. In such a case, we recommend rank ordering all covariates based on the p-values from the univariable analyses and using, for the beginning model, only the most highly significant ones. It is difficult to make a general statement about how many covariates should or can be included, but a rough guideline is to include one covariate per ten events. As an example, for the WHAS500 study where 215 events are observed, a model with fewer than 20 estimated coefficients would not be expected to cause problems of over fitting. On the other hand, a data set with fewer than 20 events cannot be expected to yield meaningful results from multivariable analyses.

5.2.1 METHODS TO EXAMINE THE SCALE OF CONTINUOUS COVARIATES IN THE LOG HAZARD

As noted above in step (5) an important but, unfortunately in practice, often ignored modeling step is to determine whether the data support the assumption of linearity in the log hazard for all continuous covariates. Methods ranging from simple to complex can now be performed in many software packages.

The simplest method is to replace the covariate with design variables formed from its quartiles (these are easily obtained from the univariable descriptive analysis). The estimated coefficients for the design variables are plotted versus the midpoints of the intervals defined by the cutpoints. At the midpoint of the first interval, a point is plotted at zero. If the correct scale is linear in the log hazard, then the polygon connecting the points should be approximately a straight line. If the polygon departs substantially from a linear trend, its form may be used to suggest a transformation of the covariate. This is often difficult as there may only be four plotted points. We refer to this method as the *quartile design variable method* and its clear advantage is that it does not require any special software. Its disadvantage is that it is not powerful enough to detect subtle, but often important, deviations from a linear trend.

Another approach is to use fractional polynomials, developed by Royston and Altman (1994), to suggest transformations. Sauerbrei and Royston (1999) and Royston and Sauerbrei (2006) study the method in some detail. Basically we wish to determine what value of p in x^p yields the best model for the covariate (e.g., the log hazard is linear in x^p). In theory, we could incorporate the power, p, as an additional parameter in the estimation procedure. However, this greatly increases the complexity of the estimation problem. Royston and Altman propose replacing full maximum likelihood estimation of the power by a search through a small but useful set of possible values. We provide a brief description of the method here and use it in the model building example in the next section.

Fractional polynomials can be used with a multivariable proportional hazards regression model, but, for sake of simplicity, we describe them using a model with a single continuous covariate. We discuss an iterative multivariable version first proposed by Royston and Ambler (1998) in Section 5.3. The univariable hazard function for the proportional hazards regression model shown in (3.7) is

$$h(t,x,\beta) = h_0(t)e^{x\beta},$$

and the log-hazard function, which is linear in the covariate, is

$$\ln\left[h(t,x,\beta)\right] = \ln\left[h_0(t)\right] + x\beta.$$

One way to generalize this log-hazard function is to specify it as a function of J terms

$$\ln\left[h(t,x,\beta)\right] = \ln\left[h_0(t)\right] + \sum_{j=1}^{J} F_j(x)\beta_j.$$

The functions $F_j(x)$ are a particular type of power function. The value of the first function is $F_1(x) = x^{p_1}$. In theory, the power, p_1, could be any number, but in most applied settings we try to use something simple. Royston and Altman (1994) propose restricting the power to be among those in the set

$$\wp = \{-2,-1,-0.5,0,0.5,1,2,3\}$$

where $p_1 = 0$ denotes the natural log of the variable. The remaining functions are defined as

$$F_j(x) = \begin{cases} x^{p_j} & , \quad p_j \neq p_{j-1} \\ F_{j-1}(x)\ln(x), & p_j = p_{j-1} \end{cases}$$

for $j = 2,\ldots,J$ and restricting powers to those in $\wp$. For example, if we chose $J = 2$ with $p_1 = 0$ and $p_2 = -0.5$, then the log–hazard function is

$$\ln\left[h(t,x,\boldsymbol{\beta})\right] = \ln\left[h_0(t)\right] + \ln(x)\beta_1 + \frac{1}{\sqrt{x}}\beta_2.$$

As another example, if we chose $J = 2$ with $p_1 = 2$ and $p_2 = 2$, then the log-hazard function is

$$\ln\left[h(t,x,\boldsymbol{\beta})\right] = \ln\left[h_0(t)\right] + x^2\beta_1 + x^2\ln(x)\beta_2.$$

This is true for all repeated powers $(p_1 = p, p_2 = p)$. The model is quadratic in x if $p_1 = 1$ and $p_2 = 2$. Again, we could allow the covariate to enter the model with any number of functions, J, but in most applied settings an adequate transformation can be found if we use $J = 1$ or 2. Implementation requires, for $J = 1$, fitting 8 models, that is, $p_1 \in \wp$. The best model is the one with the largest log partial likelihood or smallest value of what we call the Deviance, -2 times the log partial likelihood. The process is repeated with $J = 2$ by fitting the 36 models obtained from the unique possible pairs of powers (28 pairs where $p_1 \neq p_2$ and eight pairs where $p_1 = p_2$). The best model is again the one with the largest log partial likelihood. The relevant question is whether either of the two best models is significantly better than the linear model. Let $L(1)$ denote the log partial likelihood for the linear model, that is, $J = 1$ and $p_1 = 1$, let $L(p_1)$ denote the log partial likelihood for the best $J = 1$ model and let $L(p_1, p_2)$ denote the log partial likelihood for the best $J = 2$ model. Royston and Altman (1994) and Ambler and Royston (2001) suggest, and verify with simulations, that each term in the fractional polynomial model contributes approximately 2 degrees of freedom to the model, effectively one for the power and one for the coefficient. Thus, the partial likelihood ratio test comparing the linear model to the best $J = 1$ model,

$$G(1, p_1) = -2\{L(1) - L(p_1)\},$$

is approximately distributed as chi–square with 1 degree of freedom under the null hypothesis of linearity. The partial likelihood ratio test comparing the best $J = 1$ model to the best $J = 2$ model,

$$G[p_1, (p_1, p_2)] = -2\{L(p_1) - L(p_1, p_2)\},$$

is approximately distributed as chi–square with 2 degrees of freedom under the null hypothesis that the second fractional polynomial function is equal to zero. Similarly, the partial likelihood ratio test comparing the linear model to the best $J = 2$ model,

$$G[1, (p_1, p_2)] = -2\{L(1) - L(p_1, p_2)\},$$

is distributed approximately as chi–square with 3 degrees of freedom. To keep the notation simple, we have used p_1 to denote the best power both when $J = 1$ and as the first of the two powers for $J = 2$. These are not likely to be the same numeric value in practice.

    In an applied setting, these partial likelihood ratio tests can be used in one of two ways to find the best fractional polynomial model: a closed test and a sequential test procedure, see Sauerbrei, Meier-Hirmer, Benner and Royston (2006) and cited references. Sauerbrei, Meier-Hirmer, Benner and Royston also consider as a candidate for the null model, one where x is not included in the model. We do not consider this model because all covariates remaining at the end of purposeful selection step (4) have passed statistical selection criteria and thus are in the model; the null model is no longer an option.

In the closed test procedure one begins by comparing the linear model to the best two-term model via $G\big[1,(p_1,p_2)\big]$. If this test is not significant at the chosen level of significance (usually 5 percent) then we stop and assume that the log hazard is linear in x. If the test is significant then we compare the best one-term model to the best two-term model via $G\big[p_1,(p_1,p_2)\big]$. If the test is significant, then we use the best two-term model otherwise we use the best one-term model.

In the sequential test procedure, we begin by comparing the best one-term model to the best two-term model, again via $G\big[p_1,(p_1,p_2)\big]$. If the test is significant, we stop and use the best two-term model. If the test is not significant, then we compare the linear model to the best one-term model via $G(1,p_1)$. If this test is significant, then we use the best one-term model. If this test is not significant, then we use the linear model.

Ambler and Royston (2001) examined the type I error rates of the two procedures via simulation and conclude that the closed test procedure comes closer to maintaining the overall level of significance and thus is the one we use in this text.

In general, we recommend that, if either the one or two-term fractional polynomial model is selected for use, it should not only provide a statistically significant improvement, but the transformation(s) must make clinical sense.

STATA is the only software package to have fully implemented fractional polynomials. Its fractional polynomial routine offers the user considerable flexibility in expanding the number of terms, J, as well as the set of powers searched. In most settings, the default values of $J = 2$ and $\wp$ are adequate. Sauerbrei, Meier-Hirmer, Benner and Royston (2006) describe software they have developed to implement the method in the SAS package and R computer language.

Graphical methods, other than the design variable method, to check the scale of covariates may be performed in most software packages. The most easily used is similar to the added variable plot from linear regression; see Ryan (1997). A complete discussion of residuals from a fitted proportional hazards model is provided in Chapter 6. The reader wishing to know the details is welcome to read Section 6.2 before proceeding, but it is not necessary at this point.

The first plot we discuss uses as the components of the residual for the ith subject, the value of the censoring variable, c_i, and a modification of the estimator of the cumulative hazard shown in (3.42). Specifically, we use the Nelson-Aalen estimator of the log of the baseline survival function, defined as

$$\ln\big[\hat{S}_0(t)\big] = \sum_{t_i \le t} \frac{e^{x_i'\hat{\beta}}}{\sum_{l \in R_i} e^{x_l'\hat{\beta}}},$$

yielding the estimator

$$\hat{H}_i = -e^{x\hat{\beta}} \times \sum_{t_i \leq t} \frac{e^{x\hat{\beta}}}{\sum_{l \in R_i} e^{x\hat{\beta}}}.$$

These are used to calculate the estimated martingale residuals, defined as

$$\hat{M}_i = c_i - \hat{H}_i.$$

It may seem a small and unimportant detail, but the sum of the martingale residuals is not equal to zero if we use the estimator in (3.42), while they do sum to zero as defined above.

Therneau, Grambsch and Fleming (1990) suggest calculating the martingale residuals from a model that excludes the covariate of interest. One then plots these martingale residuals versus the excluded covariate. They suggest adding a lowess or other smooth to the scatterplot to aid interpretation. This plot is analogous to the added variable plot in normal errors linear regression. The smooth provides an estimate of the functional form of the covariate in the log hazard. The difficulty in using this plot is deciding what the correct functional form is if the plot looks decidedly non-linear. We refer to this plot as the *smoothed added variable plot*.

Grambsch, Therneau and Fleming (1995) expand on their earlier work to propose a plot that has greater diagnostic power to detect the functional form of a model covariate. One begins by calculating the martingale residuals from the fit of a model containing all covariates. One then calculates a lowess smooth from the scatter plot of the censoring variable, c_i, versus the covariate of interest and another smooth of the scatter plot of the estimated cumulative hazard, $\hat{H}_i$, versus the covariate of interest. Denote these smoothed values as c_{ism} and $\hat{H}_{ism}$. One uses the two sets of smoothed values to calculate

$$f_i = \ln\left(\frac{c_{ism}}{\hat{H}_{ism}}\right) + \hat{\beta}_x \times x_i,$$

where $\hat{\beta}_x$ denotes the estimator of the coefficient of the covariate of interest, denoted as x. One then plots the values of f_i versus x_i. The correct functional form of the covariate is estimated in this plot. But again, we face the same question as in the added variable martingale residual plot. Namely, what is the functional form if the plot is non-linear? We refer to the plot of f_i versus x_i as the *GTF smoothed plot*. Descriptions of applications of these and other related methods may be found in Therneau and Grambsch (2000).

In practice, our decision to transform a continuous covariate is most often based on the results of a fractional polynomial analysis. We tend to use the graphical methods to see if they support the fractional polynomial model.

Rather than illustrate the method in this section and in the next section we use and illustrate them in the model building example in the next section.

Gray (1992) suggests that spline functions may be used as a way of modeling a continuous covariate that avoids the linear scale. Ryan (1997) discusses construction and use of spline functions in linear regression. Harrell et al. (1996) and Harrell (2001) use spline functions in a variety of modeling settings, including the proportional hazards model. Because spline functions are not readily available in most packages and not as easy to use as the methods we discuss in this section, we do not consider them in this text.

5.2.2 AN EXAMPLE OF PURPOSEFUL SELECTION OF COVARIATES

Among the data sets that we have chosen to use in this text, the Worcester Heart Attack Study's WHAS500 data provides the best opportunity[1] to illustrate not only issues of variable selection including confounding and interaction but also covariates that are not linearly scaled. At the end of this exercise, you may feel that we have gone a bit overboard and the resulting model is unnecessarily complicated. However, one of our goals is to present some working rules or guidelines that you can use in your own practice when complications such as interactions and non-linear continuous covariates occur.

The results of the univariable analysis of each covariate in relation to survival time (in years) following admission to a hospital after an MI are given in Table 5.1 for the discrete covariates and in Table 5.2 for the continuous covariates defined in Table 1.2. All variables except complete heart block are significant at the 20 percent level and therefore are candidates for inclusion in the multivariable model.

In Table 5.1 the cardiogenic shock and complete heart block variables present difficulties when considered for inclusion in a multivariable model. There are only 22 and 11 subjects, respectively, with the condition present and of these 17 and 7 die, respectively. Cardiogenic shock is significant at the 1 percent level. Examination of the survival times for the 17 subjects with cardiogenic shock who died showed that nine died in the first week of follow up and five more within the first month. Thus, those having cardiogenic shock have a high rate of early death and there is little data remaining to estimate its effect beyond one month of follow up. For these reasons we are dropping this covariate as a candidate for the multivariable model. Complete heart block is not a significant univariable predictor ($p = 0.254$) but has similar "thin data" problems. Hence, it is also dropped from further consideration for the multivariable model.

---

[1] The German Breast Cancer Study is another good data set but we could add little to the excellent work illustrating modeling done on these data by Sauerbrei and Royston (1999).

Table 5.1 Estimated Median Time to Death with 95% Brookmeyer-Crowley Confidence Interval Estimates, Log-Rank Test, and Partial Likelihood Ratio Test p-values for Categorical Covariates in the WHAS500 data ($n = 500$)

Variable	Category (events, n)	Median Time to Death (95% CIE)	Log-Rank Test p-value	Partial LR Test p-value
Gender	Male (111, 300)	5.91 (4.46, .)	0.005	0.006
	Female (104, 200)	3.61 (2.37, 4.32)		
History of CVD	No (45, 125)	6.44 (4.32, .)	0.091	0.084
	Yes (170, 375)	4.32 (3.72, 6.00)		
Atrial Fibrillation	No (168, 422)	5.91 (4.32, .)	0.001	0.002
	Yes (47, 78)	2.37 (1.15, 3.66)		
Cardiogenic Shock	No (198, 478)	5.27 (4.21, .)	<0.001	<0.001
	Yes (17, 22)	0.05 (0.01, 1.22)		
Congestive Heart Complications	No (105, 345)	6.46 (5.91, .)	<0.001	<0.001
	Yes (110, 155)	0.98 (0.71, 1.51)		
Complete Heart Block	No (208, 489)	4.45 (4.12, .)	0.217	0.254
	Yes (7, 11)	5.35 (0.01, .)		
MI Order	First (125, 329)	5.91 (5.27, 6.43)	0.002	0.003
	Recurrent (90, 171)	3.37 (1.97, 4.25)		
MI Type	Non Q–wave (169, 347)	3.50 (2.61, 4.32)	<0.001	<0.001
	Q–wave (46, 153)	6.43 (6.43, .)		

Before we fit the multivariable model, we note the close agreement in Table 5.1 between the significance levels of the partial likelihood ratio test and the log–rank test. This is as expected because, for a discrete covariate, the score test from a univariable proportional hazards model is algebraically equivalent to the log–rank test, and the score test and likelihood ratio test perform similarly. This implies that the log–rank test is a perfectly acceptable choice for purposes of covariate selection for the initial multivariable model.

Table 5.3 presents the results of fitting the multivariable proportional hazards model containing all variables significant at the $p < 0.20$ level in the univariable analysis (excluding cardiogenic shock as stated above).

Examining the p-values for the Wald statistics with the goal of trying to simplify the model, we see that the two largest values are $p = 0.967$ for history of cardiovascular disease (cvd) and $p = 0.904$ for systolic blood pressure (sysbp). Deleting these two covariates and refitting the model (results shown in Table 5.4) yields a two degrees-of-freedom partial likelihood ratio test whose p-value = 0.991 (calculations not shown here). We see that the estimates of the coefficients for the covariates remaining in the model are virtually unchanged and conclude that cvd and sysbp are not confounders.

Table 5.2 Estimated Hazard Ratio for Time to Death with 95% Confidence Interval Estimates, Wald Test, and Partial Likelihood Ratio Test p-values for Continuous Co-variates in the WHAS500 data ($n = 500$)

Variable	Change	Hazard Ratio for Change (95% CIE)	Wald Test p-value	Partial LR Test p-value
Age	5 years	1.39 (1.31, 1.48)	<0.001	<0.001
Heart Rate	10 beats	1.16 (1.10, 1.23)	<0.001	<0.001
Systolic Blood Pressure	10 mmHg	0.96 (0.92, 0.99)	0.043	0.041
Diastolic Blood Pressure	10 mmHg	0.85 (0.80, 0.91)	<0.001	<0.001
Body Mass Index	5 kg/m^2	0.61 (0.53, 0.71)	<0.001	<0.001

In Table 5.4, the covariate with the largest p-value is MI order (miord) where $p = 0.758$. The results of fitting the model deleting this covariate are shown in Table 5.5 and $p = 0.758$ for the one degree-of-freedom partial likelihood ratio test comparing the model in Table 5.5 to the one in Table 5.4 (calculations not shown). The estimates of the coefficients for the covariates common to the two models are nearly the same in Table 5.4 and Table 5.5, thus, miord is not a confounder.

The covariates in Table 5.5 with the largest p-values for the Wald statistics are atrial fibrillation (afb) with $p = 0.464$ and MI type (mitype) with $p = 0.309$. The results of fitting a model deleting these two are shown in Table 5.6. The partial likelihood ratio test comparing the model in Table 5.6 to the model in Table 5.5 has $p = 0.473$ (calculations not shown). We see that the estimates of the coeffi-

Table 5.3 Estimated Coefficients, Standard Errors, z-Scores, Two-Tailed p-values, and 95% Confidence Interval Estimates for the Proportional Hazards Model Containing Variables Significant at the 20% Level in the Univariable Analysis for the WHAS500 data (n = 500)

Variable	Coeff.	Std. Err.	z	$p>|z|$	95% CIE
age	0.049	0.0068	7.12	<0.001	0.035, 0.062
hr	0.010	0.0031	3.38	0.001	0.004, 0.016
sysbp	0.0004	0.0030	0.12	0.904	−0.006, 0.006
diasbp	−0.011	0.0049	−2.16	0.031	−0.020, −0.001
bmi	−0.044	0.0164	−2.66	0.008	−0.076, −0.011
gender	−0.271	0.1457	−1.86	0.063	−0.556, 0.015
cvd	0.007	0.1781	0.04	0.967	−0.342, 0.356
afb	0.128	0.1711	0.75	0.455	−0.207, 0.464
chf	0.774	0.1499	5.16	<0.001	0.480, 1.067
miord	0.044	0.1484	0.30	0.768	−0.247, 0.335
mitype	−0.164	0.1879	−0.87	0.382	−0.532, 0.204

Table 5.4 Estimated Coefficients, Standard Errors, z-Scores, Two-Tailed p-values, and 95% Confidence Interval Estimates for the Reduced Proportional Hazards Model for the WHAS500 data (n = 500)

Variable	Coeff.	Std. Err.	z	$p>|z|$	95% CIE
age	0.049	0.0067	7.23	<0.001	0.036, 0.062
hr	0.010	0.0030	3.45	0.001	0.004, 0.016
diasbp	−0.010	0.0035	−2.87	0.004	−0.017, −0.003
bmi	−0.044	0.0163	−2.67	0.008	−0.076, −0.012
gender	−0.268	0.1447	−1.85	0.064	−0.552, 0.053
afb	0.125	0.1697	0.74	0.460	−0.207, 0.458
chf	0.776	0.1486	5.22	<0.001	0.485, 1.067
miord	0.045	0.1454	0.31	0.758	−0.240, 0.330
mitype	−0.169	0.1838	−0.92	0.357	−0.529, 0.191

cients for the covariates remaining in the model are virtually unchanged and conclude that afb and mitype are not confounders.

With the exception of gender, each of the covariates in Table 5.6 has a significant Wald test when using $\alpha = 0.05$. Because gender is such an important clinical variable and is significant at the 10 percent level, we keep it in the model. No further model reduction is possible. At this point, we would normally add any covariates not in the initial multivariable model. The only candidates from Table 5.1 are cardiogenic shock and complete heart block, which were dropped due to inadequate data. The next step is to examine the scale of the continuous covariates age, heart rate (hr), diastolic blood pressure (diasbp) and body mass index (bmi).

Before checking the scale of the continuous covariates, we note that we deleted two covariates in first and third model reductions. This reflects one of our basic modeling strategies: to delete simultaneously covariates displaying similar

Table 5.5 Estimated Coefficients, Standard Errors, z-Scores, Two-Tailed p-values, and 95% Confidence Interval Estimates for the Reduced Proportional Hazards Model for the WHAS500 data (n = 500)

Variable	Coeff.	Std. Err.	z	$p>|z|$	95% CIE
age	0.049	0.0067	7.24	<0.001	0.036, 0.062
hr	0.010	0.0030	3.49	<0.001	0.005, 0.016
diasbp	−0.010	0.0035	−2.89	0.004	−0.017, −0.003
bmi	−0.044	0.0163	−2.70	0.007	−0.076, −0.012
gender	−0.274	0.1437	−1.90	0.057	−0.555, 0.008
afb	0.124	0.1697	0.73	0.464	−0.208, 0.457
chf	0.777	0.1486	5.23	<0.001	0.486, 1.069
mitype	−0.182	0.1789	−1.02	0.309	−0.533, 0.169

Table 5.6 Estimated Coefficients, Standard Errors, z-Scores, Two-Tailed p-values, and 95% Confidence Interval Estimates for the Reduced Proportional Hazards Model for the WHAS500 data (n = 500)

Variable	Coeff.	Std. Err.	z	$p>|z|$	95% CIE	
age	0.050	0.0066	7.55	<0.001	0.037,	0.063
hr	0.011	0.0029	3.83	<0.001	0.005,	0.017
diasbp	–0.011	0.0035	–3.02	0.003	–0.017,	–0.004
bmi	–0.045	0.0163	–2.77	0.006	–0.077,	–0.013
gender	–0.270	0.1436	–1.88	0.060	–0.551,	0.011
chf	0.778	0.1467	5.30	<0.001	0.490,	1.065

statistical associations with the outcome. However, we rarely remove more than two or three at a time, and if one covariate has more clinical relevance than the others, we will remove it separately from the others. Also, if removal of more than one covariate introduces confounding for one or more remaining variables, we step back and remove them one at a time.

The first method we illustrate for checking the scale of continuous covariates uses the quartile design variables. Separately, for each of the four continuous variables, we replace the variable in the model with three design variables formed using as cutpoints the three quartiles. Table 5.7 presents a summary of the resulting coefficients and group midpoints. We next graph the coefficients against the group midpoints. These are shown in Figure 5.1.

The plots of the coefficients for age and heart rate support an assumption of linearity in the log hazard. The plot for diastolic blood pressure has a small increase from the second to third quartile. The plot of the coefficients for body mass index has a similar but larger jump. It is difficult to tell from Figure 5.1 if the plots for diastolic blood pressure and body mass index indicate a statistically significant departure from linearity or are due to random variation. Based on these plots alone, we would be reluctant to recommend any non-linear transformation of diastolic blood pressure or body mass index.

Next, we use fractional polynomials to examine the linearity assumption. The fractional polynomial analysis of age, heart rate, and diastolic blood pressure did not yield any significant transformations, thus we do not show these results. The analysis of body mass index did not support linearity in the log hazard and the summary of results from STATA is shown in Table 5.8. Unfortunately, the results do not completely conform to either the closed test or sequential test procedure, but all the required information is provided. This situation may change in later releases of STATA. We first compare the linear model to the best two-term model. The partial likelihood ratio test statistic for this test is given in the last row of the third column as $G = 10.215$. The three degrees-of-freedom p-value for this test is 0.017 (Note: this result is not currently provided in the STATA output).

Table 5.7 Estimated Coefficients for the Three Design Variables Formed from the Quartiles for the Variables Age, Heart Rate, Diastolic Blood Pressure, and Body Mass Index for the WHAS500 data (n = 500)

	Age		Heart Rate		Diastolic Blood Pressure		Body Mass Index	
Quartile Midpoint	Coeff.	Quartile Midpoint	Coeff.	Quartile Midpoint	Coeff.	Quartile Midpoint	Coeff.
44.5	0.000	52	0.000	34.5	0.000	18.1	0.000
66	0.690	77.5	0.335	71.5	−0.314	24.6	−0.453
77.5	1.428	92.5	0.483	85.8	−0.298	27.7	−0.315
93.5	1.807	143.5	0.809	145.3	−0.610	37.1	−0.592

Thus, we conclude that the best two-term model is significantly different from the linear model. We next compare the best one-term model to the best two term model. The partial likelihood ratio test statistic for this test is not provided in the table but is calculated as

$$G = 2241.668 - 2237.784 = 3.884,$$

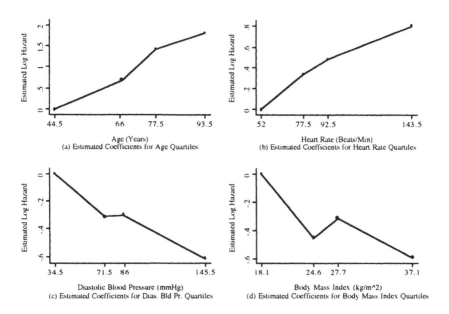

Figure 5.1 Graphs of estimated coefficients versus quartile midpoints for (a) age, (b) heart rate, (c) diastolic blood pressure, and (d) body mass index.

and its two degree-of-freedom p-value is 0.143 (Note: this p-value is provided in the last row of the fourth column of the STATA output). Because this test is not significant, we choose the one term fractional polynomial model, which states that transformation is bmi^{-2}. Before accepting this inverse squared transformation of body mass index, we need to be sure it is clinically plausible and examine whether the fractional polynomial analysis is being highly influenced by either exceptionally small or large values.

We know that both low and high body mass index are associated with poorer survival than moderate values. The fitted model (results not shown) using the inverse squared transformation of body mass index is monotonic. Hence, this transformation models the decrease in the log hazard from low to moderate body mass index but does not pick up the increase for high body mass index. A two-term model is required for any form of "quadratic like" shape in the log hazard. As noted above, the two-term model was not significantly different from the one-term model. Thus, on clinical grounds, we would choose the two-term model over the one-term model. If we use the two-term model in Table 5.8, then we will look at what the fitted (2,3) fractional polynomial looks like. Royston and Sauerbrei (2006) point out that the fractional polynomial analysis can be unduly influenced by outlying values. They propose a preliminary somewhat complicated mathematical transformation of the covariate to minimize any outlier effect. We refer the reader to their paper for the details[2]. A box plot of the distribution of body mass index, not shown here, indicates that there is one small value, 13.05, and one large value, 44.83, that have a gap of at least 1.5 from their nearest neighbor. Excluding these two values and rerunning the fractional polynomial analysis yielded models and results fully equivalent to those shown in Table 5.8. Hence, we conclude that the results in Table 5.8 are not outlier dependent.

We still have to make a choice regarding a *main effects* model, but before doing so, we consider what the smoothed added variable plot and GTF smoothed

Table 5.8 Summary of Fractional Polynomials Analysis of Body Mass Index (bmi) for WHAS500 data (n = 500)

	$-2\times$ Log-Likelihood	G for Model vs Linear	Approx. p-value	Powers
Not in model	2255.945			
Linear	2247.999	0.000	0.005*	1
$J = 1$ (2 df)	2241.668	6.331	0.012+	−2
$J = 2$ (4 df)	2237.784	10.215	0.143'	2, 3

* Compares linear model to model without bmi.
+ Compares the best $J = 1$ model to one with bmi linear.
' Compares the best $J = 2$ model to the best $J = 1$ model.

[2] We used their transformation on bmi and obtained results and models equivalent to those in Table 5.8.

plot tell us about the functional form of body mass index. The two plots are shown in Figure 5.2a and Figure 5.2b. The smoothed lines in both plots show a decrease, then an increase, on the log hazard scale, which supports the clinical knowledge about the effect of body mass index on post MI survival. The extreme increase in Figure 5.2b is caused by a few subjects with high body mass index. When we put all the results and clinical factors together, we conclude that a two-term fractional polynomial is preferred over a one-term or linear model. When using fractional polynomials, or any method for that matter, to identify the functional form of the relationship between outcome and covariate, one must take into account the fact that there is low power with small sample sizes. With time-to-event regression models, power is largely a function of the number of events, not pure sample size, a point we discussed above, and will detail more fully when discussing sample size methods.

The two-term (2, 3) fractional polynomial model has the numerically smallest value of –2log partial likelihood among the 36 two-term models fit. By using the "log" option in STATA's implementation of fractional polynomials, we are able to see what other two-term models have values of –2log partial likelihood close to the minimum of 2237.784 of the (2, 3) model.   From the log listing (not shown here), we see that there are several. In particular, the quadratic model, the two-term (1, 2) fractional polynomial has a value of 2238.103, that is only trivially different from the best model. All things being equal, we would certainly prefer the mathematically simpler quadratic model. However, the two fractional polynomial functions, (2, 3) and (1, 2), are different. The (1, 2) model is a symmetric function, while the (2, 3) model is not. The clinical implication of choosing the symmetric model states that the rate of decrease and then increase in the log hazard is the same. However, both smoothed plots in Figure 5.2 indicate an asymmetric behavior. Thus, we decide to proceed with the two-term (2, 3) fractional polynomial model. The results of fitting this model are shown in Table 5.9.

In Table 5.9 the two fractional polynomial transformations of body mass index are

$$bmifp1 = \left(\frac{bmi}{10}\right)^2$$

and

$$bmifp2 = \left(\frac{bmi}{10}\right)^3 .$$

Before we accept the model in Table 5.9 as our main effects model, we plot the fitted two-term (2, 3) fractional polynomial model and the GTF smooth versusbody mass index. That is, we form a new plot where we add a centered version of the parametric two-term fractional polynomial model to Figure 5.2b. To accomplish this, we have saved the GTF smoothed values shown in Figure 5.2b in

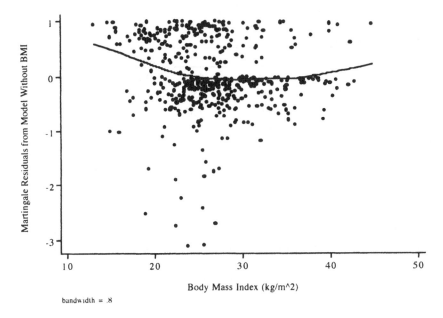

Figure 5.2a Smoothed added variable plot.

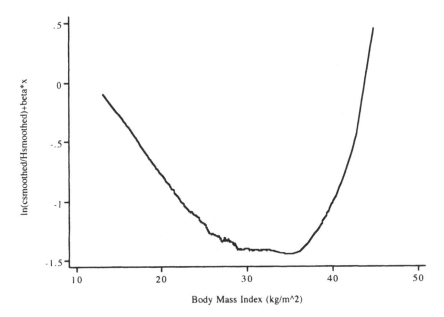

Figure 5.2b Grambsch, Therneau and Fleming (GTF) smoothed plot.
Figure 5.2 Smoothed residual plots for body mass index.

Table 5.9 Estimated Coefficients, Standard Errors, z-Scores, Two-Tailed p-values, and 95% Confidence Interval Estimates for Main Effects Proportional Hazards Model for the WHAS500 data

Variable	Coeff.	Std. Err.	z	p>|z|	95% CIE
bmifp1	−0.725	0.1726	−4.20	<0.001	−1.063, −0.386
bmifp2	0.154	0.0392	3.94	<0.001	0.078, 0.231
age	0.050	0.0066	7.53	<0.001	0.037, 0.063
hr	0.012	0.0030	3.99	<0.001	0.006, 0.018
diasbp	−0.011	0.0035	−3.05	0.002	−0.018, −0.004
gender	−0.326	0.1442	−2.26	0.024	−0.609, −0.044
chf	0.823	0.1472	5.59	<0.001	0.535, 1.111

our STATA program that produced the figure. Next we generate a new variable containing the values of the fitted two-term factional polynomial as follows

$$fp_i = -0.725 \times bmifp1_i + 0.154 \times bmifp2_i \,.$$

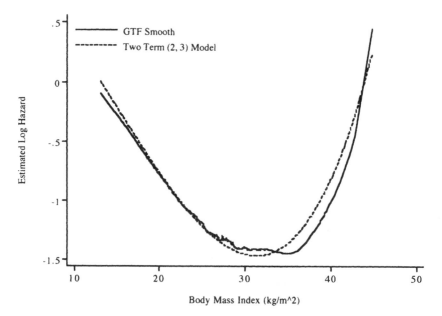

Figure 5.3 Plot of the GTF smooth and fitted two-term (2, 3) fractional polynomial model from Table 5.8 versus body mass index for the WHAS500 data.

To determine whether the two functions are similar, we add the average difference between the GTF smooth and fp_i, 0.90, to fp_i before plotting. The plot of the two functions is shown in Figure 5.3. The similarity in the two plotted functions is striking, thus adding further credence to using the (2, 3) fractional polynomial to model the effect of body mass index in the WHAS500 data.

Hence, we proceed to the final step in purposeful selection, selecting interactions, using the main effects model in Table 5.9. This step begins by creating a list of plausible interactions formed from the main effects in Table 5.9. By consulting with the Worcester Heart Attack Study investigators, we learned that only interactions involving age and gender with all other model covariates are of clinical interest. These are added, one at a time, to the main effects model and tested for significance. Table 5.10 shows the two variables forming the interaction, the degrees-of-freedom of the interaction, and the p-value for the partial likelihood ratio test comparing the models with and without the interaction. The interaction terms are formed as the arithmetic product of the pair of variables. The interactions involving body mass index are formed using the two fractional polynomial transformations, bmifp1 and bmifp2.

As an example of the calculations used in Table 5.10 we show in Table 5.11 the fitted model containing the age-by-gender interaction. The Wald statistic for the interaction coefficient has $p = 0.022$. The log partial likelihood of the fitted main effects model in Table 5.9 is $L = -1118.8921$, and for the fitted model in Table 5.11, it is $L = -1116.2793$. The partial likelihood ratio test statistic is

$$G = -2 \times \left[-1118.8921 - (-1116.2793) \right] = 5.2256,$$

yielding a p-value of 0.022 from a chi square distribution with one degree-of-freedom. The remaining p-values in Table 5.10 are determined in a similar manner.

Table 5.10 Interaction Variables, Degrees-of-Freedom (df), and p-values for the Partial Likelihood Ratio Test for the Addition of the Interaction to the Model in Table 5.9

Interaction	Variables	df	p-value
	bmi	2	0.190
	hr	1	0.132
Age	diasbp	1	0.100
	gender	1	0.022
	chf	1	0.025
	bmi	2	0.147
gender	hr	1	0.145
	diasbp	1	0.080
	chf	1	0.482

Table 5.11 Estimated Coefficients, Standard Errors, z-Scores, Two-Tailed p-values, and 95% Confidence Interval Estimates for Main Effects Proportional Hazards Model with the Interaction of Age and Gender Added for the WHAS500 data

Variable	Coeff.	Std. Err.	z	$p>|z|$	95% CIE
bmifp1	−0.673	0.1736	−3.88	<0.001	−1.013, −0.333
bmifp2	0.142	0.0394	3.60	<0.001	0.065, 0.219
Age	0.061	0.0083	7.28	<0.001	0.044, 0.077
Hr	0.012	0.0029	3.97	<0.001	0.006, 0.017
Diasbp	−0.011	0.0035	−3.08	0.002	−0.018, −0.004
Gender	1.860	0.9578	1.94	0.053	−0.022, 3.733
Chf	0.824	0.1465	5.62	<0.001	0.536, 1.111
agexgender	−0.028	0.0121	−2.30	0.022	−0.051, −0.004

As we noted when we presented the steps in purposeful selection, we believe that interactions should be significant at traditional levels. We see, in Table 5.10, that only the age-by-gender interaction and age-by-congestive-heart complications (chf) are significant at the 5 percent level. However, the age-by-diastolic-blood pressure and gender-by-diastolic-blood pressure interactions are significant at the 10 percent level. Hence, we decide to add all four to the main effects model. The results of fitting this model are shown in Table 5.12.

The log partial likelihood of the fitted model in Table 5.12 is $L = -1112.5953$. The partial likelihood ratio test statistic comparing it to the

Table 5.12 Estimated Coefficients, Standard Errors, z-Scores, Two-Tailed p-values, and 95% Confidence Interval Estimates for Main Effects Proportional Hazards Model Containing Selected Interactions for the WHAS500 data

Variable	Coeff.	Std. Err.	z	$p>|z|$	95% CIE
bmifp1	−0.643	0.1754	−3.67	<0.001	−0.987, −0.299
bmifp2	0.137	0.0400	3.44	0.001	0.059, 0.216
Age	0.034	0.0203	1.67	0.096	−0.006, 0.074
Hr	0.011	0.0230	3.77	<0.001	0.005, 0.017
diasbp	−0.052	0.0213	−2.45	0.014	−0.094, −.0110
gender	0.792	1.2196	0.65	0.516	−1.598, 4.429
chf	2.463	1.0029	2.46	0.014	0.498, 4.429
agexgender	−0.022	0.0132	−1.68	0.093	−0.048, 0.004
agexchf	−0.020	0.0127	−1.60	0.109	−0.045, 0.005
agexdiasbp	0.0005	0.0003	1.82	0.069	−0.00003, 0.001
genderxdiasbp	0.009	0.0069	1.23	0.219	−0.005, 0.022

Table 5.13 Estimated Coefficients, Standard Errors, z-Scores, Two-Tailed p-values, and 95% Confidence Interval Estimates for Main Effects Proportional Hazards Model Containing Selected Interactions for the WHAS500 data.

Variable	Coeff.	Std. Err.	z	$p>|z|$	95% CIE
bmifp1	−0.673	0.1736	−3.88	<0.001	−1.013, −0.333
bmifp2	0.142	0.0394	3.60	<0.001	0.065, 0.219
age	0.061	0.0083	7.28	<0.001	0.044, 0.077
hr	0.012	0.0029	3.97	<0.001	0.006, 0.017
diasbp	−0.011	0.0035	−3.08	0.002	−0.018, −0.004
gender	1.855	0.9578	1.94	0.053	−0.022, 3.733
chf	0.824	0.1465	5.62	<0.001	0.536, 1.111
agexgender	−0.028	0.0121	−2.30	0.022	−0.051, −0.004

main effects model in Table 5.9 is

$$G = -2 \times \left[-1118.8921 - \left(-1112.5953 \right) \right] = 12.5936 ,$$

yielding a p-value of 0.013 from a chi-square distribution with four degrees of freedom. Thus, in aggregate, the interactions contribute significantly to the main effects model. However, none of the Wald statistics for the individual interaction terms are now significant at the 5% level. At this point, we begin to reduce the model in the same manner as was used when reducing the model in Table 5.3. The least significant interaction in Table 5.12 is that of gender and diastolic blood pressure. The partial likelihood ratio test comparing the model in Table 5.12 to the model with this interaction removed yields $p = 0.196$, a value nearly identical to that of the Wald test in Table 5.12. In a similar manner, we remove the age-by-diastolic-blood-pressure interaction and the age-by-congestive-heart-complications interaction to obtain the model shown in Table 5.13.

The model in Table 5.13 is our preliminary final model. It does not become the final model until we test it for adherence to model assumptions, examine case-wise diagnostic statistics and test for goodness of fit. Before we consider these important topics in detail in Chapter 6, we discuss stepwise, best-subsets selection and the multivariable fractional polynomial method [Royston and Ambler, (1998)].

5.3 STEPWISE, BEST-SUBSETS AND MULTIVARIABLE FRACTONAL POLYNOMIAL METHODS OF SELECTING COVARIATES

Statistical algorithms for selecting covariates, such as stepwise and best-subsets selection, can be used with the proportional hazards model. They operate in an identical manner to those same methods when used in regression models such as linear or logistic regression. In addition, an iterative multivariable fractional polynomial method that combines model reduction and scale selection by fractional polynomials in a sequential manner has been proposed [Royston and Ambler, (1998)]. While the method has more user control than stepwise or best-subsets it has some of the same algorithmic elements, thus we consider it in this section rather than in the previous one.

5.3.1 STEPWISE SELECTION OF COVARIATES

Covariates may be selected for inclusion in a proportional hazards regression model using stepwise selection methods. The statistical test used as a criterion is most often the partial-likelihood ratio test. However, the score test and Wald test are often used by software packages. From a conceptual point of view, it does not matter which test is used. However, the partial-likelihood ratio test has been shown to have the best statistical testing properties of the three and should be used when there is a choice.

We assume familiarity with stepwise methods from either linear or logistic regression. Thus the presentation here will not be detailed. Detailed descriptions of stepwise selection of covariates may be found in Hosmer and Lemeshow (2000), Chapter 4, for logistic regression and in Ryan (1997), Chapter 7, for linear regression.

We begin by describing the full stepwise selection process, which consists of forward selection followed by backward elimination. The forward selection process adds to the model the covariate most statistically significant among those not in the model. The backward elimination process checks each covariate in the model for continued significance. Two variations of the full stepwise procedure available in most software packages use forward selection only or backward elimination only.

Most software packages now have the capability to create design variables for nominal scaled covariates at more than two levels and to treat these design variables as a unit when considering the covariate for entry or removal from the model. However, to keep the notation to a minimum, we describe the stepwise procedure using single degree of freedom tests for entry and removal of covariates. Thus, for this description, we assume all covariates are either continuous or dichotomous.

Step 0: Assume that there are p possible covariates, denoted $x_j, j = 1, 2, \cdots, p$. This list is assumed to include all covariates. At step 0, the partial likelihood ratio test and its p-value for the significance of each covariate is computed by comparing the log-partial likelihood of the model containing x_j to the log-partial likelihood of model zero (i.e., the model containing no covariates). This test statistic is

$$G^{(0)}(j) = -2\left[L^{(0)}(j) - L(0)\right], \quad j = 1, 2, \ldots, p,\tag{5.1}$$

where $L(0)$ is equal to the log partial likelihood of model zero, the no-covariate model, and $L^{(0)}(j)$ is equal to the log partial likelihood of the model containing covariate x_j. The test's significance level is

$$p^{(0)}(j) = \Pr\left[\chi^2(1) \geq G^{(0)}(j)\right].\tag{5.2}$$

Evaluating (5.1) and (5.2) requires fitting p separate proportional hazards models. The parenthesized superscript in (5.1) and (5.2) denotes the step, and j indexes the particular covariate. The candidate for entry into the model at step 1 is the most significant covariate and is denoted by x_{e_1}, where

$$p^{(0)}(e_1) = \min_{j}\left[p^{(0)}(j)\right].\tag{5.3}$$

For the variable x_{e_1} to be entered into the model, its p-value must be smaller than some pre-chosen criterion for significance, denoted p_E. If the variable selected for entry is significant (i.e., $p^{(0)}(e_1) < p_E$), then the program goes to step 1; otherwise it stops.

Step 1: This step begins with variable x_{e_1} in the model. Then $p - 1$ new proportional hazards models (each including one remaining variable along with x_{e_1}) are fit, and the results are used to compute the partial likelihood ratio test of the fitted two–variable model to the one–variable model containing only x_{e_1},

$$G^{(1)}(j) = -2\left[L^{(1)}(j) - L(x_{e_1})\right], \quad j = 1, 2, \ldots, p \text{ and } j \neq e_1.\tag{5.4}$$

The p-value for the test of the significance of adding x_j to the model containing x_{e_1} is

$$p^{(1)}(j) = \Pr\left[\chi^2(1) \geq G^{(1)}(j)\right].\tag{5.5}$$

The variable selected as the candidate for entry at step 2 is x_{e_2} where

$$p^{(1)}(e_2) = \min_{j \neq e_1}\left[p^{(1)}(j)\right].\tag{5.6}$$

If the selected covariate x_{e_2} is significant, $p^{(1)}(e_2) < p_E$, then the program goes to step 2; otherwise it stops.

Step 2: This step begins with both x_{e_1} and x_{e_2} in the model. During this step, two different evaluations occur. The step begins with a backward elimination check for the continued contribution of x_{e_1}. That is, does x_{e_1} still contribute to the model after x_{e_2} has been added? This is essentially an evaluation of (5.4) and (5.5) with the roles of the two variables reversed. From an operational point of view, we choose a different significance criterion for this check, denoted p_R. We choose this value such that $p_R > p_E$ to eliminate the possibility of entering and removing the same variable in an endless number of successive steps. Assume the variable entered at step 1 is still significant.

The program fits $p - 2$ proportional hazards models (each including one remaining variable along with x_{e_1} and x_{e_2}) and computes the partial likelihood ratio test and its p-value for the addition of the new covariate to the model, namely

$$G^{(2)}(j) = -2\left[L^{(2)}(j) - L\left(x_{e_1}, x_{e_2}\right) \right], \quad j = 1, 2, \ldots, p \text{ and } j \neq e_1, e_2$$

and

$$p^{(2)}(j) = \Pr\left[\chi^2(1) \geq G^{(2)}(j) \right].$$

The covariate x_{e_3} selected for entry at step 3 is the one with the smallest p-value, that is,

$$p^{(2)}(e_3) = \min_{j \neq e_1, e_2} \left[p^{(2)}(j) \right].$$

The program proceeds to step 3 if $p^{(2)}(e_3) < p_E$; otherwise it stops.

Step 3: Step 3, if reached, is similar to step 2 in that the elimination process determines whether all variables entered into the model at earlier steps are still significant. The selection process then followed is identical to the selection part of earlier steps. This procedure is followed until the last step, step S.

Step S: At this step, one of two things happens: (1) all the covariates are in the model and none may be removed or (2) each covariate not in the model has $p^{(S)}(j) > p_E$. At this point, no covariates are selected for entry and none of the covariates in the model may be removed.

The number of variables selected in any application will depend on the strength of the associations between covariates and survival time and the choice of p_E and p_R. Due to the multiple testing that occurs, it is nearly impossible to calculate the actual statistical significance of the full stepwise process. Research in linear regression by Bendel and Afifi (1977) and in discriminant analysis by Costanza and Afifi (1979) indicates that use of $p_E = 0.05$ excludes too many important covariates and one should choose a level of significance of 15 percent. In many applications, it may make sense to use 25-50 percent to allow more variables to enter than will ultimately be used and then narrow the field of selected variables using $p < 0.15$ to obtain a multivariable model for further analysis. An unavoidable problem with any stepwise selection procedure is the potential for the inclusion of "noise" covariates and the exclusion of important covariates. One must always examine the variables selected and excluded for basic scientific plausibility.

At this point, the model is likely to contain continuous covariates, and these should be examined carefully for linearity using the previously discussed methods. We then see if any interactions significantly improve the model. The stepwise selection procedure uses as candidate variables a list of plausible interactions among the main effects previously identified during the initial stepwise model building. We begin with a model containing all the main effects, and the final model is selected using usual levels of statistical significance.

As an example of stepwise selection, we consider the WHAS500 data. As in the example in the previous section, the list of candidate variables includes: age, gender, heart rate, systolic blood pressure, diastolic blood pressure, body mass index, history of cardiovascular disease, atrial fibrillation, congestive heart complications, MI order and MI type, for a total of 11 covariates.

In general, the exact order of variable selection will depend on whether we use the partial likelihood ratio test, the score test, or the Wald test as there can be small differences in the magnitude of the three test statistics. In the end, each should select nearly the same set of covariates. The amount of output available to the user at each step varies from package to package. STATA has the least, reporting only the significance level of the variable selected for entry or removal and provides only the fit of the model at the last step. Both SAS and SPSS provide more detailed output.

The results presented in Table 5.14 were obtained using SPSS and the score test. For illustrative purposes, we use entry and removal p-values of $p_E = 0.25$ and $p_R = 0.8$. Many of the covariates have quite large score test values that lead to significance levels of <0.0001, thus making it impossible to see the rank ordering. Hence, we report the score test statistics. We are able to do this in the example because each variable has a single degree of freedom. If we had a nominal scaled covariate with more than two levels, we would have to report p-values. One further complication in reporting the result is that SPSS only provides Wald chi-square statistics for covariates in the fitted model at each step.

There were a total of 7 steps, counting step 0. At step 0, is the age variable with the smallest p-value and largest score test a value of 126.26 and $p < 0.0001$. Because the p-value for age is smaller than $p_E = 0.25$ (i.e., the score test exceeds $\chi^2_{0.75}(1) = 1.32$), the variable enters the model at step 1. At step 1 congestive heart complications (chf) has the largest score statistic, 38.41, thus the smallest p-value, and it is smaller than $p_E = 0.25$. Congestive heart complications enters the model at step 2. At step 2, both age and congestive heart complications have Wald chi-square statistics that exceed the 20th percentile of the chi-square distribution with one degree of freedom, $\chi_{0.2}^2(1) = 0.0642$, and p-values to remove are less than $p_R = 0.8$. Thus they remain in the model. Among the variables not in the model, heart rate has the largest score test statistic at 9.11 and smallest p-value, $p = 0.003$. Because it is less than the criteria for entry, it enters the model. The program goes to step 3, where the three–variable model is fit. All Wald chi-square tests exceed 0.0642 and thus have p-values to remove that are less than 0.8. No variables are removed from the model. At this point the variable with the largest score test and smallest p-value for entry is diastolic blood pressure, with a score test of 9.29 and $p = 0.002$, which is less then $p_E = 0.25$. The program then goes to step 4 and fits the four-variable model.

This process of fitting, checking for continued significance, and selection continues until step 6. At this step, each of the six variables in the model has a p-value less than 0.8 to remove, and the p-values to enter for the five variables not in the model exceed 0.25 (i.e., their score tests are less than 1.32). Therefore, the program terminates the selection process at step 6.

We use the results in Table 5.14 with a significance level of 0.15 to identify the preliminary main effects model by proceeding sequentially to the next step, as long as the p-value for the variable entered is less than 0.15. At step 6 the smallest score statistic is 3.53 for the variable that entered at that step, gender. Its p-value is 0.060, less than 0.15. Thus using the 15 percent rule, we take as our preliminary

Table 5.14 Results of Stepwise Selection of Covariates, Score Test for Entry Below Solid Line, and Wald Chi-Square Test for Removal above Solid Line in Each Column for WHAS500 data (n = 500). Rows are in Order of Entry

Step	0	1	2	3	4	5	6
age	126.26	118.80	92.41	91.65	72.05	53.66	56.98
chf	84.37	38.41	36.57	26.90	25.65	26.11	28.10
hr	31.28	19.09	9.11	9.12	13.41	13.31	14.70
diasbp	23.38	5.78	5.41	9.29	9.36	8.24	9.09
bmi	44.17	7.23	8.22	8.32	7.17	7.17	7.70
gender	7.77	0.22	1.20	1.88	2.96	3.55	3.53
mitype	16.14	2.61	2.93	1.68	0.85	0.82	0.95
miord	9.55	1.85	1.89	1.19	0.72	0.50	0.27
sysbp	4.09	3.90	4.46	4.79	0.01	0.00	0.05
cvd	2.86	0.03	0.17	0.14	0.00	0.05	0.08
afb	10.87	4.13	1.06	0.60	0.95	0.52	0.45

main effects model the one fit at step 6, which is the same model found by purposeful selection.

We next check the scale of the continuous covariates in the model, following the same procedure illustrated in the previous section. Because the model is the same as the purposeful selection preliminary main effects model (Table 5.6), our stepwise main effects model is the same as the one in Table 5.9.

Stepwise selection of interactions proceeds, using as candidate variables the interactions listed in Table 5.10. At step 0, the model contains all the main effects, the model in Table 5.9. Candidate interaction variables are shown in Table 5.10. The same interactions chosen by purposeful selection are selected using a p-value to enter of 0.10. Therefore, we do not present the computational details. For this example, the preliminary model chosen by stepwise methods is also the one in Table 5.13, identified using purposeful selection.

5.3.2 BEST SUBSETS SELECTION OF COVARIATES

In the previous section, we discussed stepwise selection of covariates. Most analysts are familiar with its use from other regression modeling settings and it is available in most major software packages. However, the procedure considers only a small number of the total possible models that can be formed from the covariates. The method of best subsets selection, if available, provides a computationally efficient way to screen all possible models.

The conceptual basis for best subsets selection of covariates in a proportional hazards regression is the same as in linear regression. The procedure requires a criterion to judge a model. Given the criterion, the software screens all models containing q covariates and reports the covariates in the best, say 5, models for $q = 1, 2, ..., p$, where p denotes the total number of covariates.

Software to implement best subsets normal errors linear regression is generally, though not widely, available and has been used to provide best subsets selection capabilities for non–normal errors linear regression models such as logistic regression, see Hosmer and Lemeshow (2000, Chapter 4). There are three requirements to use the method described by Hosmer and Lemeshow: (1) It must be possible to obtain estimates of the coefficients of the model containing all p covariates from a weighted linear regression where the dependent variable is of the form

$$\mathbf{x}'\hat{\boldsymbol{\beta}} + \widehat{weight} \times (\widehat{residual}),$$

(2) the weight must be an easily computed function of the variance of the residual and (3) both weight and residual must be easily computed functions of the estimated coefficients and covariates. Only requirement 1 is satisfied in the proportional hazards regression model when fit using the partial likelihood. Even though

the partial likelihood, see (3.19), is a product of n terms, the terms are not independent of each other. Each "subject" may contribute information to more than one term in the product (i.e., "subjects" appear in every risk set until they fail or are censored). Thus, Hosmer and Lemeshow's method cannot be used to perform best subsets proportional hazards regression. We do not want to dwell on this point, but feel that it is important to explain why this easily used approach is not appropriate in this setting.

Kuk (1984) described how best subsets selection in a proportional hazards regression model may be performed with a normal errors linear regression best subsets program if the program allows data input in the form of a covariance matrix. Kuk's method is related to a general method described by Lawless and Singhal (1978). While Kuk's method is clever, none of the major software packages allows for covariance matrix input. The only best subsets program we are aware of that allowed this type of input to its regression routines is BMDP (1992) program, BMDP9R, which is no longer distributed. Hence, we do not discuss Kuk's method in this edition. Interested readers can find the details in the first edition, Hosmer and Lemeshow (1999).

An alternative method for best subset selection is to mimic the approach used in stepwise selection and choose as "best" models those in which the covariates in the model have the highest level of significance. Selection of covariates thus proceeds by inclusion rather than exclusion. The best models containing k covariates are those with the largest values of a test of the significance of the model. Theoretically, one could use any one of the three equivalent tests: partial likelihood ratio, Wald or score test. The SAS package, PROC PHREG, has implemented this selection method using the score test. Models identified are, for each fixed number of covariates, the ones with the largest value of the score test.

It is difficult to compare models of different sizes using the score test for model significance because the score test tends to increase with the number of covariates in the model. The most frequently used criterion to compare normal errors liner regression models containing different numbers of covariates is Mallow's C. See Mallows (1973) and Ryan (1997 Chapter 7) for a discussion of the use of Mallow's C in normal errors linear regression modeling. Good models are those with small values of Mallow's C. In the context of the proportional hazards model Mallow's C is defined as

$$C = W_q + (p - 2q), \tag{5.7}$$

where p is the number of variables under consideration and q denotes the number of covariates not included in the subset model. The quantity W_q is the value of the multivariable Wald statistic testing that the coefficients for the q covariates are simultaneously equal to zero and is obtained from a fit of the model containing all p covariates. We use score tests, as follows, to approximate the value of W_q in (5.7). Let the score test for the model containing all p covariates be denoted S_p

and the score test for the model containing a particular set of k ($= p - q$) covariates be denoted S_k. The value of the score test for the exclusion of the q covariates from the full p variable model is approximately $S_q = S_p - S_k$. Because the Wald and score tests are asymptotically equivalent, this suggests that an approximation to Mallow's C for a fitted model containing $p - q$ covariates is

$$C = S_q + (p - 2q). \tag{5.8}$$

Using SAS's PROC PHREG with METHOD = BEST to perform the computations to obtain S_p and S_k, we show in Table 5.15 the five best models from the WHAS500 data. We note that we must compute (5.8) by hand or use a spreadsheet program, which simplifies sorting to find the models with the smallest values of C.

As an example, consider model 1 in Table 5.15, with $k = 6$ covariates in the model. The value of the score test for the significance of the 11-covariate model is $S_{11} = 208.6223$ and the value of the score test for the significance of the 6-covariate model is $S_6 = 206.4896$. The approximation to the score test for the addition of the 5 covariates to the 6–covariate model is

$$S_5 \cong S_{11} - S_6 = 208.6223 - 206.4896 = 2.1327.$$

The value of the approximation to Mallow's C is

$$C = 2.1327 + (11 - 2 \times 5) = 3.1327$$

The advantage of best subsets over stepwise is illustrated in table 5.15 where we see that all good models, by Mallow's C, contain age, hr, diasbp, bmi and chf. The covariate gender is in four of the five models. Adding sysbp, mitype or miord does not improve the models. With stepwise, we are able to examine only progressively larger models and not ones with the same number of covariates. At

Table 5.15 Five Best Models Identified Using the Score Test Approximation to Mallow's C. Model Covariates, Approximate Mallow's C, and the Approximate Score Test for the Excluded Covariates for the WHAS500 data ($n = 500$)

Model	Model Covariates	C	S_q
1	age, gender, hr, diasbp, bmi, chf,	3.13	2.13
2	age, gender, hr, diasbp, bmi, chf, mitype	3.58	0.58
3	age, hr, diasbp, bmi, chf	4.95	5.95
4	age, gender, hr, diasbp, bmi, chf, sysbp	4.77	1.77
5	age, gender, hr, diasbp, bmi, chf, miord	4.99	1.99

this point, one strategy would begin by fitting one of the larger models (e.g., the second best containing age, gender, hr, diasbp, bmi, chf, and mitype) and then use Wald tests and confounding considerations to simplify it. Another possibility is to begin with a model containing the nine different covariates in the five best models. In work not shown, this process leads to the same model found by both purposeful selection and stepwise. Complete agreement in the covariates in the models selected by the three methods may not always occur. However, it is our experience that the three methods select a similar set of covariates.

When using procedures such as stepwise or best subsets selection to identify possible model covariates, we must remember the results should be taken only as suggestions for models to be examined in more detail. One cannot rule out the possibility that these methods may reveal new and interesting associations, but the collection of covariates must make clinical sense to the researchers. The statistical selection procedures suggest, but do not dictate, the model.

5.3.3 SELECTING COVARIATES AND CHECKING THEIR SCALE USING MULTIVARIABLE FRACTIONAL POLYNOMIALS

Sauerbrei, Meier–Hirmer, Brenner and Royston (2006) describe software for SAS, STATA and R that implements a multivariable fractional polynomial method, referred to here as mfp, that Royston and Ambler (1999) first wrote for the STATA package. The algorithm combines elements of backward elimination of non-significant covariates with an iterative examination of the scale of all continuous covariates using either the closed or sequential test procedures described in Section 5.2.1.

The mfp procedure begins by fitting a multivariable model that contains the user-specified covariates. All variables are modeled linearly, and the significance level of their respective Wald tests defines the order in which they are processed in all following steps. This initial collection, ideally, would include all study covariates. However, we may have a setting where there is an inadequate number of events to allow inclusion of all covariates and, in this case, we might choose, as a subset, the clinically important covariates and those significant at, say, the 25 percent level on univariable analysis. In the example below, using the WHAS500 data, we include all covariates except cardiogenic shock and complete heart block, which are excluded for reasons of inadequate data (described previously). The initial model includes all covariates as linear terms in the log hazard. In subsequent fits, each covariate is modeled according to a specified number of degrees of freedom. All dichotomous and design variables have one degree of freedom, meaning they are not candidates for fractional polynomial transformation. Continuous covariates may be forced to be modeled linearly by specifying one degree of freedom, or may be candidates for a one-or two-term fractional polynomial by specifying two or four degrees of freedom, respectively.

Following the initial multivariable linear fit, variables are considered in descending order of their Wald statistics. For covariates modeled with one degree of freedom, a partial likelihood ratio test is used to assess their contribution to the model, and its significance relative to a chosen alpha level is noted. Continuous covariates are modeled using either the closed or sequential test method, noting if the covariate should be removed, kept linear, or transformed. This completes the first cycle.

The second cycle begins with a fit of a multivariable model containing the model from cycle one (i.e., the model with covariates transformed or deleted). All covariates are considered again for possible transformation, inclusion or exclusion from the model. Covariates are examined in descending order of the Wald statistics. Continuous covariates with a significant fractional polynomial transformation are entered transformed, which becomes their null model. The point of this step is two fold: (1) does the transformation "linearize" the covariate in the log hazard, and (2) does the transformation affect scaling of other covariates. Each covariate's level of significance is noted as well as the need to transform. This completes the second cycle.

The mfp procedure stops when the results of two consecutive cycles are the same. The minimum number is two. More than two cycles occur if additional transformations of continuous covariates are suggested in cycle two and beyond or if the level of significance of the partial likelihood ratio test for contribution to the model changes the decision to include or exclude a covariate.

We use the mfp method on a model for the WHAS500 data that begins with all categorically scaled model covariates in Table 5.1, except cardiogenic shock and complete heart block, and all continuous variables in Table 5.2. The dichotomous covariates in Table 5.1 are each modeled with one degree of freedom. The continuous covariates in Table 5.2 are each modeled with up to four degrees of freedom. The process took two cycles to converge, using the 15 percent level of significance for both inclusion and transformation. The results from cycle 2 are shown in Table 5.16.

In this table, the first covariate processed is age so, we know it had the largest Wald statistic. Because age is continuous and we allow up to four degrees of freedom the first test, line[3] 1, compares a model not containing age to one where age is transformed by the $(3,3)$ transformation. The value in the Deviance column of 2301.581 is for the model that excludes age. The value in the G column, 67.477, is the difference between 2301.581 and the Deviance for the best two-term fractional polynomial model. The value in the p column in line 1 is the significance level using four degrees of freedom, $p = \Pr\left[\chi^2(4) \ge 67.477\right]$. The superscripted "*" means that the test is significant at the user-specified significance level for inclusion, 0.15 in this example, in the model. Because the test is

---

[3] The Stata output does not include line numbers. We included them in Table 5.16 to help in discussing the results.

significant, the procedure then compares the best two-term fractional polynomial model to the linear model. Hence, the value of 2237.784 in the Deviance column is for a linear model including age. The difference between 2237.784 and the Deviance for the two-term fractional polynomial model is 3.680 and its p-value computed, using 3 degrees of freedom, is $0.298 = \Pr\left[\chi^2(3) \geq 3.680\right]$. Because this is not significant at our chosen alpha level, 0.15, the processing of age stops and the final model is shown in line 3 as age linear in the log hazard.

The second covariate processed is congestive heart complication, chf; it had the second largest Wald statistic. This variable is dichotomous and, as such, we modeled it with a single degree of freedom. Thus, for this covariate there are only two choices. It is either not in the model or in the model and modeled linearly. The Deviance in line 4, 2268.808, is for a model that excludes chf. The test is $G = 31.023$, which is equal to the difference between 2268.808 and the Deviance from the model including chf, and its p-value computed using a chi-square distribution with one degree of freedom is reported as 0.000^*, indicating that it is significant at the 15 percent level. The value of "1" in the transformation column means that chf is not transformed (i.e., modeled linearly). Hence the final model for chf is to include chf modeled linearly.

The third variable processed is heart rate. Its results are similar to those for age, except the best two-term fractional polynomial is $(-2,-2)$.

The results for body mass index, bmi, are different and warrant elaboration. The results in line 9 are similar in terms of models being compared with those for age in line 1 except the two-term fractional polynomial is $(2,3)$. The results in line 10 are similar to those for age in line 2. However, in this case, the test is significant, at the 15 percent level, so processing continues. The results in line 11 compare the best two-term to the best one-term, (-2), fractional polynomial model. The p-value for this comparison is 0.143, which is significant at the 15 percent level, denoted by a "+". Hence the final model for bmi is the two-term fractional polynomial $(2,3)$, shown in line 12.

Processing of diastolic blood pressure is similar to age and that of gender is similar to chf.

You will note that two different significance levels are being used. One controls the fractional polynomial processing. We chose a value of 0.15. If we had used 0.05, then processing of bmi would have chosen a one-term fractional polynomial model as the p-value comparing the two to one-term models is 0.143 in line 11. Tests significant at this level are denoted by an "+" following the p-value. The second significance level controls the inclusion and exclusion of covariates from the model. For example, if the p-value in line 1 for age was greater than 0.15, then age would have been tagged for removal. Significant results at this level are denoted by an "*" following the p-value. Examples of variables tagged for removal begin with MI type (mitype), in line 18 and continue to history of cardiovascular disease in line 27. In STATA, the user may choose values or use

Table 5.16 Results from the Final Cycle of MFP Applied to the WHAS500 data ($n = 500$)

Line	Cov.	Scale	Comp.	Deviance	G	p	df	Transf.
1	age	null	FP2	2301.581	67.477	0.000*	.	3 3
2		lin.		2237.784	3.680	0.298	1	
3		Final		2237.784			1	
4	chf	null	lin.	2268.808	31.023	0.000*	.	1
5		Final		2237.784			1	
6	hr	null	FP2	2253.103	18.116	0.001*	.	−2 −2
7		lin.		2237.784	2.797	0.424	1	
8		Final		2237.784			1	
9	bmi	null	FP2	2255.945	18.106	0.001*	.	2 3
10		lin.		2247.999	10.215	0.017+	1	
11		FP1		2241.668	3.884	0.143+	−2	
12		Final		2237.784			2 3	
13	diasbp	null	FP2	2247.368	12.275	0.015*	.	3 3
14		lin.		2237.784	2.691	0.442	1	
15		Final		2237.784			1	
16	gender	null	lin.	2242.906	5.122	0.024*	.	1
17		Final		2237.784			1	
18	mitype	null	lin.	2237.784	0.852	0.356	.	1
19		Final		2237.784			.	
20	afb	null	lin.	2237.784	0.234	0.629	.	1
21		Final		2237.784			.	
22	miord	null	lin.	2237.784	0.153	0.695	.	1
23		Final		2237.784			.	
24	sysbp	null	FP2	2237.784	3.095	0.542	.	−.5 −.5
25		Final		2237.784			.	
26	cvd	null	lin.	2237.784	0.052	0.820	.	1
27		Final		2237.784			.	

*: $p <$ chosen significance level for inclusion
+: $p <$ chosen significance level for transformation

program defaults. The rationale for our choice of 0.15 for both is two fold: we wanted to include main effects that had the possibility to be confounders and we can see if one-and two-term transformations are marginally different. We prefer to put the user in control of making important final modeling decisions. We discuss this in greater detail below.

All variables are processed until all transformations and decisions to include or exclude are the same for each covariate at two consecutive cycles. The results in Table 5.16 show that the final mfp model contains age, chf, hr, bmi transformed using (2,3), diasbp, and gender. In this case, the mfp method identified the same main effects model as the other methods, but also identifies that among the continuous covariates, only bmi needs to be transformed.

The mfp method is clearly an extremely powerful analytic modeling tool, which, on the surface, would appear to relieve the analyst of having to think too hard about model content. This is not the case, of course. We recommend that, if one uses mfp, then its model be considered as a suggestion for a possible main effects model, much in the way that stepwise and best subsets identify possible models. The model needs a thorough evaluation to be sure all covariates and transformations make clinical sense, that transformations are not caused by a few extreme observations and, quite importantly, that excluded covariates are not confounders of model covariate estimates of effect. We highly recommend you spend time with Royston and Sauerbrei (2006), Sauerbrei, Meier-Hirmer, Benner and Royston (2006) and the host of other excellent papers cited that describe, in detail, the development and use of both fractional polynomials and the mfp procedure.

In summary, stepwise, best subsets and mfp have their place as covariate selection methods, but it is always the responsibility of the user to choose the content and form of the final model.

5.4 NUMERICAL PROBLEMS

The software available in the major statistical packages for fitting the proportional hazards model is easy to use and, for the most part, contains checks and balances that warn the user of impending numerical disasters. However, there are certain data configurations that cause numerical difficulties that may not produce a suitable warning to the user. The problem of *monotone likelihood* described by Bryson and Johnson (1981) is one such problem. This problem in a survival analysis is similar to the occurrence of a zero frequency cell in a two-by-two contingency table or when the distributions of a continuous covariate are completely separated by the binary outcome variable in logistic regression. The problem occurs in a proportional hazards regression when the rank ordering of the covariate and the survival times are the same. That is, at each observed survival time, the subject who fails has the largest (smallest) value of one of the covariates among the subjects in the risk set.

To illustrate the problem, we created a hypothetical data set containing 100 observations of survival time in days, truncated at one year with approximately 30 percent of the observations censored. We created a dichotomous covariate whose

Table 5.17 Estimated Coefficient, Standard Error, z-Score, Two-Tailed p-value, and 95% Confidence Intervals for a Proportional Hazards Model Containing a Monotone Likelihood Covariate ($n =100$)

Variable	Coeff.	Std. Err.	z	$p>|z|$	95% CIE
x	37.08	9.7E6	0.00	1.00	−1.92E7, 1.92E7

Table 5.18 Estimated Coefficients, Standard Errors, z-Scores, Two-Tailed p-values, and 95% Confidence Intervals for a Proportional Hazards Model Containing Two Highly Correlated Continuous Covariates ($n = 100$)

Variable	Coeff.	Std. Err.	z	$p > |z|$	95% CIE
x1	18.00	41.44	0.43	0.66	−63.2, 99.2
x2	−17.72	41.44	−0.43	0.66	−98.9, 63.5

value is equal to one if the observed survival time was less than the median and zero otherwise. The results of fitting the proportional hazards model are shown in Table 5.17, where the notation "9.7E6" means 9.7×10^6.

The estimated coefficient and its standard error are unreasonably large. The software also required 25 iterations to obtain this value. As in the case of logistic regression, any implausibly large coefficient and standard error is a clear indication of numerical difficulties. In this case, a graph of the covariate versus time would indicate the problem.

The example in Table 5.17 is a simple one because it involves a single covariate. In practice, the situation is likely to be more complex, with a combination of multiple covariates inducing the same effect. Bryson and Johnson (1981) show that certain types of linear combinations (e.g., a simple sum of the covariates) may yield monotone likelihood. In these situations, the problem will manifest itself with unreasonably large coefficients and standard errors.

Extreme collinearity among the covariates is another possible problem. Most software packages contain diagnostic checks for highly correlated data, but clinically implausible results may be produced before the program's diagnostic switch is tripped. The results of fitting a proportional hazards model when the relationship between the two covariates is $x_2 = x_1 + u$, where u is the value of a uniformly distributed random variable on the interval (0, 0.01), are shown in Table 5.18. The correlation between the covariates is effectively 1.0, yet the program prints a result. Similar results were obtained until $u \sim U(0, 0.0001)$, at which point one of the covariates was dropped from the model by the program.

The bottom line is that it is ultimately the user of the software who is responsible for the results of an analysis. Any analysis producing "large" effect(s) or standard error(s) should be treated as a "mistake" until the involved covariate(s) are examined critically.

EXERCISES

1. An important step in any model building process is assessing the scale of continuous variables in the model. There are two continuous variables, age and bmi, in the WHAS100 data. Use the methods discussed in this chapter to assess the scale of both in a model containing age and bmi.

2. In this problem, use the ACTG320 data with covariates (see Table 1.5) tx, sex, ivdrug, karnof, cd4, priorzdv, and age. Using the methods for model building discussed in this chapter, find the best model for estimating the effect of the covariates on survival time to AIDS diagnosis or death. This process should include the following steps: variable selection, assessment of the scale of continuous variables, and selection of interactions.

Note: Save any work done for Exercise 2 as there are exercises in Chapter 6 dealing with this model.

3. Without referring to the work by Sauerbrei and Royston (1999) use the methods in this Chapter to find the best model for the GBCS data for time to recurrence. Is the same model appropriate for modeling time to death?

CHAPTER 6

Assessment of Model Adequacy

6.1 INTRODUCTION

Model-based inferences depend completely on the fitted statistical model. For these inferences to be "valid" in any sense of the word, the fitted model must provide an adequate summary of the data upon which it is based. Hence a complete and thorough examination of model adequacy is just as important as careful model development.

The goal of statistical model development is to obtain the model that best describes the "middle" of the data. The specific definition of "middle" depends on the particular type of statistical model, but the idea is basically the same for all statistical models. In the normal errors linear regression model setting, we can describe the relationship between the observed outcome variable and one of the covariates with a scatterplot. This plot of points for two or more covariates is often described as the "cloud" of data. In model development, we find the regression surface (i.e., line, plane, or hyperplane) that best fits/splits the cloud. The notion of "best" in this setting means that we have equal distances from observed points to fitted points above and below the regression surface. A "generic" main effects model with some nominal covariates, which treats continuous covariates as linear, may not have enough tilts, bends, or turns to fit/split the cloud. Each step in the model development process is designed to tailor the regression surface to the observed cloud of data.

In most, if not all, applied settings, the results of the fitted model will be summarized for publication using point and interval estimates of clinically interpretable measures of the effect of covariates on the outcome. Examples of summary measures include the mean difference (for linear regression), the odds ratio (for logistic regression) and the hazard ratio (for proportional hazards regression). Because any summary measure is only as good as the model it is based on, it is vital that one evaluate how well the fitted regression surface describes the data cloud. This process is generally referred to as *assessing the adequacy of the model*; like model development, it involves a number of steps. Performing these in a thorough and conscientious manner assures us that our inferential conclusions based on the fitted model are the best and most valid possible.

The methods for assessing the adequacy of a fitted proportional hazards model are essentially the same as for other regression models. We assume that the reader has had some experience with these methods, particularly with those for the logistic regression model [see Hosmer and Lemeshow (2000, Chapter 5)]. In the current setting, these include methods for: (1) examining and testing the proportional hazards assumption, (2) evaluating subject-specific diagnostic statistics that measure leverage and influence on the fit of the proportional hazards model and (3) computing summary measures of goodness-of-fit.

6.2 RESIDUALS

Central to the evaluation of model adequacy in any setting is an appropriate definition of a residual. As we discussed in Chapter 1, a regression analysis of survival time is set apart from other regression models, the fact that the outcome variable is time to an event and the observed values may be incomplete or censored. In earlier chapters, we suggested that the semiparametric proportional hazards model is a useful model for data of this type and we described why and how it may be fit using the partial likelihood. This combination of data, model and likelihood makes definition of a residual much more difficult than is the case in other settings.

Consider a logistic regression analysis of a binary outcome variable. In this setting, values of the outcome variable are "present" ($y = 1$) or "absent" ($y = 0$) for all subjects. The fitted model provides estimates of the probability that the outcome is present (i.e., the mean of Y). Thus, a natural definition of the residual is the difference between the observed value of the outcome variable and that predicted by the model. This form of the residual also follows as a natural consequence of characterizing the observed value of the outcome as the sum of a systematic component and an error component. The two key assumptions in this definition of a residual are: (1) the value of the outcome is known and (2) the fitted model provides an estimate of the "mean of the outcome variable." Because assumption 2 and, more than likely, assumption 1 are not true when using the partial likelihood to fit the proportional hazards model to censored survival data, there is no obvious analog to the usual "observed minus predicted" residual used with other regression models.

The absence of an obvious residual has led to the development of several different residuals, each of which plays an important role in examining some aspect of a fitted proportional hazards model. Most software packages provide access to one or more of these residuals.

We assume, for the time being, that there are p covariates and that the n independent observations of time, covariates and censoring indicator are denoted by the triplet $(t_i, \mathbf{x}_i, c_i)$, $i = 1, 2, \ldots, n$, where $c_i = 1$ for uncensored observations and $c_i = 0$ otherwise. Schoenfeld (1982) proposed the first set of residuals for use with a fitted proportional hazards model and packages providing them refer to them as the "Schoenfeld residuals." These are based on the individual contributions to the derivative of the log partial likelihood. This derivative for the kth covariate is shown in (3.22) and is repeated here as

$$\frac{\partial L_p(\boldsymbol{\beta})}{\partial \beta_k} = \sum_{i=1}^{n} c_i \left\{ x_{ik} - \frac{\displaystyle\sum_{j \in R(t_i)} x_{jk} e^{\mathbf{x}_j' \boldsymbol{\beta}}}{\displaystyle\sum_{j \in R(t_i)} e^{\mathbf{x}_j' \boldsymbol{\beta}}} \right\} \qquad (6.1)$$

$$= \sum_{i=1}^{n} c_i \left\{ x_{ik} - \overline{x}_{w_i k} \right\},$$

where

$$\overline{x}_{w_i k} = \frac{\displaystyle\sum_{j \in R(t_i)} x_{jk} e^{\mathbf{x}_j' \boldsymbol{\beta}}}{\displaystyle\sum_{j \in R(t_i)} e^{\mathbf{x}_j' \boldsymbol{\beta}}} . \qquad (6.2)$$

The estimator of the Schoenfeld residual for the ith subject on the kth covariate is obtained from (6.1) by substituting the partial likelihood estimator of the coefficient, $\hat{\boldsymbol{\beta}}$, and is

$$\hat{r}_{ik} = c_i \left(x_{ik} - \hat{\overline{x}}_{w_i k} \right) \qquad (6.3)$$

where

$$\hat{\overline{x}}_{w_i k} = \frac{\displaystyle\sum_{j \in R(t_i)} x_{jk} e^{\mathbf{x}_j' \hat{\boldsymbol{\beta}}}}{\displaystyle\sum_{j \in R(t_i)} e^{\mathbf{x}_j' \hat{\boldsymbol{\beta}}}}$$

is the estimator of the risk set conditional mean of the covariate. Because the partial likelihood estimator of the coefficient, $\hat{\boldsymbol{\beta}}$, is the solution to the equations obtained by setting (6.1) equal to zero, the sum of the Schoenfeld residuals is zero. The Schoenfeld residuals are equal to zero for all censored subjects and thus contain no information about the fit of the model. Hence, software packages set the value of the Schoenfeld residual to missing for subjects whose observed survival time is censored.

Grambsch and Therneau (1994) suggest that scaling the Schoenfeld residuals by an estimator of its variance yields a residual with greater diagnostic power than the unscaled residuals. Denote the vector of p Schoenfeld residuals for the ith subject as

$$\hat{\mathbf{r}}_i' = (\hat{r}_{i1}, \hat{r}_{i2}, \dots, \hat{r}_{ip}) ,$$

where $\hat{r}_{ik}$ is the estimator in (6.3), with the convention that $\hat{r}_{ik}$ = missing if $c_i = 0$. Let the estimator of the $p \times p$ covariance matrix of the vector of residuals for the ith subject, as reported in Grambsch and Therneau (1994), be denoted by $\widehat{\text{Var}}(\hat{r}_i)$, and the estimator is missing if $c_i = 0$. The vector of scaled Schoenfeld residuals is the product of the inverse of the covariance matrix times the vector of residuals, namely

$$\hat{r}_i^* = \left[\widehat{\text{Var}}(\hat{r}_i)\right]^{-1} \hat{r}_i. \qquad (6.4)$$

The elements in the covariance matrix $\widehat{\text{Var}}(\hat{r}_i)$ are, in the current setting, a weighted version of the usual sum-of-squares matrix computed using the data in the risk set. For the ith subject, the diagonal elements in this matrix are

$$\widehat{\text{Var}}(\hat{r}_i)_{kk} = \sum_{j \in R(t_i)} \hat{w}_{ij} \left(x_{jk} - \hat{\bar{x}}_{w,k}\right)^2,$$

and the off-diagonal elements are

$$\widehat{\text{Var}}(\hat{r}_i)_{kl} = \sum_{j \in R(t_i)} \hat{w}_{ij} \left(x_{jk} - \hat{\bar{x}}_{w,k}\right)\left(x_{jl} - \hat{\bar{x}}_{w,l}\right)$$

where

$$\hat{w}_{ij} = \frac{e^{x'_j \hat{\beta}}}{\sum_{l \in R(t_i)} e^{x'_l \hat{\beta}}}.$$

Grambsch and Therneau (1994) suggest using an easily computed approximation for the scaled Schoenfeld residuals. This suggestion is based on their experience that the matrix, $\widehat{\text{Var}}(\hat{r}_i)$, tends to be fairly constant over time. This occurs when the distribution of the covariate is similar in the various risk sets. Under this assumption, the inverse of $\widehat{\text{Var}}(\hat{r}_i)$ is easily approximated by multiplying the estimator of the covariance matrix of the estimated coefficients by the number of events (i.e., the observed number of uncensored survival times, m),

$$\left[\widehat{\text{Var}}(\hat{r}_i)\right]^{-1} = m\widehat{\text{Var}}(\hat{\beta}).$$

The approximate scaled Schoenfeld residuals are the ones computed by software packages, namely

$$\hat{\mathbf{r}}_i^* = m\widehat{\text{Var}}\left(\hat{\boldsymbol{\beta}}\right)\hat{\mathbf{r}}_i. \tag{6.5}$$

Subsequent references to the scaled Schoenfeld residuals, $\hat{\mathbf{r}}_i^*$, will mean the approximation in (6.5), not the true scaled residuals in (6.4). We demonstrate the use of the scaled Schoenfeld residuals to assess the proportional hazards assumption in Section 6.3.

The next collection of residuals comes from the counting process formulation of a time-to-event regression model. This is an extremely useful and powerful mathematical tool for studying the proportional hazards model. However, most descriptions of it, including those in statistical software manuals, are difficult to understand without knowledge of calculus. In this section and those that follow, we try to present the counting process results in an intuitive and easily understood manner. An expanded introduction to the counting process approach is given in Appendix 2. A complete development of the theory as well as applications to other settings may be found in Fleming and Harrington (1991) and Andersen, Borgan, Gill and Keiding (1993).

Assume that we follow a single subject with covariates denoted by $\mathbf{x}$ from time "zero" and that the event of interest is death. We could use as the outcome any other event that can occur only once or the first occurrence of an event that can occur multiple times, such as cancer relapse. The counting process representation of the proportional hazards model is a linear-like model that "counts" whether the event occurs (e.g., the subject dies) at time t. The basic model is

$$N(t) = \Lambda(t, \mathbf{x}, \boldsymbol{\beta}) + M(t) \tag{6.6}$$

where the function $N(t)$ is the "count" that represents the observed part of the model, the function $\Lambda(t, \mathbf{x}, \boldsymbol{\beta})$ is the "systematic component" of the model, and the function $M(t)$ is the "error component."

The function $N(t)$ is defined to be equal to zero until the exact time the event occurs and is equal to one thereafter. If the total length of follow-up is one year, and our subject dies on day 200, then

$$N(t) = \begin{cases} 0 \text{ for } t < 200 \\ 1 \text{ for } t \geq 200 \end{cases}.$$

If the subject does not die during the one year of follow-up, then the count is always zero, $N(t) = 0$. Hence, the maximum value of the count function occurs at

the end of follow-up of the subject and is equal to the value of the censoring indicator variable.

The systematic component of the model is, as we show in Appendix 2, equal
to the cumulative hazard at time t under the proportional hazards model,

$$\Lambda(t,\mathbf{x},\boldsymbol{\beta}) = H(t,\mathbf{x},\boldsymbol{\beta}),$$

until follow-up ends on the subject, and it is equal to zero thereafter. Thus, the
value of the function for a subject who either dies or is censored on day 200 is

$$\Lambda(t,\mathbf{x},\boldsymbol{\beta}) = \begin{cases} e^{\mathbf{x}^{\prime}\boldsymbol{\beta}} H_0(t) & \text{for } t \leq 200 \\ 0 & \text{for } t > 200 \end{cases},$$

where $H_0(t)$ is the cumulative baseline hazard function. It follows that the
maximum value for the systematic component also occurs at the end of follow-up,
regardless of whether the event occurred. The function $M(t)$ in (6.6) is, under
suitable mathematical assumptions, a martingale and plays the role of the error
component. It has many of the same properties that error components in other
models have, in particular its mean is zero under the correct model. If we rearrange (6.6), $M(t)$ may be expressed in the form of a "residual" as

$$M(t) = N(t) - \Lambda(t,\mathbf{x},\boldsymbol{\beta}). \tag{6.7}$$

The quantity in (6.7) is called the *martingale residual*. In theory, it has a value at
each time t, but the most useful choice of time at which to compute the residual is
the end of follow-up, yielding a value for the ith subject of

$$M(t_i) = N(t_i) - H(t_i,\mathbf{x},\boldsymbol{\beta}), \tag{6.8}$$

because $\Lambda(t_i,\mathbf{x},\boldsymbol{\beta}) = H(t_i,\mathbf{x},\boldsymbol{\beta})$. For ease of notation, let $M_i = M(t_i)$. The estimator, obtained by substituting the value of the partial likelihood estimator of the
coefficients, $\hat{\boldsymbol{\beta}}$, is

$$\hat{M}_i = c_i - \hat{H}(t_i,\mathbf{x},\hat{\boldsymbol{\beta}}) \tag{6.9}$$

since $N(t_i) = c_i$ and the estimator $\hat{H}(t_i,\mathbf{x},\hat{\boldsymbol{\beta}})$ is defined in (3.42). We mentioned
in Chapter 5 that this residual, (6.9), can be used for a graphical method to assess
the scale of a continuous covariate. We use the martingale residuals in Section 6.5
to provide a tabular display of model fit.

The residual in (6.9) is also called the Cox–Snell or modified Cox–Snell residual (see Cox and Snell (1968) and Collett (2003)). This terminology is due to the work of Cox and Snell, who showed that the values of $\hat{H}\left(t_i, \mathbf{x}, \hat{\boldsymbol{\beta}}\right)$ may be thought of as observations from a censored sample with an exponential distribution and parameter equal to 1.0. In our experience, this distribution theory is not as useful for model evaluation as the theory derived from the counting process approach.

Using the counting process approach, the expressions in (6.7) and (6.8) are a completely natural way to define a residual. To see why it also makes sense to consider (6.8) as a residual in the proportional hazards regression model, assume for ease of notation, that there are no ties and that the value of the baseline hazard at time t_i is

$$
h_0\left(t_i\right) = \frac{c_i}{\displaystyle\sum_{j \in R(t_i)} e^{\mathbf{x}_j'\boldsymbol{\beta}}} \tag{6.10}
$$

and that the cumulative baseline hazard is

$$
H_0\left(t_i\right) = \sum_{t_j \le t_i} h_0\left(t_j\right). \tag{6.11}
$$

The Breslow estimator of the cumulative baseline hazard is obtained from (6.11) by substituting the value of the partial likelihood estimator of the coefficients, $\hat{\boldsymbol{\beta}}$. Under these assumptions, the derivative in (6.11) may be expressed as

$$
\frac{\partial L_p(\boldsymbol{\beta})}{\partial \beta_k} = \sum_{i=1}^n x_{ik}\left[c_i - H\left(t_i, \mathbf{x}, \boldsymbol{\beta}\right)\right]. \tag{6.12}
$$

The expression in (6.12) is similar to likelihood equations obtained for other models, such as linear and logistic regression, in that it expresses the partial derivative as a sum of the value of the covariate times an "observed minus expected" residual.

The next set of residuals are obtained by expressing the martingale residuals, (6.12), in a slightly different form. The score equation for the kth covariate may be expressed as

$$
\frac{\partial L_p(\boldsymbol{\beta})}{\partial \beta_k} = \sum_{i=1}^n L_{ik}. \tag{6.13}
$$

The expression for L_{ik} is somewhat complex. Readers who are willing to accept without further elaboration that the estimator of L_{ik} is the *score residual* provided by software packages may skip the next paragraph where we describe L_{ik} in greater detail.

The score residual for the ith subject on the kth covariate in (6.13) may be expressed as

$$L_{ik} = \sum_{j=1}^{n} \left(x_{ik} - \bar{x}_{w,k} \right) dM_i \left(t_j \right). \tag{6.14}$$

The mean in the expression, $\bar{x}_{w,k}$, is the value of (6.2) computed at t_j. The quantity $dM_i\left(t_j \right)$ is the change in the martingale residual for the ith subject at time t_j and is

$$dM_i\left(t_j \right) = dN_i\left(t_j \right) - Y_i\left(t_j \right) e^{\mathbf{x}\boldsymbol{\beta}} h_0\left(t_j \right). \tag{6.15}$$

The first part of (6.15), $dN_i\left(t_j \right)$, is the change in the count function for the ith subject at time t_j. This will always be equal to zero for censored subjects. For uncensored subjects, it will be equal to zero except at the actual observed survival time, when it will be equal to one. That is, $dN_i\left(t_i \right) = 1$ for uncensored subjects. In the second part of (6.15), the function $Y_i\left(t_j \right)$ is called the *at risk process* and is defined as follows:

$$Y_i\left(t_j \right) = \begin{cases} 1 \text{ if } t_i \geq t_j \\ 0 \text{ if } t_i < t_j \end{cases}$$

and $h_0\left(t_j \right)$ is the value of (6.10) evaluated at t_j. An expanded computational formula yields the estimator

$$\hat{L}_{ik} = c_i \times \left(x_{ik} - \hat{\bar{x}}_{w,k} \right) - x_{ik} \times \hat{H}\left(t_i, \mathbf{x}, \hat{\boldsymbol{\beta}} \right) + e^{\mathbf{x}\hat{\boldsymbol{\beta}}} \sum_{t_j \leq t_i} \hat{\bar{x}}_{w,k} \frac{c_j}{\sum_{l \in R_j} e^{\mathbf{x}\hat{\boldsymbol{\beta}}}}. \tag{6.16}$$

Let the vector of p score residuals for the ith subject be denoted as

$$\hat{\mathbf{L}}_i' = \left(\hat{L}_{i1}, \hat{L}_{i2}, \ldots, \hat{L}_{ip} \right). \tag{6.17}$$

A scaled version of the score residuals in (6.17) is also used in model evaluation. These are defined as

$$\hat{\mathbf{L}}_i^{*'} = \widehat{\text{Var}}(\hat{\boldsymbol{\beta}})\hat{\mathbf{L}}_i \qquad (6.18)$$

where $\widehat{\text{Var}}(\hat{\boldsymbol{\beta}})$ is the estimator of the covariance matrix of the estimated coefficients. These are commonly referred to as the *scaled score residuals* and their values may be obtained from some software packages.   We use the score and scaled score residuals to measure the leverage and influence, respectively, of particular subjects.

Before moving on, we provide a brief summary of residuals. The martingale residual, $\hat{M}_i$, in (6.9) has the form typically expected of a residual in that it resembles the difference between an observed outcome and a predicted outcome. The other four residuals (Schoenfeld, scaled Schoenfeld, score, and scaled score) are covariate-specific. Every subject has a value of the score residual for the kth covariate, $\hat{L}_{ik}$ in (6.16) and for the scaled score residual, $\hat{L}_{ik}^{*}$ from (6.18), but the Schoenfeld residual in (6.3) and the scaled Schoenfeld residual in (6.5) are defined only at the observed survival times. Thus, there are only m subjects with values for these residuals. Each of these residuals provides a useful tool for examining one or more aspects of model adequacy.

Next we consider methods for assessing the proportional hazards assumption.

6.3   ASSESSING THE PROPORTIONAL HAZARDS ASSUMPTION

The proportional hazards assumption is vital to the interpretation and use of a fitted proportional hazards model. As discussed in detail in Chapter 4, the estimated hazard ratios do not depend on time. Specifically, the proportional hazards model has a log-hazard function of the form

$$\ln\left[h(t,\mathbf{x},\boldsymbol{\beta})\right] = \ln\left[h_0(t)\right] + \mathbf{x}'\boldsymbol{\beta} . \qquad (6.19)$$

This function has two parts, the log of the baseline hazard function, $\ln\left[h_0(t)\right]$, and the linear predictor, $\mathbf{x}'\boldsymbol{\beta}$. Methods for building the linear predictor part of the model are discussed in detail in Chapter 5. The proportional hazards assumption characterizes the model as a function of time, not of the covariates *per se*. Assume for the moment that the model contains a single dichotomous covariate. A plot of the log-hazard, (6.19), over time would produce two continuous curves, one for $x = 0$, $\ln\left[h_0(t)\right]$, and the other for $x = 1$, $\ln\left[h_0(t)\right] + \beta$. It follows that the difference between these two curves at any point in time is β, regardless of how simple or complicated the baseline hazard function is. This is the reason the estimated hazard ratio, $\hat{HR} = \exp\left(\hat{\beta}\right)$, has such a simple and useful interpretation.

As a second example, suppose age is the only covariate in the model and that it is scaled linearly. Consider the plots over time of the log-hazard function for age a and age $a+10$. If the coefficient, β, is positive, then the difference between the two plotted functions is 10β at every point in time. Assessing the proportional hazards assumption is an examination of the extent to which the two plotted hazard functions are equidistant from each other over time.

There are, effectively, an infinite number of ways the model in (6.19) can be changed to yield non-proportional hazard functions or log-hazard functions that are not equidistant over time. As a result, a large number of tests and procedures have been proposed. However, work by Grambsch and Therneau (1994) and simulations by Ng'andu (1997) show that one easily performed test and an associated graph yield an effective method for examining this critical assumption.

Grambsch and Therneau (1994) consider an alternative to the model in (6.19) originally proposed by Schoenfeld (1982), that allows the effect of the covariate to change over time as follows:

$$\beta_j(t) = \beta_j + \gamma_j g_j(t), \tag{6.20}$$

where $g_j(t)$ is a specified function of time. The rationale for this model is that the effect of a covariate could change continuously or discretely over the period of follow-up. For example, the baseline value of a specific covariate may lose its relevance over time. The opposite could also occur, namely the baseline measure is more strongly associated with survival later in the follow-up. Under the model in (6.20), Grambsch and Therneau show that the scaled Schoenfeld residuals in (6.4), and their approximation in (6.5), have, for the jth covariate, a mean at time t of approximately

$$E\left[r_j^*(t)\right] \cong \gamma_j g_j(t). \tag{6.21}$$

The result in (6.21) suggests that a plot of the scaled Schoenfeld residuals over time may be used to assess visually whether the coefficient γ_j is equal to zero and, if not, what the nature of the time dependence, $g_j(t)$, may be. Grambsch and Therneau derive a generalized least-squares estimator of the coefficients and a score test of the hypothesis that they are equal to zero, given specific choices for the functions $g_j(t)$. In addition, they show that specific choices for the function yield previously proposed tests. For example, using $g(t) = \ln(t)$ yields a model first suggested by Cox (1972) and a test by Gill and Schumacher (1987) discussed by Chappell (1992). With this function, the model in (6.20) is

$$\beta_j(t) = \beta_j + \gamma_j \ln(t),$$

and the linear predictor portion of the model in (6.20) is

$$\beta_j x_j + \gamma_j x_j \ln(t). \tag{6.22}$$

The form of the linear predictor in (6.22) suggests that we can test the hypothesis that $\gamma_j = 0$ via the partial likelihood ratio test, score test, or Wald test obtained when the time varying interaction $x_j \ln(t)$ is added to the proportional hazards model. The advantage of this approach over the generalized least-squares score test proposed by Grambsch and Therneau is that it may be done using the model fitting software in many statistical software packages. One should note that when the interaction term, $x_j \ln(t)$, is included in the model, the partial likelihood becomes much more complicated. The interaction is a function of follow up time, its value must be recomputed for each term in the risk set at each observed survival time. The interaction term is not simply the product of the covariate and the subject's observed value of time, $x_j \ln(t_j)$.

Other functions of time have been suggested, for example Quantin et al. (1996) suggest using $g(t) = \ln\left[H_0(t)\right]$. Based on simulations reported in their paper, this test appears to have good power, but it is not as easy to compute as the test based on $g(t) = \ln(t)$. Because the Breslow estimator of $H_0(t)$ must be computed and must be accessible at each observed survival time. The STATA package allows us to use, in addition to $g(t) = \ln(t)$, the functions $g(t) = t$, $g(t) = \hat{S}_{KM}(t)$ and $g(t) = rank(t)$. Simulations in Quantin et al. (1996) and Ng'andu (1997), show that the test based on $g(t) = \ln(t)$ has power nearly as high or higher than other commonly used functions to detect reasonable alternatives to proportional hazards. While this is generally true, our experience is that, in specific cases, the significance level of the tests may vary with the function from highly significant with one choice to marginal or non-significant with another choice. For this reason, we tend to perform the tests with a variety of functions. Using more than one test certainly increases the chance of making a Type I error for each covariate, but finding a "significant" time varying effect may lead to a more informative model. In any case, if the test for any covariate is significant, then its time varying effect must make clinical sense.

In most settings, we recommend the following two-step procedure for assessing the proportional hazards assumption: (1) calculate covariate specific tests and (2) plot the scaled and smoothed scaled Schoenfeld residuals obtained from the model. The results of the two steps should support each other. Methods for han-

Table 6.1 Score Tests and p-values for Proportional Hazards for Each of the Covariates as Well as the Global Test for the Model in Table 5.13 Fit to the WHAS500 Data

Covariate	df	$g(t) = t$		$g(t) = \ln(t)$		$g(t) = \hat{S}_{KM}(t)$		$g(t) = \text{rank}(t)$	
		chi2	p	chi2	p	chi2	p	chi2	p
bmifp1	1	1.66	0.198	0.01	0.914	0.35	0.554	0.17	0.679
bmifp2	1	1.24	0.265	0.00	0.957	0.18	0.671	0.06	0.814
age	1	1.41	0.236	4.29	0.038	3.29	0.070	3.86	0.049
hr	1	0.08	0.777	1.03	0.310	0.57	0.452	0.91	0.340
diasbp	1	0.00	0.997	0.53	0.467	0.35	0.555	0.41	0.523
gender	1	0.23	0.630	2.05	0.153	1.32	0.251	1.65	0.200
chf	1	0.44	0.507	0.33	0.564	0.03	0.873	0.09	0.767
agexgender	1	0.18	0.672	2.24	0.135	1.35	0.245	1.73	0.189
Global	8	3.65	0.887	7.47	0.487	5.10	0.747	6.36	0.607

dling nonproportional hazards are discussed in Chapter 7, where we consider extensions of the proportional hazards model.

We now turn to evaluating the model developed in Chapter 5 for the WHAS500 data, shown in Table 5.13. This model is relatively complex in that it contains 8 terms: three main effects without interactions, an interaction and its main effects, and two terms that model nonlinear effects of a continuous covariate. Our first step is to evaluate the score test based on the scaled Schoenfeld residuals using each of the four functions of time available in STATA. The results are shown in Table 6.1.

The results in Table 6.1 indicate that there is some evidence, for three of the four functions of time, of the hazard being nonproportional in age. Nevertheless, the evidence for this is weak. Age is involved in an interaction with gender, which does not have a significant score test. If the evidence were stronger, this would have implied that the nonproportional hazard in age may be for males in the multivariable model because the main effect for age corresponds to the age effect for males (gender = 0). The global 8 degrees-of-freedom tests are not significant. We also point out the importance of using the covariate specific tests because, if we do not, we might miss a possible non-proportionality in any of the individual covariates. There is no strong evidence of nonproportional hazards for any of the terms in the model. We obtained similar results when we added time varying interactions of the form g(t)*x to the model and assessed significance using Wald statistics for individual terms and the partial likelihood ratio test for the global test of proportional hazards. At this point, it makes sense to look at a scatterplot of the scaled Schoenfeld residuals to see whether they support the results of the score tests.

It is our experience that these plots are difficult to interpret, as any departure from proportional hazards may be subtle and difficult to see, even with a smooth

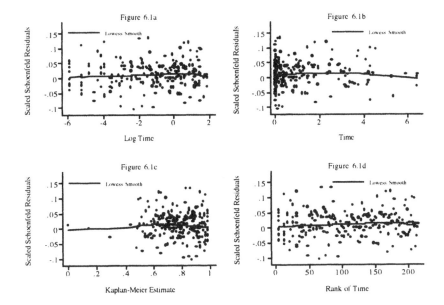

Figure 6.1 Scatterplot of scaled Schoenfeld residuals for heart rate and their lowess smooth versus the natural log of follow up time (years), follow up time, the Kaplan-Meier estimate, and the rank of follow up time.

added to the plot. Rather than begin with age, we illustrate the plot for heart rate (hr) in Figure 6.1 to provide an example of what the plot should look like for a continuous covariate when the score test fails to reject the null hypothesis of no time varying effect [i.e., $H_0 : \gamma_j = 0$ in (6.21)].

In Figure 6.1, we plot the scaled Schoenfeld residuals versus each of the four functions of time used in Table 6.1. In Figure 6.1a we plot versus log of time. This plot emphasizes the first year of follow up, as 75 percent of the plot is devoted to this time interval. This plot shows no discernable pattern, appearing to be "randomly" scattered about zero. The lowess smooth has a slight positive slope. The slight downturn at the far right is likely due to the effect of the two small values in the lower right of the plot. In Figure 6.1b, the scaled Schoenfeld residuals are plotted versus follow up time. About 75 percent of the plot is devoted to the time interval from one to six years. This plot places a high visual emphasis on a few subjects with follow up times that exceed three years. In particular, we see that the downturn in the far right of Figure 6.1b is much more visible and likely due to the effect on the lowess smooth of the subjects with the four longest follow up times. Overall the lowess smooth displays a slight rise and then fall, which by the score test is not a significant departure from a slope of zero. In Figure 6.1c, the scaled Schoenfeld residuals are plotted versus the Kaplan-Meier estimate of the

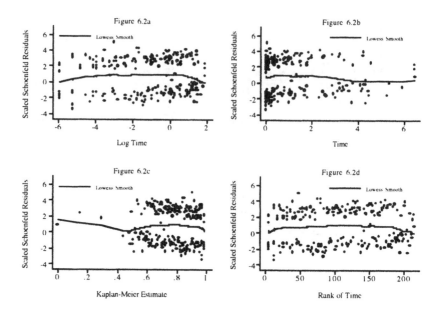

Figure 6.2 Scatterplot of scaled Schoenfeld residuals for congestive heart complications and their lowess smooth versus the natural log of follow up time (years), follow up time, the Kaplan-Meier estimate, and the rank of follow up time.

survival function. The plot places undue emphasis on the four subjects with the longest follow up times (i.e., Kaplan-Meier estimates $\leq .4$). In the remainder of the plot, to the right of 0.4, the points appear to be randomly scattered about the lowess smooth, which appears to have a slope equal to zero. In this case, a better plot would be one over the interval $[0.4, 1]$, which we leave as an exercise. The scaled Schoenfeld residuals are plotted in Figure 6.1d versus the rank of survival time in the sample of 500. The plot looks similar to Figure 6.1c, but with better resolution for shorter follow up times (i.e., ones with rank ≤ 100). Like the other three plots, there is no obvious departure from the points being randomly distributed about the lowess smooth, which has a slight bend. In summary, the four plots support the proportional hazards assumption.

Next we examine the same four scatterplots of the scaled Schoenfeld residuals for congestive heart complications (chf) in Figure 6.2. Congestive heart complications is a dichotomous covariate and each of the four score tests fails to reject the hypothesis of proportional hazards. We first note the two bands of points. The upper band corresponds to the 110 subjects who had complications and subsequently died. The points in the lower band correspond to the 105 subjects with no complications who died. This band-like behavior is typical of the scaled score residuals for dichotomous covariates that appear in the model as a main effect only. When dichotomous covariates are involved in an interaction with a continuous covariate, the scatterplot of the scaled score residuals for the main effect and its interaction tend to look more like those of a fully continuous covariate.

The lowess smooth in Figure 6.2a has a vaguely parabolic shape in that it rises, levels, and then drops. The rise occurs during the first seven days, $6.69 = 365 \times \exp(-4)$. The lowess smooth has slope about zero from 7 days to one year, $0 = \ln(1)$, and then drops. The overall effect is that a straight line would have slope zero. It is not clear at this point if the early and late departures from zero slope are meaningful so, for the time being, we proceed as if the plot supports the score tests. The other three plots display these trends, but, as noted above in the discussion of Figure 6.1, with a focus on different intervals of follow up time. However, we return to this point and explore the possibility of a time varying effect in more detail in Chapter 7 where we discuss time varying covariates.

The scatterplots and lowess smooths of the scaled Schoenfeld residuals for the two fractional polynomial transformations of body mass index (bmifp1 and bmifp2), diastolic blood pressure (diasbp), gender, and the gender by age interaction support the score test results. Hence we proceed, treating the hazard in these covariates as being proportional.

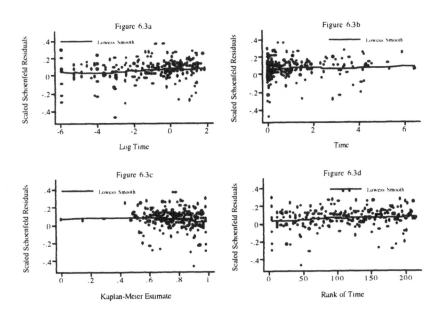

Figure 6.3 Scatterplot of scaled Schoenfeld residuals for age and their lowess smooth versus the natural log of follow up time (years), follow up time, the Kaplan-Meier estimate, and the rank of follow up time.

Next we show, in Figure 6.3, four scatterplots of the scaled Schoenfeld residuals and their lowess smooth for age. In Figure 6.3a, we see that the lowess smooth has slope zero for the first week of follow up; from this point on, the trend is slightly upward. The upward trend is easier to see in Figure 6.1b and Figure 6.1d. As we noted above, due to the inclusion of the age-by-gender interaction, we believe that non-proportionality may be among males only. As with the case of congestive heart complications, we are going to proceed with further model evaluation assuming that the main effect age has a proportional hazard, returning to reexamine the issue in Chapter 7.

In closing, we note two points: (1) The score tests and scatterplots based on the scaled Schoenfeld residuals with various functions of follow up time are the primary diagnostic test and descriptive statistics for assessing whether the hazard is proportional in each covariate separately as well as overall, and (2) Application of the tests and plots, in general, supports treating the model in Table 5.13 as adhering to the proportional hazards assumption.

6.4   IDENTIFICATION OF INFLUENTIAL AND POORLY FIT SUBJECTS

Another important aspect of model evaluation is a thorough examination of regression diagnostic statistics to identify which, if any, subjects: (1) have an unusual configuration of covariates, (2) exert an undue influence on the estimates of the parameters, and/or (3) have an undue influence on the fit of the model. Statistics similar to those used in linear and logistic regression are available to perform these tasks with a fitted proportional hazards model. There are some differences in the types of statistics used in linear and logistic regression and proportional hazards regression, but the essential ideas are the same in all three settings.

Leverage is a diagnostic statistic that measures how "unusual" the values of the covariates are for an individual. In some sense it is a residual in the covariates. In linear and logistic regression, leverage is calculated as the distance of the value of the covariates for a subject to the overall mean of the covariates [see Hosmer and Lemeshow (2000), Kleinbaum, Kupper, Muller and Nizam (1998), and Ryan (1997)]. It is proportional to $(x - \bar{x})^2$. The leverage values in these settings have nice properties in that they are always positive and sum over the sample to the number of parameters in the model. While it is technically possible to break the leverage into values for each covariate, this is rarely done in linear and logistic regression. Leverage is not quite so easily defined nor does it have the same nice properties in proportional hazards regression. This is due to the fact that subjects may appear in multiple risk sets and thus may be present in multiple terms in the partial likelihood.

The score residuals defined in (6.16) and (6.17) form the nucleus of the proportional hazards diagnostics. The score residual for the ith subject on the kth covariate, see (6.14), is a weighted average of the distance of the value, x_{ik}, to the risk set means, $\bar{x}_{w,k}$, where the weights are the change in the martingale residual, $dM_i(t_j)$. The net effect is that, for continuous covariates, the score residuals have the linear regression leverage property that the further the value is from the mean, the larger the score residual is, but "large" may be either positive or negative. Thus, the score residuals are sometimes referred to as the leverage or partial leverage residuals.

The graphs of the score residuals for the covariates bmifp1, bmifp2, heart rate, and diastolic blood pressure obtained from the fitted model in Table 5.13 are shown in Figure 6.4a to Figure 6.4d. These four terms were chosen because they are continuous variables and not involved in an interaction in the fitted model. The graphs for remaining model terms are in Figure 6.5a to Figure 6.5d.

To aid in the interpretation of the plots in this section, we have used the diamond to highlight the points that we feel lie further from the remainder of the data than we would expect. These represent subjects whose data we will want to investigate further.

In Figure 6.4, we observe three extreme points for body mass index, one for heart rate and two for diastolic blood pressure. In Figure 6.5, we see one extreme point for age and one for the age-by-gender interaction. For dichotomous covariates, it is more informative to use a box plot at each level of the covariate. In the plot for congestive heart complications, we see one for chf = 0 and two for chf = 1. In the plot for gender, there are two values for male and one for female that warrant further attention.

In linear and logistic regression, high leverage is not necessarily about a concern. However, a subject with a high value for leverage may contribute undue influence to the estimate of a coefficient. The same is true in proportional hazards regression. To examine influence in the proportional hazards setting, we need statistics analogous to Cook's distance in linear and logistic regression. The purpose of Cook's distance is to obtain an easily computed statistic that approximates the change in the value of the estimated coefficients if a subject is deleted from the data. This is denoted as

$$\Delta\hat{\beta}_{ki} = \hat{\beta}_k - \hat{\beta}_{k(-i)}, \tag{6.23}$$

where $\hat{\beta}_k$ denotes the partial likelihood estimator of the coefficient computed using the entire sample of size n and $\hat{\beta}_{k(-i)}$ denotes the value of the estimator if the ith subject is removed. Cain and Lange (1984) show that an approximate estimator of (6.23) is the kth element of the vector of coefficient changes

$$\Delta\hat{\beta}_i = \left(\hat{\beta} - \hat{\beta}_{(-i)}\right) = \hat{Var}(\hat{\beta})\hat{L}_i, \tag{6.24}$$

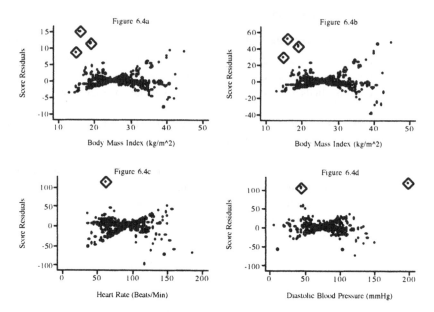

Figure 6.4 Graphs of the score residuals computed from the model in Table 5.13 for (a) bmifp1, (b) bmifp2, (c) heart rate, and (d) diastolic blood pressure.

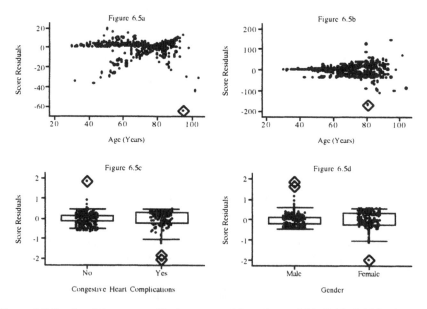

Figure 6.5 Graphs of the score residuals computed from the model in Table 5.13 for (a) age, (b) age by gender interaction, (c) congestive heart complications, and (d) gender.

where $\hat{\mathbf{L}}_i$ is the vector of score residuals, (6.17), and $\widehat{\text{Var}}(\hat{\boldsymbol{\beta}})$ is the estimator of the covariance matrix of the estimated coefficients. These are commonly referred to as the *scaled score residuals* and their values may be obtained from some software packages, for example, SAS, and easily computed in STATA.

Graphs of the scaled score residuals, (6.24), are presented in Figure 6.6 for the covariates whose score residuals are graphed in Figure 6.4. and in Figure 6.7 for the variables whose score residuals are plotted in Figure 6.5. The plots in Figures 6.4 and 6.6 look different. Nevertheless, the same three points are identified as being influential for bmifp1 in Figures 6.4a and Figure 6.6a. However, it appears that three different points are identified as being influential for bmifp2. Similarly, we see a single influential point in the plots for heart rate and diastolic blood pressure.

In Figure 6.7 we see two points that may have influence on the coefficient for age and two points for the interaction of age and gender. The box plot for congestive heart complications shows two possibly influential subjects with chf = 1. The plot for gender identifies perhaps three male subjects with influence. Note that two male subjects with very small influence values that are so close together they are indistinguishable on the graph.

Cook's distance in linear and logistic regression may be used to provide a single overall summary statistic of the influence a subject has on the estimators of

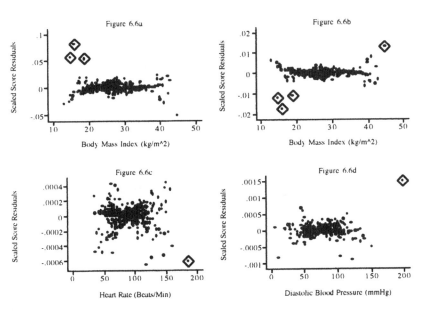

Figure 6.6 Graphs of the scaled score residuals computed from the model in Table 5.13 for (a) bmifp1, (b) bmifp2, (c) heart rate, and (d) diastolic blood pressure.

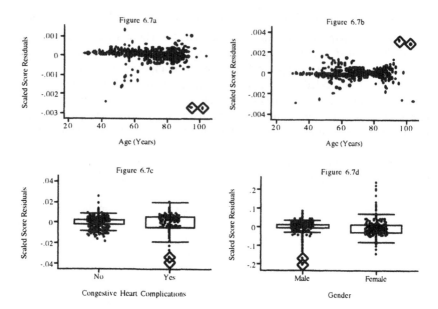

Figure 6.7 Graphs of the scaled score residuals computed from the model in Table 5.13 for (a) age, (b) age-by-gender interaction, (c) congestive heart complications, and (d) gender.

all the coefficients. The overall measure of influence is

$$\left(\hat{\boldsymbol{\beta}}-\hat{\boldsymbol{\beta}}_{(-i)}\right)'\left[\hat{\text{Var}}\left(\hat{\boldsymbol{\beta}}\right)\right]^{-1}\left(\hat{\boldsymbol{\beta}}-\hat{\boldsymbol{\beta}}_{(-i)}\right),$$

and using (6.24) it may be approximated using

$$ld_i = \left(\Delta\hat{\boldsymbol{\beta}}_i\right)'\left[\hat{\text{Var}}\left(\hat{\boldsymbol{\beta}}\right)\right]^{-1}\left(\Delta\hat{\boldsymbol{\beta}}_i\right)$$

$$= \left(\hat{\mathbf{L}}_i\right)'\left[\hat{\text{Var}}\left(\hat{\boldsymbol{\beta}}\right)\right]\left[\hat{\text{Var}}\left(\hat{\boldsymbol{\beta}}\right)\right]^{-1}\left[\hat{\text{Var}}\left(\hat{\boldsymbol{\beta}}\right)\right]\left(\hat{\mathbf{L}}_i\right)$$

so

$$ld_i = \left(\hat{\mathbf{L}}_i\right)'\left[\hat{\text{Var}}\left(\hat{\boldsymbol{\beta}}\right)\right]\left(\hat{\mathbf{L}}_i\right). \tag{6.25}$$

The statistic in (6.25) has been shown by Pettitt and Bin Daud (1989) to be an approximation to the amount of change in the log partial likelihood when the ith subject is deleted. In this context, the statistic is called the *likelihood displacement statistic*, hence the rationale for labeling it *ld* in (6.25), thus

$$ld_i \cong 2\left[L_p\left(\hat{\beta}\right) - L_p\left(\hat{\beta}_{(-i)}\right)\right]. \tag{6.26}$$

We feel it makes the most sense to plot ld_i in (6.25) versus the martingale residuals.

The plots of the values of the likelihood displacement statistic versus the martingale residuals are shown in Figure 6.8. The plot has an asymmetric "cup" shape with the bottom of the cup at zero. In linear and logistic regression, the influence diagnostic, Cook's distance, is a product of a residual measure and leverage. While the same concise representation does not hold in proportional hazards regression, it is approximately true in the sense that an influential subject will have a large residual and/or leverage. Thus, the largest values of the likelihood displacement form the sides of the cup and correspond to poorly fit subjects (ones with either large negative or large positive martingale residuals).

The next step in the modeling process is to identify explicitly the subjects with the extreme values, refit the model deleting these subjects, and calculate the change in the individual coefficients. The final decision on the continued use of a subject's data to fit the model will depend on the observed percentage change in the coefficients that results from deleting the subject's data and, more importantly, the clinical plausibility of that subject's data.

By examining the values of the covariates and diagnostic statistics, we find 10 subjects with high leverage, high influence or large Cook's distance. These subjects are listed, with their data, in Table 6.2. The subjects are generally older, with low body mass index. At this stage of the analysis, we do nothing, delaying further action until we examine influence on parameter estimates.

Table 6.2 Nine Subjects with High Leverage, High Influence or Large Cook's Distance from the Fitted Model in Table 5.13

Study ID	Body Mass Index	Age	Heart Rate	Diastolic Blood Pressure	Gender	CHF
51	22.45	80	105	72	Male	Yes
89	15.93	95	62	45	Male	No
112	14.84	87	105	104	Female	No
115	18.90	81	118	70	Female	Yes
153	39.94	32	102	83	Female	No
194	24.21	43	47	90	Male	Yes
251	22.27	102	89	60	Male	Yes
256	44.84	53	96	99	Female	No
416	28.55	80	64	198	Male	No
472	25.40	72	186	84	Male	No

We leave it as an exercise to verify that, when we fit the model in Table 5.13, deleting the 10 subjects listed in Table 6.2, the percentage change in the eight estimated coefficients is 33.7, 31.2, 14.9, 17.7, 19.9, 11.2, 2.8, and 14.7, respectively. The greatest effect of the deletion is on the coefficients for the two fractional polynomial variables for body mass index. The change is largely due to deletion of subjects 89, 112, 115, and 256. This is not unexpected because these four subjects are among those with the lowest and highest values of bmi. The changes in the other coefficients are less than 20 percent, though the change in the estimate of the coefficient for diastolic blood pressure is 19.9 percent.

We consulted with the Worcester Heart Attack Study team on the plausibility of the data for subjects 89, 11, 115, 256, and 416. The bmi values for subjects influential for the estimates of the coefficients (89, 112, 115 and 256) for the two fractional polynomial variables were judged to be reasonable and should be kept in the analysis. However, they felt that a diastolic blood pressure of 198, while clinically possible, was so unusual relative to the other subjects in the study that this subject should be removed from the analysis.

As a result of the deletion, we fit the model in Table 5.13 after deleting subject 416, and the results are displayed in Table 6.3. Other than a change in the estimated coefficient for diastolic blood pressure by about 15 percent, all other model summary statistics are essentially unchanged. The results of model evaluation were also essentially unchanged.

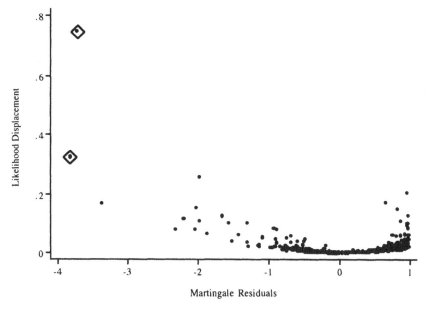

Figure 6.8 Graphs of the likelihood displacement or Cook's distance statistic computed from the model in Table 5.13 versus the martingale residual.

Table 6.3 Estimated Coefficients, Standard Errors, z-Scores, Two-Tailed p-values, and 95% Confidence Interval Estimates for the Preliminary Final Proportional Hazards Model for the WHAS500 data, $n = 499$

Variable	Coeff.	Std. Err.	z	$p>|z|$	95% CIE
bmifp1	−0.685	0.1741	−3.94	<0.001	−1.026, −0.344
bmifp2	0.145	0.0395	3.66	<0.001	0.067, 0.222
age	0.060	0.0083	7.15	<0.001	0.043, 0.076
hr	0.012	0.0029	4.13	<0.001	0.006, 0.018
diasbp	−0.012	0.0035	−3.48	<0.001	−0.019, −0.005
gender	1.838	0.9579	1.92	0.055	−0.039, 3.716
chf	0.830	0.1469	5.65	<0.001	0.542, 1.118
agexgender	−0.027	0.0121	−2.28	0.023	−0.051, −0.004

In summary, we feel it is important to examine plots of the score residuals, scaled score residuals, and the likelihood displacement statistic. The first two statistics are useful for identifying subjects with high leverage or who influence the value of a single coefficient. The latter provides useful information for assessing influence on the vector of coefficients. Each statistic portrays an important aspect of the effect a particular subject has on the fitted model. One always hopes that major problems are not uncovered. However, if the model does display abnormal sensitivity to the subjects deleted, this is a clear indication of fundamental problems in the model and we recommend going back to "square-one" and repeating each step in the modeling process, perhaps with these subjects deleted. The next step in the modeling process is to compute an overall goodness-of-fit test.

6.5   ASSESSING OVERALL GOODNESS-OF-FIT

Until quite recently, all the proposed tests for the overall goodness-of-fit of a proportional hazards model were difficult to compute in most software packages. For example, the test proposed by Schoenfeld (1980) compares the observed number of events with a proportional hazards regression model-based estimate of the expected number of events in each of G groups formed by partitioning the time axis and covariate space. Unfortunately, the covariance matrix required to form a test statistic comparing the observed to expected number of events is quite complex to compute. The test proposed by Lin, Wei and Ying (1993) is based on the maximum absolute value of partial sums of martingale residuals. This test requires complex and time-consuming simulations to obtain a significance level. Other tests [e.g., O'Quigley and Pessione (1989) and Pettitt and Bin Daud (1990)] require that the time axis be partitioned and interactions between covariates and interval-specific, time-dependent covariates be added to the model. Overall goodness-of-fit is based on a significance test of the coefficients for the added variables.

Grønnesby and Borgan (1996) propose a test similar to the Hosmer-Lemeshow test [Hosmer and Lemeshow (2000)] used in logistic regression. They suggest partitioning the data into G groups based on the ranked values of the estimated risk score, $\mathbf{x}'\hat{\boldsymbol{\beta}}$. The test is based on the sum of the martingale residuals within each group, and it compares the observed number of events in each group to the model-based estimate of the expected number of events. Using the counting process approach, they derive an expression for the covariance matrix of the vector of G sums. They show that their quadratic form test statistic has a chi-square distribution with $G-1$ degrees of freedom when the fitted model is the correct model and the sample is large enough that the estimated expected number of events in each group is large. As presented in their paper, the calculations of Grønnesby and Borgan (1996) are not a trivial matter.

May and Hosmer (1998), following the method used by Tsiatis (1980) to derive a goodness-of-fit test in logistic regression, prove that Grønnesby and Borgan's test is the score test for the addition of $G-1$ design variables, based on the G groups, to the fitted proportional hazards model. Thus, the test statistic may be calculated in any package that performs score tests. Using the asymptotic equivalence of score tests and likelihood ratio tests, one may approximate the score test with the partial likelihood ratio test, which may be done in any package.

One may be tempted to define groups based on the subject-specific estimated survival probabilities,

$$\hat{S}\left(t_i, \mathbf{x}_i, \hat{\boldsymbol{\beta}}\right) = \left[\hat{S}_0\left(t_i\right)\right]^{\exp\left(\mathbf{x}_i'\hat{\boldsymbol{\beta}}\right)}.$$

This should not be done because the values of time differ for each subject. If groups are to be based on the survival probability scale, they should be computed using the risk score and a fixed value of time for each subject. For example, in the WHAS500 we could use the estimated one-year survival probability

$$\hat{S}\left(1, \mathbf{x}_i, \hat{\boldsymbol{\beta}}\right) = \left[\hat{S}_0\left(1\right)\right]^{\exp\left(\mathbf{x}_i'\hat{\boldsymbol{\beta}}\right)}.$$

Because the choice of a time is arbitrary, one cannot interpret the probability as a prediction of the number of events in each risk group. It merely provides another way to express the risk score.

May and Hosmer's (1998) result greatly simplifies the calculation of the test, and also suggests that a two-by-G table presenting the observed and expected numbers of events in each group is a useful way to summarize the model fit. The individual observed and expected values in the table may be compared by appealing to counting process theory. Under this theory, the counting function is approximately a Poisson variate with mean equal to the cumulative hazard function. Sums of independent count functions will be approximately Poisson distributed, with mean equal to the sum of the cumulative hazard function. This suggests considering the observed counts within each risk group to be distributed approximately Poisson, with mean equal to the estimated expected number of counts. Furthermore, the fact that the Poisson distribution may be approximated by the normal for large values of the mean suggests that an easy way to compare the observed and expected counts is to form a z-score by dividing their difference by the square root of the expected. The two-tailed p-value is obtained from the standard normal distribution. There are obvious dependencies in the counts due to the fact that the same estimated parameter vector is used to calculate the individual expected values and some dependency due to grouping of subjects into risk groups. The effect of these dependencies has not been studied, but it is likely to smooth the counts toward the expected counts. Thus, the proposed cell-wise z-score comparisons should, if anything, be a bit conservative.

Due to the similarity of the Grønnesby and Borgan and the Hosmer and Lemeshow test for logistic regression, May and Hosmer as well as Parzen and Lipsitz (1999) suggest using 10 risk score groups. Nevertheless, based on simulation results, May and Hosmer (2004) show that, for small samples or samples with a large percentage of censored observations, the test rejects too often. They suggest the number of groups be chosen such that G = integer of {maximum of [2 and minimum of (10 and the number of events divided by 40)]}. With this grouping strategy, the test is shown to have acceptable size and power. There are 214 deaths observed for the model in Table 6.3. Thus, the number of events divided by 40 is 5.35 and G would be chosen as five groups. When we perform the overall goodness-of-fit test with five groups, the value of the partial likelihood ratio test for the inclusion of four quintile-of-risk design variables is 9.42 which, with 4 degrees of freedom, has a p-value of 0.0514; this is borderline statistically significant.

Table 6.4 presents the observed and estimated expected numbers of events, the z-score and two-tailed p-value within each quintile of risk for the fitted model in Table 6.3. The results in the observed and expected columns of Table 6.4 are obtained as follows: (1) Following the fit of the model in Table 6.3, we saved the martingale residuals and risk score; (2) We sorted the risk score and created a grouping variable with values $1 - 5$ based on the quintiles of the risk score; (3) We calculated the observed number of events in each quintile by summing the censoring variable over the subjects in each quintile. For example, the sum of the follow up status (censoring) variable over the 100 subjects in the first quintile is 6; (4) We created the model cumulative hazard by subtracting the martingale residual from the follow up status (censoring) variable; and (5) We calculated the expected number of events in each quintile by summing the cumulative hazard over the subjects in each quintile. For example, the sum of the cumulative hazard over the 100 subjects in the first quintile is 8.2. We note that, unlike the goodness of fit test in logistic regression, the value of the test statistic is cannot be obtained by summing over the five rows in Table 6.4. It must be calculated using either the score or likelihood ratio test for the inclusion of four reference cell design variables formed from the quintile grouping variable. Any one of the five groups may be used as the reference value.

The numbers in Table 6.4 are large enough for all the five quintiles of risk and we feel comfortable using the normal approximation to the Poisson distribution. With a p-value equal to 0.084, only the fourth quintile has a borderline significant difference between the observed and model-based expected count. We conclude that there is sufficient agreement between observed and expected number of events within each of the five quintiles of risk. The model displayed in Table 6.3 has passed the test for a good fitting model.

As in all regression analyses, some measure analogous to R^2 may be of interest as a measure of model performance. As shown in a detailed study by Schemper and Stare (1996), there is not a single, simple, useful, easy to calculate and easy to interpret measure for a proportional hazards regression model. In particular, most measures depend on the proportion of censored values. A perfectly adequate model may have what, at face value, seems a low R^2 due to a high percentage of censored data. In our opinion, further work needs to be done before we can recommend one measure over another. However, if one must compute such a measure, then

$$R_p^2 = 1 - \left\{ \exp\left[\frac{2}{n}\left(L_0 - L_p\right) \right] \right\}$$

Table 6.4 Observed Number of Events, Estimated Number of Events, z-Scores, and Two-Tailed p-values within Each Quintile of Risk Based on the Model in Table 6.3

Quintile	Cut Point	Count	Observed	Expected	z	p
1	1.37	100	6	8.2	-0.76	0.448
2	2.17	100	15	22.5	-1.58	0.115
3	2.80	100	41	37.6	0.56	0.574
4	3.53	100	66	53.4	1.73	0.084
5	5.66	99	86	92.4	0.67	0.504

is perhaps the easiest and best one to use, where L_p is the log partial likelihood for the fitted model with p covariates, and L_0 is the log partial likelihood for model zero, the model with no covariates. For the fitted model in Table 6.3, the value is

$$R_p^2 = 1 - \left(\exp\left\{ \left[\frac{2}{499} \right] \times \left[(-1211.3649) - (-1108.4149) \right] \right\} \right) = 0.36 .$$

R_p^2 has been suggested by Nagelkerke (1991). Two other measures that extend R_p^2 and are easy to calculate have been suggested by O'Quigley, Xu and Stare (2005) and Royston (2006). The measure suggested by O'Quigley et al. replaces n in R_p^2 by the number of events and is thus less dependent on the percentage of censored observations. This measure is termed "measure of explained randomness"

$$R_{p,e}^2 = 1 - \left\{ \exp\left[\frac{2}{m}(L_0 - L_p) \right] \right\} ,$$

where m is the number of events observed. To obtain a measure that more closely resembles the measure of explained variation for linear regression, Royston (2006) suggests using

$$R_{p,v}^2 = \frac{R_{p,e}^2}{R_{p,e}^2 + \frac{\pi^2}{6}\left(1 - R_{p,e}^2\right)} .$$

For the fitted model in Table 6.3, these two measures yield $R_{p,e}^2 = 0.65$ and $R_{p,v}^2 = 0.53$. This illustrates that different measures of explained variation or randomness can yield quite different values for the same model.

We are now in a position to discuss the interpretation of this model and how best to present the results to the audience of interest.

6.6 INTERPRETING AND PRESENTING RESULTS FROM THE FINAL MODEL

The model fit to the WHAS500 data, shown in Table 6.3, is reported again in Table 6.5. It is an excellent model for teaching purposes, as it contains examples of many of the complications that we are likely to encounter in practice. The model contains a simple dichotomous covariate (chf), two continuous linear covariates (hr and diasbp), a continuous non-linear covariate (bmi) and an interaction between a continuous and a dichotomous covariate (age and gender). In this section, when we refer to "the model", it is the one in Table 6.5.

We begin by discussing how to prepare point and interval estimates of hazard ratios for the covariates. Note that we have avoided including any exponentiated coefficients in tables of estimated coefficients in Chapters 5 and 6. While most software packages automatically provide these quantities, they are likely to be useful summary statistics for only a few model covariates. We feel it is best not to attempt estimating any hazard ratios until one has completed all steps in both model development and model checking (i.e., we want to be sure that the model fits, that it satisfies the proportional hazards assumption, and that any and all highly influential subjects have been dealt with in a scientifically appropriate manner).

Only the covariates for heart rate and diastolic blood pressure appear as linear main effects, and congestive heart problems is the only categorical covariate not involved in an interaction. As a result, these have hazard ratios that may be estimated by exponentiating their estimated coefficients. It is convenient to display these estimated hazard ratios and their confidence intervals in a table similar to Table 6.6.

The estimated hazard ratio for a 10-beat/min increase in heart rate is $1.13 = \exp(10 \times 0.012)$. This means that subjects with a 10-beat/min higher heart rate are dying at a 13 percent higher rate than are subjects at the lower heart rate. The 95 percent confidence interval in Table 6.6 suggests that an increased rate of dying as high as 20 percent or as little as a 7 percent is consistent with the data.

Table 6.5 Estimated Coefficients, Standard Errors, z-Scores, Two-Tailed p-values, and 95% Confidence Interval Estimates for the Final Proportional Hazards Model for the WHAS500 data, $n = 499$

Variable	Coeff.	Std. Err.	z	$p > |z|$	95% CIE
bmifp1	−0.685	0.1741	−3.94	<0.001	−1.026, −0.344
bmifp2	0.145	0.0395	3.66	<0.001	0.067, 0.222
age	0.060	0.0083	7.15	<0.001	0.043, 0.076
hr	0.012	0.0029	4.13	<0.001	0.006, 0.018
diasbp	−0.012	0.0035	−3.48	<0.001	−0.019, −0.005
gender	1.838	0.9579	1.92	0.055	−0.039, 3.716
chf	0.830	0.1469	5.65	<0.001	0.542, 1.118
age×gender	−0.027	0.0121	−2.28	0.023	−0.051, −0.004

Because the model is linear in heart rate, this interpretation holds over the observed range of heart rate.

The estimated hazard ratio for a 10-mm/Hg increase in diastolic blood pressure is $0.89 = \exp(10 \times -0.012)$. Thus, subjects with a 10-mm/Hg higher blood pressure are dying at a rate 11 percent lower than are subjects with lower blood pressure. The 95 percent confidence interval in Table 6.6 suggests that a decrease in the rate of dying could be as much as 17 percent or as little as 5 percent with 95 percent confidence. Because the model is linear in diastolic blood pressure, this interpretation holds over the observed range of diastolic blood pressure.

The estimated hazard ratio for congestive heart complications is $2.29 = \exp(0.830)$. Subjects who have congestive heart complications at study entry are dying at a rate 2.29 times higher than those subjects who do not have congestive heart complications. The 95 percent confidence interval in Table 6.6 indicates that the rate could actually be as much as a 3.06-fold or as little as a 1.72-fold increase in the rate of dying.

When a study is aimed at the effect of a single treatment or risk factor of interest, the hazard ratio is often presented for only this covariate, with the other covariates in the model relegated to footnote status. We feel that this is not good statistical or scientific practice. With such an oversimplified summary, the reader has no way of evaluating whether an appropriate model building and model checking paradigm has been followed or what the actual fitted model contains. We feel that the full model should be presented in a table similar to Table 6.5 at some point in the results section.

Age and gender are present in the model, with both main effects and their interaction. Because gender is dichotomous, we present hazard ratios for gender at various ages and then the hazard ratio for increasing age for each gender. The process is essentially the same for both. We first write the equation for the log hazard as a function of the variables of interest, holding all the others fixed,

$$g(age, gender, \mathbf{z}) = \beta_1 age + \beta_2 gender + \beta_3 age \times gender + \boldsymbol{\beta}'\mathbf{z},$$

Table 6.6 Estimated Hazard Ratios and 95% Confidence Interval Estimates for Heart Rate and Congestive Heart Complications for the WHAS500 Study, $n = 499$

Variable	Hazard Ratio	95% CIE
Heart Rate	1.13*	1.07, 1.20
Diastolic Blood Pressure	0.89'	0.83, 0.95
Congestive Heart Complications	2.29	1.72, 3.06

* Hazard ratio for a 10 beat/min increase.

Hazard ratio for a 10 mm/Hg increase.

Table 6.7 Estimated Hazard Ratios and 95% Confidence Interval Estimates for the Effect of Female Gender at the Stated Values of Age

Age	40	50	60	70	80	90
HR	2.13	1.63	1.24	0.95	0.72	0.55
95% CIE	(0.81, 5.45)	(0.77, 3.31)	(0.72, 2.04)	(0.65, 1.30)	(0.53, 0.93)	(0.36, 0.78)

where $\boldsymbol{\beta}'\mathbf{z}$ denotes the contribution to the log hazard of the other five model covariates.

We then write the expression for the difference of interest, in this case, female versus male with age fixed:

$$
\begin{aligned}
g\left(female, age = a, \boldsymbol{\beta}'\mathbf{z}\right) &- g\left(male, age = a, \boldsymbol{\beta}'\mathbf{z}\right) \\
&= \left(\beta_1 a + \beta_2 \times 1 + \beta_3 a \times 1 + \boldsymbol{\beta}'\mathbf{z}\right) \\
&\quad - \left(\beta_1 a + \beta_2 \times 0 + \beta_3 a \times 0 + \boldsymbol{\beta}'\mathbf{z}\right) \\
&= \beta_2 + \beta_3 a .
\end{aligned}
\tag{6.27}
$$

Next, choose a value for age, say 50, and estimate the hazard ratio using the exponentiated value of (6.27) with the estimated coefficient of gender from Table 6.5, $\hat{\beta}_2 = 1.838$, and the estimated coefficient of the interaction of age and gender, $\hat{\beta}_3 = -0.027$. The estimated hazard ratio at age 50 is

$$
\widehat{HR}\left(female \text{ versus } male, age = 50\right) = e^{1.838 - 0.027 \times 50} = 1.63 .
$$

The endpoints of the $100(1-\alpha)$ percent confidence interval estimator of the hazard ratio are computed by exponentiating the endpoints of the confidence interval of the estimator of (6.27), which are

$$
\hat{\beta}_2 + \hat{\beta}_3 a \pm z_{1-\alpha/2} \widehat{SE}\left(\hat{\beta}_2 + \hat{\beta}_3 a\right),
\tag{6.28}
$$

where

$$
\widehat{SE}\left(\hat{\beta}_2 + \hat{\beta}_3 a\right) = \left[
\begin{aligned}
&\widehat{Var}\left(\hat{\beta}_2\right) + a^2 \times \widehat{Var}\left(\hat{\beta}_3\right) \\
&+ 2a \times \widehat{Cov}\left(\hat{\beta}_2, \hat{\beta}_3\right)
\end{aligned}
\right]^{0.5} .
\tag{6.29}
$$

The values of the variances and covariance needed to compute the standard error are available from software packages. In this example, these are

$$\hat{\text{Va}}\text{r}\left(\hat{\beta}_2\right) = 0.91766349,$$

$$\hat{\text{Va}}\text{r}\left(\hat{\beta}_3\right) = 0.00014526,$$

and

$$\hat{\text{Co}}\text{v}\left(\hat{\beta}_2,\hat{\beta}_3\right) = -0.01141769.$$

We present many decimal places for the variances and covariance as a reminder that rounding should be done at the final step if values are calculated manually. Using these values, the 95 percent confidence interval at age 50 is $(0.77, 3.31)$. Confidence interval estimates at the other values of age in Table 6.7 are computed in a similar manner. Because the value 1.0 is contained in the confidence interval, the estimated increase in the rate of dying is not significant. The value 1.0 is also contained in all the confidence intervals for ages 40, 60, and 70. At age 80, the model estimates that females are dying at a rate 28 percent lower than males. The estimated decrease is significant, as 1.0 is not in the confidence interval and could be much as 47 percent or as little as 7 percent, with 95 percent confidence. By age 90, females are estimated to be dying at a rate 45 percent less than males. However, only 29 of the 499 subjects are 90 or older.

The results in Table 6.7 show that, by including the significant age by gender interaction in the model, we are able to refine the estimate of the gender effect to be significant only for age 80 or older. Had we not included this interaction, we would have incorrectly concluded that females have a significantly decreased rate at all ages (e.g., fit the main effect model in Table 5.9 excluding the subject with id number 416).

The estimated gender-specific hazard ratios for a 10-year increase in age are computed following the same procedure. For males the difference in the log hazards is

$$g(age = a + 10, male, \boldsymbol{\beta}'\mathbf{z}) - g(age = a, male, \boldsymbol{\beta}'\mathbf{z})$$
$$= \left(\beta_1(a+10) + \beta_2 \times 0 + \beta_3(a+10) \times 0 + \boldsymbol{\beta}'\mathbf{z}\right)$$
$$- \left(\beta_1 a + \beta_2 \times 0 + \beta_3 a \times 0 + \boldsymbol{\beta}'\mathbf{z}\right) = \beta_1 10.$$

For females the difference in the log hazard is

$$g(age = a + 10, female, \boldsymbol{\beta}'\mathbf{z}) - g(age = a, female, \boldsymbol{\beta}'\mathbf{z})$$
$$= \left(\beta_1(a+10) + \beta_2 \times 1 + \beta_3(a+10) \times 1 + \boldsymbol{\beta}'\mathbf{z}\right)$$
$$- \left(\beta_1 a + \beta_2 \times 1 + \beta_3 a \times 1 + \boldsymbol{\beta}'\mathbf{z}\right)$$
$$= \left(\beta_1 + \beta_3\right)10.$$

The estimated hazard ratios using the fitted model in Table 6.5 are $1.82 = \exp(0.060 \times 10)$ for males and $1.39 = \exp[(0.060 - 0.027) \times 10]$ for females. Because the hazard ratio for males only involves the main effect coefficient, the end points of its 95 percent confidence interval are easily obtained by multiplying the end points in Table 6.5 for the coefficient by 10 and then exponentiating, yielding the interval $(1.54, 2.14)$. The required standard error of the log hazard ratio for females is

$$\widehat{SE}\left[\left(\hat{\beta}_1 + \hat{\beta}_3\right) \times 10\right] = 10 \times \left[\widehat{Var}\left(\hat{\beta}_1\right) + \widehat{Var}\left(\hat{\beta}_3\right) + 2\widehat{Cov}\left(\hat{\beta}_1, \hat{\beta}_3\right)\right]^{0.5}.$$

The estimate of $\widehat{Var}\left(\hat{\beta}_3\right)$ is shown above and other estimates are $\widehat{Var}\left(\hat{\beta}_1\right) = 0.00006937$ and $\widehat{Cov}\left(\hat{\beta}_1, \hat{\beta}_3\right) = -0.00006033$. Using these values, the 95 percent confidence intervals are $(1.54, 2.14)$ for males and $(1.14, 1.67)$ for females.

This means, that for each 10-year increase in age, the rate of dying among males increases 1.82 fold; this increase could be as little as 1.54 fold or as much as 2.14 fold with 95 percent confidence. For females the effect of increasing age is less, 1.39 fold, but is still significant. In practice, the estimates and their confidence intervals could be included in a table similar to Table 6.6, in a separate table, or simply described in the results section. Whichever format is used, one must be sure to include the age increment in the presentation.

Body mass index is modeled with two non-linear terms, so any hazard ratio will depend on the values of body mass index being compared. The graph in Figure 5.3 of the log hazard using the two non-linear terms shows a decrease in the log hazard until the minimum is reached at about 31.5 kg/m^2 followed by an asymmetric increase. The most logical and informative presentation in this case would compare the hazard ratio relative to the minimum value. These hazard ratios could either be tabulated or presented graphically, along with their confidence limits. Both are illustrated here.

One must proceed carefully when calculating hazard ratios for nonlinear functions of a covariate. First, write down the expression for the log-hazard function, keeping all other covariates constant. For ease of presentation, let the log-hazard function computed at a particular value of body mass index, bmi, holding all other covariates fixed and denoted as $\mathbf{z}$, be

$$g(bmi, \mathbf{z}) = \beta_1 bmifp1 + \beta_2 bmifp2 + \boldsymbol{\beta}'\mathbf{z},$$

where

$$bmifp1 = (bmi/10)^2$$

and

$$bmifp2 = (bmi/10)^3.$$

The next step is to write down the equation for the difference of interest in the log hazard function. For any fixed value of bmi ($bmi = bmi_c$) it is

$$g(bmi = bmi_c, \mathbf{z}) - g(bmi = 31.5, \mathbf{z}) = a\beta_1 + b\beta_2,$$

where

$$a = (bmi_c/10)^2 - 9.9225$$

and

$$b = (bmi_c/10)^3 - 31.25588.$$

The estimator of the hazard ratio is

$$\widehat{HR}(bmi = bmi_c \text{ versus } bmi = 31.5) = e^{a\hat{\beta}_1 + b\hat{\beta}_2}. \tag{6.30}$$

The estimator of the endpoints of the $100(1-\alpha)$ percent confidence interval for the difference in the log-hazard functions is

$$\left(a\hat{\beta}_1 + b\hat{\beta}_2\right) \pm z_{1-\alpha/2}\widehat{SE}\left(a\hat{\beta}_1 + b\hat{\beta}_2\right), \tag{6.31}$$

where

$$\widehat{SE}\left(a\hat{\beta}_1 + b\hat{\beta}_2\right) = \left[a^2\widehat{Var}\left(\hat{\beta}_1\right) + b^2\widehat{Var}\left(\hat{\beta}_2\right) + 2ab\widehat{Cov}\left(\hat{\beta}_1, \hat{\beta}_2\right)\right]^{0.5}. \tag{6.32}$$

The estimators of the variances and covariance in (6.32) are obtained from output of the covariance matrix of the estimated coefficients from software packages. In the current example these values are $\widehat{Var}\left(\hat{\beta}_1\right) = 0.0303041$, $\widehat{Var}\left(\hat{\beta}_2\right) = 0.00156365$, and $\widehat{Cov}\left(\hat{\beta}_1, \hat{\beta}_2\right) = -0.0068076$. The endpoints of the confidence interval estimator for the hazard ratio are obtained by exponentiating the estimators in (6.31).

We calculated the value of the hazard ratio in (6.30) for the entire range of bmi and have graphed it, along with its 95 percent confidence bands, in Figure 6.9. One subject with $bmi = 44.84$ is excluded from the plot, as the upper confidence limit is 16.3, which when included, greatly distorts the appearance of the plot and hinders interpretation.

The plot in Figure 6.9 clearly demonstrates that, in the WHAS500 data, the rate of dying relative to the model-based minimum at 31.5 decreases and then in creases in an asymmetric manner. While difficult to see in Figure 6.9 a listing of the values shows that 1.0 is contained in the confidence limits for body mass index between the values of 26.9 and 39.9. Thus, there is a significant increase in the rate of dying for body mass index less than 26.9 and greater than 39.9.

The plot in Figure 6.9 provides an easily understood description of the overall change in the estimated hazard ratios. However, it is not possible to read details at specific values of body mass index; for this we need a table. As an example, we show in Table 6.8 the estimated hazard ratios and 95 percent confidence limits for selected values of body mass index. The results in Table 6.8 show that a body mass index of 20 or less increases by more than two-fold the estimated rate of dy ing compared with a body mass index of 31.5. Results similar to those in Figure 6.9 and Table 6.8 can easily be obtained using a different referent value, for exam ple 25.0, by replacing 31.5 in all expressions with the new value.

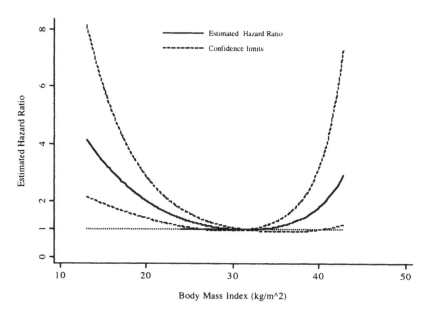

Figure 6.9 Estimated hazard ratio and 95 percent confidence bands comparing each value of body mass index to the model-based minimum-risk value of 31.5 with a referent line at 1.0 added for interpretation.

Before moving on, we want to emphasize the fact that, in this section, we have had to describe both the calculation and interpretation of the estimated hazard ratios. In practice, the estimated hazard ratios and their confidence intervals would likely be tabulated or graphed with no computational details presented and thus lend themselves to a discussion with more continuity than was possible here. However, for a complicated nonlinear variable like the body mass index, inclusion of an appendix providing an outline of how the graphed (or tabulated) hazard ratios and their confidence intervals have been computed can be a helpful addition to a paper.

We also note that we were somewhat surprised that the lowest hazard ratio was estimated to occur for a body mass index of 31.5. Individuals with a body mass index of 30 or larger are considered obese (underweight if bmi < 18.5, normal weight if $18.5 \le$ bmi < 25, overweight if $25 \le$ bmi < 30) and would typically not be at reduced risk for most health outcomes. This particular sample might be biased because body mass index was not recorded on all patients and thus a selection bias could have occurred. Nevertheless, the non-linearity in the log hazard of bmi provides a good example of how to detect and model non-linearity.

We conclude our presentation of the fitted model in Table 6.5 with graphs of the covariate-adjusted survival functions. In the WHAS500 data, no one variable can be regarded as the most important risk factor. Thus, with these data, we might choose to provide covariate adjusted survival functions at various quantiles of the risk score, as illustrated in Figure 4.7. However, for demonstration purposes we consider an example of plotting that is a bit more complicated than that of a dichotomous covariate. Suppose that we would like the covariate adjusted survival functions for 72-year-old males and 72-year-old females. Because the model is complicated and includes the gender-by-age interaction, it is not clear what we could use for a mean or median subject, so we use the modified risk score method discussed in Section 4.3 and illustrated in (4.28) and (4.29). The modified risk score is calculated for each subject as

$$r\hat{m}_i = \hat{r}_i - 0.060 \times age_i - 1.838 \times gender_i - (-0.027) \times age_i \times gender_i$$

and the median is $r\hat{m}_{50} = -1.75464$. The plotted points for the covariate-adjusted survival function for 72-year-old males are

Table 6.8 Estimated Hazard Ratios and 95% Confidence Interval Estimates for the Effect of Body Mass Index (BMI) Compared with Body Mass Index = 31.5

BMI	15	20	25	30	35	40
HR	3.38	1.99	1.29	1.02	1.09	1.78
95% CIE	(1.90, 6.03)	(1.39, 2.85)	(1.07, 1.55)	(0.97, 1.07)	(0.93, 1.29)	(1.00, 3.17)

$$\hat{S}\left(t_i, \hat{rm}_{50}, age = 72, male\right) = \left[\hat{S}_0\left(t_i\right)\right]^{\exp(-1.175464 + 0.060 \times 72)}$$

and for 72-year-old-females they are

$$\hat{S}\left(t_i, \hat{rm}_{50}, age = 72, female\right) = \left[\hat{S}_0\left(t_i\right)\right]^{\exp(-1.75464 + 0.060 \times 72 + 1.838 \times 1 - 0.027 \times 72 \times 1)} .$$

Graphs of these two functions are shown in Figure 6.10 over the first 6 years of follow up. The survival functions in Figure 6.10 are consistent with the estimated hazard ratios in Table 6.7, which indicate a slightly reduced and not significant rate of dying at age 72. Actual calculation shows that the estimated hazard ratio at 72 years is 0.87, or a 13 percent reduction in the rate of dying. The curves are each plotted over the same subjects and are constrained to have this hazard ratio at all plotted values.

The modified risk score adjusted 75th percentiles may be estimated, albeit crudely, from the plots in Figure 6.10 or from a time-sorted list of the functions. The values are 1.92 years for 72-year-old females and 1.5 years for 72-year-old males. As noted in Section 4.5, there is no easily computed confidence interval for

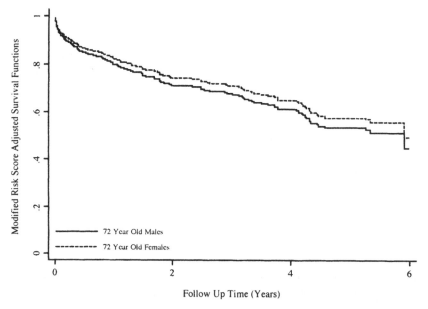

Figure 6.10 Graphs of the modified risk score adjusted survival functions for 72-year-old males and 72-year-old females using the fitted model in Table 6.5.

the estimator of the percentiles time from a modified risk-score-adjusted survival function.

In conclusion, the fitted model, shown in Table 6.5, has allowed description of a number of interesting relationships between time to death following an admission to the hospital after an MI and patient characteristics on admission. The notable results include significant effects due to heart rate, diastolic blood pressure, and congestive heart complications, differential effects of age within each gender, differential effect of gender for age, and the nonlinear effect of the body mass index.

In the next chapter, we consider alternative methods for modeling study covariates. These methods are of interest in themselves, but they also provide alternatives to models that are inadequate due to poor fit or violations of the proportional hazards assumption.

EXERCISES

1. Using WHAS100 data, assess the fit of the proportional hazards model containing age, body mass index, gender, and the age-by-gender interaction. This assessment of fit should include the following steps: evaluation of the proportional hazards assumption for each covariate, examination of diagnostic statistics, and an overall test of fit. If the model does not fit or adhere to the proportional hazards assumption what would you do next? Note: the goal is to obtain a model to estimate the effect of each covariate.

2. Using the model obtained at the conclusion of Problem 1, present a table of estimated hazard ratios, with confidence intervals. Present graphs of the modified risk score adjusted survival functions at the three quartiles $(25^{th}, 50^{th}, and 75^{th})$ of body mass index. Use the estimated survival functions to estimate the median survival time for each of the three risk groups

3. In Section 6.4 diagnostic statistics were plotted and 10 subjects, shown in Table 6.2, were identified as being possibly influential. Fit the model shown in Table 6.5, deleting these subjects one at a time and then, collectively, calculate the percentage change in all coefficients with each deletion. Do you agree or disagree with the conclusion to delete subject 416? Explain the rationale for your decision.

4. An alternative model considered but not used in Section 5.2 is one that contains an age-by-congestive heart problem interaction in place of the age-by-gender interaction. Perform all the model evaluation and fit steps performed in problem 1 on the alternative model.

5. Repeat problem 2 using the model from problem 5.

6. Repeat problems 1 and 2 for the ACTG320 model from Problem 2 in Chapter 5. Plot modified risk score adjusted survival functions for the two levels of treatment.

CHAPTER 7

Extensions of the Proportional Hazards Model

7.1 INTRODUCTION

Up to this point, we have made several simplifying assumptions in developing and interpreting proportional hazards models. We have used a model with a common unspecified baseline hazard function where all the study covariates had values that remained fixed over the follow-up period. Additionally, we have assumed that the observations of the time variable were continuous and subject only to right censoring. In some settings, one or more of these assumptions may not be appropriate.

We may have data from a study in which subjects were randomized within study sites. If we account for site by including it as a covariate, the model forces the baseline hazards to be proportional across study sites. This may not be justified and, if it is not, a careful analysis of the proportional hazards assumption (as discussed in Chapter 6) for site may reveal the problem. One possible solution is to use site as a stratification variable, whereby each site would have a separate baseline hazard function. This same line of thought might apply to cohort year in the Worcester Heart Attack Study. Also, stratification can sometimes be employed with fixed covariates that, on testing, show evidence of non-proportional hazards.

When study subjects are observed on a regular basis during the follow-up period, the course of some covariates over time may be more predictive of survival experience than were the original baseline values. For example, continued survival of intensive care unit patients may depend more on changes in covariates that measure their physiologic condition since admission than on their values at admission. Covariates whose values change over time are commonly called *time-varying* or *time-dependent* covariates. These may include measurements on individual subjects or measurements that record study conditions and apply to a number of study subjects.

Suppose that, in the process of model checking, we determine that the hazard function is non-proportional in one or more of the covariates. We may include in the model an explicit function of the covariate and time, which is essentially the test for non-proportional hazards described in Chapter 6. In some settings, this may provide a useful solution to the problem. A similar approach is to partition the time axis and to fit different functional forms for the covariate within time intervals. We could use the smoothed plots of the scaled Schoenfeld residuals to identify the intervals where the "slope" was the same. In general, we would not attempt such an analysis unless there was strong evidence for it from subject matter considerations, statistical tests, and plots of the type discussed in Chapter 6.

While right censoring is by far the most frequently encountered censoring mechanism, there may be settings in which incomplete observations arise from other types of censoring. Thus, it may be necessary to model the data taking into account a variety of different censoring patterns.

In settings in which subjects are not under continual observation, but rather their follow-up status is determined at "fixed" intervals, another problem may arise. For example, if we are studying survival of patients admitted to a coronary intensive care unit who were discharged alive, we may contact subjects at 3-month intervals. All that may be known on the subjects is their vital status at these interval points, and the recorded values of time would be 3, 6, 12, and so on. Such data are highly discrete and, in this setting, we should consider using an extension of the proportional hazards model designed to handle interval censored data.

These and other topics that extend the basic proportional hazards model are discussed in some detail in this chapter. We begin with the stratified proportional hazards model.

7.2 THE STRATIFIED PROPORTIONAL HAZARDS MODEL

The rationale for creating a stratified proportional hazards model is the same as that for other stratified analyses. We assume there are variables known to affect the outcome, but we consider obtaining estimates of their effects to be of secondary importance to those of other covariates. These covariates might be fixed by the design of the study or they might have been identified in earlier analyses. For example, in the Worcester Heart Attack Study, patients are identified by the calendar year of their admission. In previous chapters, we ignored cohort year. The stratified proportional hazards model is also sometimes used to accommodate non-proportional hazards in a covariate.[1]

The stratified proportional hazards model is, in spirit, quite similar to the one used in a matched logistic regression analysis [see Hosmer and Lemeshow (2000, Chapter 7)]. The effect of all covariates whose values are constant within each

---

[1]Note that, if the hazard function for a continuous covariate has been identified as being nonproportional using the methods in Chapter 6, one could create a grouped or categorized version of the covariate, treat it as if it were a nominal scale covariate, and stratify on it.

stratum is incorporated into a stratum-specific baseline hazard function. The effects of other covariates may be modeled either with a constant slope across strata or with different slopes. For example, in the model developed for the WHAS500 data in Chapters 5, we assumed that covariate effects were constant over cohort years. Because cohort year is not of interest by itself, we could stratify on it and then include cohort year by covariate interactions to determine whether there is evidence of a change in effect over calendar years. In general, this modeling decision, based on the slopes being equal or unequal, may be made based on subject matter considerations or by using the methods for selecting interactions discussed in Chapter 5.

We now describe the stratified proportional hazards model using constant slopes. We note that the non-constant slopes model may be handled simply by specifying an interaction between one of the covariates and the stratification variable. The proportional hazard function for stratum s is

$$h_s(t,\mathbf{x},\boldsymbol{\beta}) = h_{s0}(t)e^{\mathbf{x}'\boldsymbol{\beta}}, \qquad (7.1)$$

where we assume there are $s = 1, 2, \ldots, S$ strata. In the WHAS500 data, there are $S = 3$ strata denoting the three years data were collected.

Hazard ratios are computed using the estimated coefficients and apply to each stratum. For example, in a stratified model, suppose that the estimated coefficient for a dichotomous covariate is $\ln(2)$, hence the stratum-specific estimated hazard ratio is 2. The interpretation of this hazard ratio is the same as in the unstratified model, that is, the hazard rate in the $x = 1$ group is twice the hazard rate in the $x = 0$ group, and this interpretation applies to each stratum.

The form of the partial likelihood for the sth stratum is identical to the partial likelihood used in earlier chapters, see (3.19), but it includes an additional subscript, s, indicating the stratum. The contribution to the partial likelihood for the sth stratum is

$$l_{sp}(\boldsymbol{\beta}) = \prod_{i=1}^{n_s}\left[\frac{e^{\mathbf{x}'_{si}\boldsymbol{\beta}}}{\sum_{j \in R(t_{si})} e^{\mathbf{x}'_{sj}\boldsymbol{\beta}}}\right]^{c_{si}}, \qquad (7.2)$$

where n_s denotes the number of observations in the sth stratum, t_{si} denotes the ith observed value of time in the sth stratum, c_{si} is the value of the 0/1 censoring variable associated with t_{si}, $R(t_{si})$ denotes the subjects in stratum s in the risk set at time t_{si}, and $\mathbf{x}_{si}$ is the vector of p covariates. The full stratified partial likelihood, is obtained by multiplying the contributions to the likelihood, namely

$$l_{Sp}(\boldsymbol{\beta}) = \prod_{s=1}^{S} l_{sp}(\boldsymbol{\beta}). \tag{7.3}$$

The subscript s is used in (7.3) to differentiate the stratified partial likelihood from the unstratified partial likelihood, $l_p(\boldsymbol{\beta})$, used in previous chapters. The maximum stratified partial likelihood estimator of the parameter vector, $\boldsymbol{\beta}$, is obtained by solving the p equations obtained by differentiating the log of (7.3) with respect to the p unknown parameters and setting the derivatives equal to zero. We do not provide these equations because they are quite similar in form to those in (3.31). The only difference is that the weighted risk set covariate means are based on the data within each stratum. The estimator of the covariance matrix of the estimated coefficients is obtained from the inverse of the observed information matrix in a manner similar to the unstratified setting, see (3.32)–(3.34).

The general steps in model building and assessment are the same for the stratified model as for the unstratified model, the only difference is that the stratified analysis is based on the partial likelihood in (7.3). The stratified analysis of the WHAS500 data using year as a stratification variable would require that we repeat all the steps in Chapters 5 and 6 relevant to model building and assessment. Repeating these steps would not demonstrate anything new. While providing a convenient conceptual example, a fit of the model in Table 6.3 stratifying on year yields estimated coefficients that differ by less than 10 percent from the estimates in Table 6.3. Hence, little would be gained by further consideration of the WHAS500 data. Instead we turn to the ACTG320 study.

Using the purposeful selection paradigm in Chapter 5, we obtain a model containing the following covariates in Table 1.5: treatment indicator (tx), IV drug history dichotomized (ivdrug_d: 0 = never, 1 = ever), two design variables for Karnofsky performance scale using the value of 100 as the reference and pooling the subjects in the two categories $karnof = 70$ and $karnof = 80$ as only 32 subjects have a value of 70, age, and CD4 count. There is no evidence of non-linearity in the log hazard for age and CD4 count. Also, there are no significant interactions among the model covariates. Checking the assumption of a proportional hazard for each model covariate shows that there is some evidence of a non-proportional hazard in CD4 with p-values ranging from 0.07 to 0.12 for the four tests discussed in Section 6.3. The effect of CD4 count on survival among AIDS patients is well known. In these data, we do not have continuing measures of CD4 count, only its value at baseline. Thus we create a categorical variable, based on the observed CD4 quartiles, and stratify on it. While the categorical variable is constant within strata, the measured values are not. Thus, we could include CD4 in the stratified model as well. When it is included, its estimated coefficient is not significant with a Wald test $p = 0.22$. The results of the fitted stratified model are shown in Table 7.1.

Table 7.1 Estimated Coefficients, Standard Errors, z-Scores, Two-Tailed p-values, and 95% Confidence Intervals for the Proportional Hazards Model Stratified by CD4 Quartile for the ACTG320 data $(n = 1151)$

Variable	Coeff.	Std. Err.	z	$p > |z|$	95% CIE
tx	−0.668	0.2155	−3.10	0.002	−1.090, −0.245
ivdrug_d	−0.546	0.3226	−1.69	0.090	−1.179, 0.086
karnof_70_80	1.191	0.2963	4.02	<0.001	0.610, 1.772
karnof_90	0.412	0.2927	1.41	0.159	−0.162, 0.986
age	0.022	0.0112	2.01	0.045	0.001, 0.044

Log-likelihood = −506.7552

After a stratified model has been fit, the methods described in Section 3.5 may be used to estimate stratum-specific baseline survival functions. These functions may then be used to estimate covariate-adjusted, stratum-specific, survival functions using the methods described in Section 4.5.

In the current example, we denote the estimators of the stratum-specific baseline survival function as $\hat{S}_{s0}(t)$, $s = 1, 2, 3, 4$ because CD4 was coded into quartiles. The fitted model in Table 7.1 is modestly complicated; we choose to use the modified risk score approach to obtain graphs to describe the effect of treatment within each stratum [see (4.30)–(4.31)]. Because this estimate is to be made within strata, and because the distribution of the risk score could be different across strata, we favor using stratum-specific median modified risk scores. The median values, based on the fitted model in Table 7.1, are $\hat{rm}_{1\,50} = 1.2176$ for quartile 1, $\hat{rm}_{2\,50} = 1.1761$ for quartile 2, $\hat{rm}_{3\,50} = 1.0862$ for quartile 3, and $\hat{rm}_{450} = 1.0937$ for quartile 4.

It follows that the estimators for the stratum-specific modified risk-score-adjusted survival functions for the two treatments within each stratum are described by the equations

$$\hat{S}(t, Stratum = s, \text{tx} = 0, \hat{rm}_{s50}) = \left[\hat{S}_{s0}(t)\right]^{\exp(\hat{rm}_{s50})} \qquad (7.4)$$

and

$$\hat{S}(t, Stratum = s, \text{tx} = 1, \hat{rm}_{s50}) = \left[\hat{S}_{s0}(t)\right]^{\exp[\hat{rm}_{s50} + (-0.668)]}, \qquad (7.5)$$

where $\hat{rm}_{s50}$ is the value of the median modified risk score within stratum s and −0.668 is the estimated coefficient of treatment from Table 7.1.

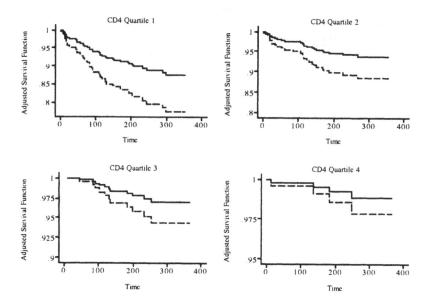

Figure 7.1 Graphs of the stratum-specific modified risk-score-adjusted survival functions for control (---) and treatment (——). Note the differences in scales.

In Figure 7.1 we present the graphs of the treatment by stratum-modified risk-score-adjusted survival functions. The range of the estimated survival functions is different for each stratum and the scales have been adjusted accordingly. In each of the four figures, the lower function corresponds to the modified risk-score-adjusted survival function for the control treatment while the upper curve is that of the "treatment," which is the same as the control plus IDV (see Section 1.6). The distance between the two curves for each stratum is such that the estimated hazard ratio for treatment versus control is

$$\hat{HR} = \exp(-0.668) = 0.51$$

with a 95 percent confidence interval estimate of $(0.336, 0.782)$. Thus the that inclusion of IDV reduces the rate of death and/or time to AIDS diagnosis by almost 50 percent; the reduction could be as little as 22 percent or as much as 66 percent with 95 percent confidence.

The modified risk-adjusted survival functions may be used in the same manner illustrated in Section 6.6 to obtain estimates of adjusted quantiles of time to death or AIDS diagnosis. Because the ranges are different within each stratum and none include even the 75th percentile, one would question the value of this application in this example.

As we have noted, the stratified proportional hazards model may be the best model to use in a setting in which covariates have values fixed by the design of the study. As we illustrate with the ACTG320 data, using a stratified analysis can provide the possibility for a simple solution to non-proportional hazards in a covariate. In all cases, one must pay attention to the number of observations and survival times within each stratum. Small numbers within any stratum will result in an estimated baseline survival function with greater variance than the estimates from strata with more data. However, the variance of the estimates of the coefficients in a stratified model is, as before, a function of the total sample size and total number of survival times.

7.3 TIME-VARYING COVARIATES

Until now we have assumed that the values of all covariates were determined at the point when follow-up began on each subject (time zero) and that these values did not change over the period of observation. There may be situations where one or more of the covariates are measured during the period of follow up and their values change. In these settings, it may be the case that the value of the hazard for the event depends more on the current values of these covariates than on their values at time zero.

It is not difficult to generalize the proportional hazards regression model and its partial likelihood to include time-varying covariates. However, from a conceptual point of view, the model becomes much more complicated, and one should give serious consideration to the nature of any time-varying covariate before including it in the model. Specifically, one must pay close attention to the definition of when the analysis time is zero (i.e., when the "clock starts"), because the start of analysis time may occur at different calendar times for different subjects. However, the value of any time-varying covariate must depend only on study time, not on calendar time. Another concern is the potential to overfit a model when using time-varying covariates. In all instances, inclusion of time-varying covariates should be based on strong clinical evidence. One of the earliest applications of the use of time-varying covariates in a biomedical setting may be found in Crowley and Hu's (1977) analysis of the Stanford heart transplant data. In a summary paper, Andersen (1992) illustrates the use of time-varying covariates in several examples and discusses some of the problems we may encounter when including them in a model. Fisher and Lin (1999) also provide illustrations of the use of time-varying covariates and discuss related conceptual issues and potential problems and biases. Collett (2002) and Marubini and Valsecchi (1995) discuss time-varying covariates at a level comparable to this text, while Fleming and Harrington (1991), Andersen, Borgan, Gill and Keiding (1993) and Kalbfleisch and Prentice (2002) present the topic from the counting process point of view.

Time-varying (or time-dependent) covariates are usually classified as being either *internal* or *external*. An internal time-varying covariate is one whose value is subject-specific and requires that the subject be under periodic observation. For example, consider a clinical trial for a new cancer treatment in which the endpoint is death from the cancer. Suppose that we have a covariate measured at baseline, but whose value can change over time. It may be the case that the hazard depends on a more recent value than on the baseline value. For values of this covariate to be measured during the follow up period, the subjects in this study must be under direct observation. In contrast, an external time-varying covariate is one whose value at a particular time does not require subjects to be under direct observation. Typically, these covariates are study or environmental factors that apply to all subjects under observation. For example, consider a study of a new medication for relief from symptoms of hay fever in which the time variable for the outcome records the number of hours until self-perceived relief from symptoms. In this study, an example of an external covariate is the average hourly pollen count. A subject-specific external covariate is the subject's age. If we follow subjects for a long enough period of time, their current age may have more of an effect on survival than their age when the study began. However, once we know a subject's birth date, age may be computed at any point in time, regardless of whether the subject is still under observation. Another important external time-varying covariate is time itself. We made extensive use of this time-varying covariate in Chapter 6, where it was used to test the assumption of proportional hazards in fixed covariates via the inclusion of the interactions of the form $x \times g(t)$ in the model. In the remainder of this section, we will not differentiate between internal and external time-varying covariates.

The reader might wonder why neither age nor analysis time were modeled as a time-varying covariate in previous chapters. Age and analysis time advance in parallel if linear functions of age (or analysis time) are considered. If we were to include age as a time-varying covariate, the estimate of its effect would not change because any effects relating to the advancement of age would be "absorbed" into the baseline hazard function.

We need to generalize the notation to include time-varying covariates in the model. Let $x(t)$ denote the value of the covariate x measured at time t. Assume, as we have up to this point, that we have adjusted each subject's follow-up time to begin at zero as opposed to using real or calendar time. Thus, we assume that t determines the value of $x(t)$ even though the same t may arise from different calendar times. For example, suppose we define a time-varying covariate as the length of stay in a hospital. Subject 1 may be admitted to a hospital on May 1 and stay in the hospital for 60 days. Subject 2 may be admitted to a hospital on July 1 and also stay in the hospital for 60 days. It is important that both subjects were in the hospital for 60 days, not that they were admitted at different times. To include such a covariate in the partial likelihood [(3.19) or (3.20)] and their multivariable equivalents, we need to account for the subject as well as for the specific time. Let $x_l(t_i)$ denote the value of the covariate for subject l at time t_i. To allow for multiple covariates, we let $x_{lk}(t_i)$, $k = 1, 2, \ldots, p$ denote the value of the kth covariate for subject l at time t_i and denote the vector of covariates as

$$\mathbf{x}_l'(t_i) = \left[x_{l1}(t_i), x_{l2}(t_i), \ldots, x_{lp}(t_i) \right]. \tag{7.6}$$

The notation in (7.6) is completely general in the sense that, if a particular covariate, x_k, is fixed (i.e., not time-varying) then

$$x_{lk}(t_i) = x_{lk}(t = 0) = x_{lk}$$

and this has led some authors, for example, Andersen, Borgan, Gill and Keiding (1993), to use the time-dependent notation in (7.6) exclusively. The generalization of the proportional hazards regression function (3.7) to include possibly multiple time-varying covariates is

$$h(t, \mathbf{x}(t), \boldsymbol{\beta}) = h_0(t) \exp\left[\mathbf{x}'(t) \boldsymbol{\beta} \right]. \tag{7.7}$$

Because the hazard function in (7.7) may depend on time in ways other than through the baseline hazard function, it is no longer proportional in the same way as when only baseline covariates are used. In most settings where time-varying covariates are included, the model will also contain fixed covariates (e.g., gender). Suppose we have a model containing the subject's blood pressure at time t, denoted $x_1(t)$ and gender denoted x_2. The hazard function for this model is, from (7.7),

$$h(t, \mathbf{x}(t), \boldsymbol{\beta}) = h_0(t) \exp\left[x_1(t)\beta_1 + x_2\beta_2 \right].$$

The hazard ratio for gender is

$$\text{HR}(t, x_2 = 1, x_2 = 0 \mid x_1(t)) = \frac{h_0(t) \exp\left[x_1(t)\beta_1 + \beta_2 \right]}{h_0(t) \exp\left[x_1(t)\beta_1 \right]},$$
$$= \exp(\beta_2)$$

which does not depend on time. So in a sense, the hazard has a proportionality property, but the component relating to time is $h_0(t) \exp\left[x_1(t)\beta_1 \right]$. This difference has led some authors [e.g., Collett (2003)] to drop the term "proportional" when using the model in (7.7). However, we think this might confuse the reader and, as a result, we will continue to call it the proportional hazards model because it is still proportional to a function of time, albeit one potentially much more complicated than the baseline hazard function.

A serious bias can occur when we include a time-varying covariate in the model, and the effect of a treatment on the outcome is mediated by this time-varying covariate. For example, blood pressure varies over time and could be a mediator of the effect of the treatment on outcome. In this case, inclusion of blood pressure as a time-varying covariate might bias our estimate of treatment effect because we may fail to identify a treatment effect, even if it were present. This potential problem also illustrates why modeling of time-varying covariates can be conceptually complicated.

An important assumption of the model in (7.7) is that the time-varying covariate effect, as measured by its coefficient, does not depend on time. Models with time-varying coefficients are discussed in the context of additive models in Chapter 9.

The generalization of the partial likelihood function in (3.19) is

$$l_p(\boldsymbol{\beta}) = \prod_{i=1}^{n} \left[\frac{e^{\mathbf{x}_i'(t_{(i)})\boldsymbol{\beta}}}{\displaystyle\sum_{l \in R(t_{(i)})} e^{\mathbf{x}_l'(t_{(i)})\boldsymbol{\beta}}} \right]^{c_i} . \tag{7.8}$$

The estimators of the coefficients and their associated standard errors are obtained in a manner identical to the one described in Chapter 3, using (7.8) in place of (3.19) and (3.20). Often the biggest problem in practice is the data management necessary to describe to the software the values of the time-varying covariates. We strongly suggest that, before data collection actually begins, one consult with experts in data management for whatever software package is going to be used for model development. There is considerable variability among software packages with respect to the ease with which time-varying covariates are handled.

We illustrate modeling a time-varying covariate with two examples. The first comes from the UMARU Impact Study (UIS) described in Section 1.3 and Table 1.3. These data were used extensively in the first edition of this text. In this study, subjects were randomized to one of two residential treatment programs of different durations that were designed to prevent return to drug use. Subjects were free to leave the program at any time, and the time to event was self-reported return to drug use. We discovered that treatment appeared to have a time dependent effect. We hypothesized that the treatment effect may simply be housing a subject where he/she has no access to drugs. Here, for purposes of illustrating a time varying covariate, we begin with a univariable model containing treatment. Although we don't present the detailed results here, the estimated hazard ratio from a fit of this model for the longer versus the shorter duration of treatment is 0.79 (95 percent confidence limits are 0.67, 0.94). Based on this model, we would conclude that longer duration of treatment significantly reduces the rate of returning to drug use. To examine the "under treatment" hypothesis, we create a time-varying dichotomous subject specific time varying covariate OFF_TRT(t), where

$$OFF\_TRT(t) = \begin{cases} 0 \text{ if } t \le LOT \\ 1 \text{ if } t > LOT \end{cases},$$

where LOT stands for the number of days the subject was on treatment. For example, consider one of the terms in (7.8) and suppose the survival time indexing the risk set is 30 days. Subjects in the risk set would have $OFF\_TRT(30) = 0$ if their value of LOT is greater than 30, meaning that after 30 days of follow-up they were still in a treatment facility. Once the length of follow-up, t, exceeds the duration of treatment, LOT, a subject is "off treatment" and the value of OFF_TRT changes to one and remains at one as long as they are being followed. There is a considerable amount of computation involved when fitting a model with time-varying covariates. Not only must the composition of each risk set be determined, the actual values of the time-varying covariates also need to be computed. In the first edition of this text, we fit a model containing treatment and $OFF\_TRT(t)$. To provide a different example using these data, we fit a model containing $TREAT$, $OFF\_TRT(t)$ and their interaction. The results of this fit are shown in Table 7.2.

The results in Table 7.2 demonstrate a dramatic effect due to the time-varying covariate, $OFF\_TRT(t)$. We note that all three coefficients are significant. With the inclusion of the time-varying covariate and its interaction with treatment assignment, we must proceed carefully when estimating a hazard ratio. The log-hazard for the fitted model is

Table 7.2 Estimated Coefficients, Standard Errors, z-Scores, Two-Tailed p-values, and 95% Confidence Intervals for the Model Adding the Time-Varying Covariate OFF_TRT to Model Containing Treatment ($n = 628$)

Variable	Coeff.	Std. Err.	z	$p > \lvert z \rvert$	95% CIE
TREAT	−0.524	0.2258	−2.32	0.020	−0.967, −0.081
OFF_TRT	2.270	0.1865	12.17	<0.001	1.905, 2.636
TREATxOFF_TRT	0.621	0.2463	2.52	0.012	0.138, 1.104

$$\ln\{h[t, TREAT, OFF\_TRT(t)]\} = \ln[h_0(t)] + \hat{\beta}_1 TREAT + \hat{\beta}_2 OFF\_TRT(t)$$
$$+ \hat{\beta}_3 TREAT \times OFF\_TRT(t).$$

Using this model, we can estimate four different hazards ratios: the effect of treatment assignment for subjects who are still under treatment and those off treatment and the effect of going off treatment within treatment assignment.

The log hazard ratio at time t for the effect of treatment assignment, $TREAT = 1$ vs, $TREAT = 0$, among those still on the treatment program, $OFF\_TRT(t) = 0$, is

$$\ln\left\{\widehat{HR}\left[t, TREAT = 1, TREAT = 0 | OFF\_TRT(t) = 0\right]\right\}$$
$$= \ln\left\{h[t, TREAT = 1, OFF\_TRT(t) = 0]\right\}$$
$$- \ln\left\{h[t, TREAT = 0, OFF\_TRT(t) = 0]\right\}$$
$$= \left\{\ln[h_0(t)] + \hat{\beta}_1 \times 1 + \hat{\beta}_2 \times 0 + \hat{\beta}_3 \times 0 \times 1\right\}$$
$$- \left\{\ln[h_0(t)] + \hat{\beta}_1 \times 0 + \hat{\beta}_2 \times 0 + \hat{\beta}_3 \times 0 \times 0\right\}$$
$$= \hat{\beta}_1 \ .$$

We obtain expressions for the other three log hazard ratios by evaluating the respective differences in the log hazards. The log hazard at time t comparing treatment assignment, long versus short, for subjects off treatment is

$$\ln\left\{\widehat{HR}\left[t, TREAT = 1, TREAT = 0 | OFF\_TRT(t) = 1\right]\right\} = \hat{\beta}_1 + \hat{\beta}_3 .$$

The log hazard at time t comparing subjects on and off treatment within the shorter treatment, $TREAT = 0$, is

$$\ln\left\{\widehat{HR}\left[t, OFF\_TRT(t) = 1, OFF\_TRT(t) = 0 | TREAT = 0\right]\right\} = \hat{\beta}_2 .$$

The log hazard at time t for subjects on the longer treatment, $TREAT = 1$, is

$$\ln\left\{\widehat{HR}\left[t, OFF\_TRT(t) = 1, OFF\_TRT(t) = 0 | TREAT = 1\right]\right\} = \hat{\beta}_2 + \hat{\beta}_3 .$$

The four estimated hazard ratios and their 95 percent confidence limits are shown in Table 7.3.

Table 7.3 Estimated Hazard Ratios and 95% Confidence Limit Estimates (CIE) for the Effect of Treatment and Being Off or On Treatment

Hazard Ratio for	Within Those	$\hat{\text{HR}}$	95% CIE
Long vs. Short	On Treatment	0.59	0.380, 0.922
Treatment Assignment	Off Treatment	1.10	0.910, 1.335
Off vs. On	Shorter Tx Duration	9.68	6.718, 13.955
Treatment	Longer Tx Duration	18.02	12.055, 26.927

The results in Table 7.3 show that, among subjects still on treatment, those randomized to the longer of the two treatments are returning to drug use 41 percent less than subjects randomized to the shorter treatment, and this decrease is significant. Once subjects leave active treatment, there is no significant difference between the rate of returning to drug use for the longer and shorter durations of treatment. The effect of leaving treatment significantly increases the rate of returning to drug use within both levels of treatment assignment. Because the interaction effect in Table 7.2 is significant, we know that the estimated hazard ratios of 9.68 and 18.02 are significantly different.

In summary, by using a time-varying covariate that measures whether a subject has left the treatment program, we are able to obtain a much clearer picture of when the longer duration treatment is effective in reducing the rate of return to drug use as well as how the rate of return to drug use increases once subjects leave active treatment. We see clearly that this increase depends on treatment assignment. Interpretations and conclusions comparing $TREAT = 1$ versus $TREAT = 0$ do not depend on a particular value of follow up time. Instead, the value presented (i.e., the hazard ratio) is appropriate for the stated comparison (i.e., at a value of follow up time where subjects in the two programs are actively in treatment).

The stated interpretations and conclusions comparing $OFF\_TRT(t) = 1$ versus $OFF\_TRT(t) = 0$ require that the comparison is made for the same time t. If all patients were on treatment for exactly the same length of time and thus would go off treatment at exactly the same time, there would be no time point for which $OFF\_TRT(t) = 1$ for some patients and $OFF\_TRT(t) = 0$ for other patients. In such a case, it would not make sense to estimate and interpret the hazard ratios presented in the last two rows of Table 7.3. Nevertheless, for the UMARU Impact Study, the time points at which patients go off treatment vary greatly and the stated hazard ratios are valid for those time points where some patients are on and others are off treatment.

An alternative to the time-varying covariate analysis presented here is to fit a model with a time-dependent effect for treatment. There are four possible parameterizations:

the standard PH model with fixed covariates,

$$h(t,x) = h_0(t)\exp(\beta x),$$

the PH model with time-varying covariates (this is the model described above using $OFF\_TRT(t)$),

$$h(t,x) = h_0(t)\exp(\beta x(t)),$$

the PH model where the effect depends on time but x does not change, (i.e., the setting where patients are randomized to treatment but its effect changes over time),

$$h(t,x) = h_0(t)\exp(\beta(t)x),$$

and the PH model where both, effect and covariate values, change over time,

$$h(t,x) = h_0(t)\exp(\beta(t)x(t)).$$

We illustrate the use of the third model in Chapter 9 where we discuss a linear additive model for time to event data. We do not consider the fourth model in this book.

Data for our second example of time-varying covariates have been provided to us by Dr. Frederick Anderson, Jr, Director of the Center for Outcomes Research (COR) at the University of Massachusetts / Worcester and come from the Global Registry of Acute Coronary Events (GRACE). Data for the registry have been collected for 7.5 years from 113 Coronary Care Units (or equivalent) in 14 Countries. The registry now contains data on nearly 60,000 subjects with an acute coronary syndrome. Data from GRACE have been analyzed and reported in over 50 publications. For a paper relevant to the current example see Granger et al (2003). A complete list of GRACE publications may be found at the Center for Outcomes Research web site, www.outcomes-umassmed.org/grace.

The data we use are a blinded, specially selected sample of 1000 subjects. We thank Dr. Gordon FitzGerald of COR for his help in obtaining the sample and for discussing the use of time-varying covariates in this data set with us. A key variable for some subjects is whether they underwent a revascularization procedure such as coronary artery bypass surgery and when during their hospitalization this procedure took place. Some subjects do not have a procedure performed; some have it performed on admission, while others have it performed some days after their admission. Of interest here is whether revascularization is associated with survival after admission. To be able to demonstrate effects, our sample of data

Table 7.4 Description of Variables in the GRACE Data, 1000 Subjects

Variable	Description	Values
id	Patient Identification Number	1 - 1000
days	Follow Up Time	0.5* - 180
death	Death During Follow Up	1= Death, 0 = Censored
revasc	Revascularization Performed	1 = Yes, 0 = No
revascdays	Days to Revascularization After Admission	0 – 14 if revasc = 1 and equals the value of days if revasc = 0
los	Length of Hospital Stay	Days
age	Age at Admission	Years
sysbp	Systolic Blood Pressure on Admission	mm Hg
stchange	ST-segment deviation on index ECG	1= Yes, 0 = No

* Subjects who died or were discharged on the day they were admitted have been assigned a value of 0.5.

contains proportionally more deaths (32 versus about 8 percent) and revascularized subjects (52 versus 38 percent) than in the full GRACE database. Hence, results presented here may not be indicative of what would be obtained if we fit the same models on the full GRACE data. The variables in our data set, called GRACE1000 are described in Table 7.4. The data set contains three baseline covariates: age, systolic blood pressure, and an indicator of whether the baseline electrocardiogram (ECG) showed evidence of a deviation from normal in the ST segment.

The naïve approach to fitting a model is to treat revascularization status, *revasc*, as a fixed or baseline covariate. The results of fitting this model are shown in Table 7.5. Fractional polynomial analysis showed that, for these data, the log hazard is linear in the inverse of age and the square root of systolic blood pressure. Thus, in Table 7.4, we have $age\_inv = (1/age) \times 1000$ and $sysbp\_sqrt = \sqrt{sysbp}$. The estimated hazard ratio for revascularization is 0.59 with 95 percent confidence limits $(0.468, 0.741)$. Controlling for age, systolic blood pressure, and ST segment change, the model estimates that subjects who undergo a revascularization procedure have a rate of death during the follow up period that is 41 percent less than subjects who do not under go such a procedure.

Table 7.5 Estimated Coefficients, Standard Errors, z-Scores, Two-Tailed p-values, and 95% Confidence Interval Estimates for the Fitted Proportional Hazards Model Treating Revascularization as a Baseline Covariate (n = 1000)

Variable	Coeff.	Std. Err.	z	$p > |z|$	95% CIE
revasc	−0.530	0.1172	−4.52	<0.001	−0.759, −0.300
age_inv	−0.189	0.0225	−8.41	<0.001	−0.233, −0.145
sysbp_sqrt	−0.207	0.0387	−5.36	<0.001	−0.283, −0.131
stchange	0.513	0.1189	4.32	<0.001	0.280, 0.746

The problem with the naïve approach is that revascularization status is not known at admission for all subjects. For subjects who have $revasc = 1$ and $revascdays = 0$, we could argue its value is known at admission. For subjects who have $revasc = 0$, the fact that they did not undergo this procedure is only known at discharge from the hospital or at the time of death, if death occurs during hospitalization.

The correct way to model revascularization is through a time-varying covariate. As a first step, we treat revascularization as a dichotomous time-varying covariate similar to $OFF\_TRT(t)$ in the previous example, namely

$$\text{revasc\_t}(t) = \begin{cases} 0 \text{ if } t <= revascdays \text{ or } revasc = 0 \\ 1 \text{ if } t > revascdays \text{ and } revasc = 1 \end{cases}.$$

The results of fitting this model are shown in Table 7.6. We see that the estimated coefficient for the time-varying effect of revascularization is significant with $p = 0.035$. The estimated hazard ratio at time t for $revasc\_t(t) = 1$ versus $revasc\_t(t) = 0$ is $0.77 = \exp(-0.261)$ with 95 percent confidence limits of $(0.604, 0.982)$. The interpretation is that the rate of death among subjects who had undergone a revascularization procedure some time prior to t are dying at a rate that is 23 percent less than subjects who had not undergone a revascularization procedure prior to t, a reduction much smaller than the 41 percent from the naïve model. It is important to note that the comparison group of subjects with $revasc\_t(t) = 0$ includes subjects who never had the procedure, $revasc = 0$, as well as those who had the procedure performed after t. Because we used a dichotomous time-varying covariate, the estimate holds over all t for which comparing $revasc\_t(t) = 1$ to $revasc\_t(t) = 0$ is valid, i.e., $t \geq 1$.

We see that the time varying estimate in Table 7.6 is approximately 50 percent smaller than the naïve estimate in Table 7.5. In the naïve analysis, days of

Table 7.6 Estimated Coefficients, Standard Errors, z-Scores, Two-Tailed p-values, and 95% Confidence Intervals for the Fitted Proportional Hazards Model Treating Revascularization as a Time-Varying Covariate ($n = 1000$)

Variable	Coeff.	Std. Err.	z	$p > |z|$	95% CIE
revasc_t	−0.261	0.1237	−2.11	0.035	−0.503, −0.018
age_inv	−0.202	0.0228	−8.85	<0.001	−0.247, −0.157
sysbp_sqrt	−0.215	0.0392	−5.48	<0.001	−0.291, −0.138
stchange	0.501	0.1191	4.20	<0.001	0.267, 0.734

follow up are incorrectly attributed to survival after revascularization from time zero to the end of follow up. For example, suppose a subject underwent revascularization on day 4 and died on day 10. In the naïve analysis, all 10 days of follow up are attributed to survival after revascularization. In the correct time-varying approach, days 0 to 4 are counted toward survival without revascularization and 5 to 10 days are counted toward survival with revascularization (i.e., $revasc(t) = 0$ for $t \le 4$ and $revasc(t) = 1$ for $t > 4$). The naïve analysis, in a sense, over-counts the days of survival due to revascularization.

Table 7.7 Frequency Distribution of Days to Revascularization

Days	Freq.	Percent
0	151	28.9
1	81	15.5
2	38	7.3
3	30	5.8
4	17	3.3
5	13	2.5
6	11	2.1
7	14	2.7
8	37	7.1
9	33	6.3
10	31	5.9
11	22	4.2
12	17	3.3
13	21	4.0
14	6	1.2
Total	522	100

As a follow up question, suppose the clinicians on the GRACE study wanted to determine whether the effect depended on the number of days from admission to revascularization. To answer this question, we begin by examining the frequency distribution of days to revascularization (revascdays) among those who had a revascularization procedure performed. This is shown in Table 7.7. Based on these frequencies and clinical considerations, we choose to create six time-varying covariates based on having a revascularization performed on days 0, 1, 2-3, 4-7, 8-10, or 11-14. The time-varying covariates are defined as follows:

$$\text{revasc\_t0}(t) = \begin{cases} 1 \text{ if } t > revascdays \text{ and } revascdays = 0 \text{ and } revasc = 1 \\ 0 \text{ Otherwise} \end{cases},$$

$$\text{revasc\_t1}(t) = \begin{cases} 1 \text{ if } t > revascdays \text{ and } revascdays = 1 \text{ and } revasc = 1 \\ 0 \text{ Otherwise} \end{cases},$$

$$\text{revasc\_t2\_3}(t) = \begin{cases} 1 \text{ if } t > revascdays \text{ and } 2 \leq revascdays \leq 3 \text{ and } revasc = 1 \\ 0 \text{ Otherwise} \end{cases},$$

$$\text{revasc\_t4\_7}(t) = \begin{cases} 1 \text{ if } t > revascdays \text{ and } 4 \leq revascdays \leq 7 \text{ and } revasc = 1 \\ 0 \text{ Otherwise} \end{cases},$$

$$\text{revasc\_t8\_10}(t) = \begin{cases} 1 \text{ if } t > revascdays \text{ and } 8 \leq revascdays \leq 10 \text{ and } revasc = 1 \\ 0 \text{ Otherwise} \end{cases},$$

and

$$\text{revasc\_t11\_14}(t) = \begin{cases} 1 \text{ if } t > revascdays \text{ and } 11 \leq revascdays \leq 14 \text{ and } revasc = 1 \\ 0 \text{ Otherwise} \end{cases},$$

where t stands for days of follow up.

The results of fitting the model containing the six time-varying covariates are shown in Table 7.8; we see that only the time-varying covariates denoting revascularization on days 0 and 1 are significant. Using Wald tests (analyses not explicitly shown here), we find that the estimated coefficients for days 0 and 1 are not significantly different from each other, nor are the estimated coefficients for the other four time-varying covariates different from each other. The Wald tests suggest that a much more parsimonious model would be one with two time-varying covariates: One denoting days 0 and 1 and the other for days 2-14. The results of fitting the reduced model are shown in Table 7.9.

Table 7.8 Estimated Coefficients, Standard Errors, z-Scores, Two-Tailed p-values, and 95% Confidence Interval Estimates for the Fitted Proportional Hazards Model Treating Revascularization as a Time-Varying Covariate at Six Levels ($n = 1000$)

Variable	Coeff.	Std. Err.	z	$p > |z|$	95% CIE
revasc_t0	−0.611	0.1939	−3.15	0.002	−0.991, −0.231
revasc_t1	−0.719	0.3267	−2.20	0.028	−1.360, −0.079
revasc_t2_3	0.012	0.2644	0.05	0.963	−0.506, 0.531
recasc_t_4_7	0.024	0.2914	0.08	0.935	−0.547, 0.595
recasc_t_8_10	−0.107	0.2379	−0.45	0.652	−0.574, 0.359
recasc_t_11_14	0.029	0.2689	0.11	0.915	−0.498, 0.556
age_inv	−0.199	0.0228	−8.72	<0.001	−0.244, −0.154
sysbp_sqrt	−0.221	0.0393	−5.62	<0.001	−0.298, −0.144
Stchange	0.552	0.1208	4.57	<0.001	0.315, 0.789

Using the results in Table 7.9, we would be tempted to exponentiate the estimated coefficients for the two time-varying covariates and interpret them as estimating a hazard ratio in a manner similar to using the results in Table 7.6. However, the definition of the two time-varying covariates are linked because both cannot have a value of 1 simultaneously. Hence, we have to consider carefully which subjects have a value of zero. Suppose we let $t = 5$ days. At this value of time, we effectively have a categorical covariate at three levels with two design variables as described in Table 7.10. Similar coding would apply at other values of follow up time.

Based on the coding in Table 7.10 and the discussions in Section 4.2 about modeling nominal scaled covariates using reference cell coding, the reference group for the two design variables includes subjects who never had a revasculari-

Table 7.9 Estimated Coefficients, Standard Errors, z-Scores, Two-Tailed p-values, and 95% Confidence Interval Estimates for the Fitted Proportional Hazards Model Treating Revascularization as a Time-Varying Covariate at Two Levels ($n = 1000$)

Variable	Coeff.	Std. Err.	z	$p > |z|$	95% CIE
revasc_t0_1	−0.638	0.1733	−3.68	<0.001	−0.978, −0.298
revasc_t2_14	−0.020	0.1522	−0.13	0.897	−0.318, 0.278
age_inv	−0.199	0.0228	−8.74	<0.001	−0.244, −0.155
sysbp_sqrt	−0.221	0.0392	−5.63	<0.001	−0.297, −0.144
stchange	0.556	0.1199	4.64	<0.001	0.321, 0.791

Table 7.10 Coding the Two Time-Varying Covariates at $t = 5$

Status	$revasc\_t0\_1(5)$	$revasc\_t2\_14(5)$
{ $revasc = 0$ } or { $revasc = 1$ and $revascdays \geq 15$ }	0	0
$revasc = 1$ and $revasdays = 0$ or 1	1	0
$revasc = 1$ and $2 \leq revascdays \leq 14$	0	1

zation performed and subjects who had a revascularization performed after day 4. This latter group decreases in number up to day 14, after which all revascularizations had been performed. Hence, the least complicated interpretation of the estimated hazard ratios applies to $days \geq 15$ when the reference group includes only those subjects who did not have a revascularization procedure preformed, $revasc = 0$. These estimated hazard ratios are presented in Table 7.11.

The interpretations at any time after 15 days of follow up are as follows: Subjects who had a revascularization performed on admission or one day after admission are dying at a rate that is 47 percent less than subjects who did not undergo revascularization. This difference is significant and could be as much as 62 percent less or as little as 26 percent less with 95 percent confidence. Subjects who had revascularization performed between 2 and 14 days after hospital admission are dying at a rate that is not significantly different from subjects who did not have revascularization performed. Estimates of hazard ratios at follow up times less than 15 days are the same as those in Table 7.11, but are complicated by the fact the reference group contains subjects who have not yet had a revascularization procedure, but will sometime before day 15.

In summary, by using time-varying covariates that designate revascularization status and the day on which it took place, we are able to provide correct estimates

Table 7.11 Estimated Hazard Ratios and 95 Percent Confidence Limit Estimates for the Time-Varying Effect of Revascularization at 15 or More Days of Follow Up

Revascularization Performed On	$\hat{HR}$	95% CIE
Days 0 or 1	0.53	0.376, 0.742
Days 2 - 14	0.98	0.728, 1.321

of its effect on long-term survival.

Before leaving the example using the GRACE data, we want to remind the reader that we have used a select subset of only 1000 subjects. Thus, the results presented here do not apply to the larger GRACE database.

In each of the two examples, we used dichotomous time-varying covariates. We did not illustrate a setting in which the covariate varies continuously over time, as would be the case with a measured physiologic variable such as blood pressure. Inclusion of such a covariate in the partial likelihood in (7.8) is rather straightforward. The data management task of keeping track of the value(s) presents a bigger challenge. In particular, with multiple measurements, we have several choices for assigning covariate values at event times where actual values are not observed (e.g., the last measured value, the maximum of the previously measured values etc.). Hence, it is clear that, in these settings, clinical considerations of relevance to the event are vital.

Another approach to allowing the hazard function in (7.7) to change over time is to modify the baseline hazard so that it changes over time. For example, if follow up was for two years, measured in days, one might use two time-interval-specific baseline hazards defined as

$$h_0(t) = \begin{cases} h_{10}(t), t \le 365 \\ h_{20}(t), t > 365 \end{cases}.$$

It is not easy to fit such a model with coefficients that do not depend on the time interval. One way around the problem is to model the baseline hazard completely parametrically or through cubic spline functions as suggested by Royston (2001).

In Chapter 4, we discussed presentation and interpretation of covariate-adjusted survival curves. These methods were used in Section 6.6 and in the previous section. For models containing time-varying covariates, it is possible to estimate the baseline survivorship function because it does not depend on the covariates. However, it is not feasible to present individual covariate-adjusted survivorship functions; these are explicit functions of time, which is changing.

In closing, we note that time-varying covariates can provide a useful and powerful adjunct to the covariate composition of a survival time regression model. However, one should carefully consider all the implications of adding them to the model before doing so.

7.4 TRUNCATED, LEFT CENSORED, AND INTERVAL CENSORED DATA

Another simplifying assumption we have made up to this point is that the data are subject only to right censoring. That is, each observation of time begins at a well-defined and known zero value, and follow-up continues until the event of interest occurs or until observation terminates for a reason unrelated to the event of interest (e.g., the subject moves away or the study ends). In practice, this is the most frequently encountered type of survival data; however, other reasons for incomplete observation of survival time do occur. In this section, we consider some of these reasons, as well as methods for extending the proportional hazards model to address them.

Imagine the time scale for a study as a horizontal line. Incomplete observation of time can occur anywhere, but it is most common at either the beginning (i.e., on the left) or at the end (i.e., on the right) of the time scale. Censoring and truncation are the two most common causes of incomplete observation. Thus, when we consider an observation of time, we must evaluate whether the observation is subject to left censoring or left truncation and/or right censoring or right truncation. In practice, it is unlikely that an observation will be both censored and truncated on the same end of the time scale; however, an event time can be subject to incomplete observation on both sides (e.g., left truncated and right censored).

We begin with left truncation as it is, after right censoring, the next most common source of incomplete observation of survival time. To illustrate, suppose that, in the WHAS500 data, we were only interested in the survival time of patients who were discharged alive from the hospital. We define the beginning of survival time as the time the subject was admitted to the hospital. In this study, a selection process will take place in the sense that only those subjects who are discharged alive are eligible to be included in the analysis. As a result, their minimum survival time would be the length of their particular hospital stay. Observations of time that do not exceed the minimum survival time are left truncated. In this setting, all follow up times considered for the analysis must exceed some fixed value (which can be different for each individual); those subjects whose follow up times do not exceed this value are excluded from the analysis. In other words, observations subject to left truncation are not considered for the analysis.

Delayed entry is a closely related concept. Recall that the hazard rate at any time is, in the Nelson–Aalen sense, estimated by the ratio of the number of events to the number at risk. The survival experiences of subjects with delayed entry do not contribute to the analysis until time exceeds an intermediate event (being discharged alive from the hospital in the above example). Their entry into the risk sets is delayed until this intermediate event occurs. Once entered into the analysis, subjects remain at risk until they die or are right censored. The intermediate event is not reached for left-truncated values.

From a model fitting point of view, left truncation or delayed entry is difficult to handle unless the statistical software package allows counting process type data. In this data structure, each subject's follow-up time is described by a beginning time (which need not be zero), an end time, and a right-censoring indicator variable. Currently, most of the major statistical software packages have this capability. In practice, a particular study may contain follow up times that represent all four possible combinations of left truncation and right censoring, and these are handled by the counting process style of data description. Once accounted for in the data setup, the analysis proceeds exactly as described in the previous chapters.

We use the WHAS500 data to provide an example of analysis with left truncation and delayed entry. In this sample, 461 subjects were discharged alive from the hospital. One subject is recorded as having been discharged alive but has length of follow-up equal to length of hospital stay. Thus, when delayed entry is considered, this subject does not contribute to the analysis. To illustrate the effect of delayed entry, we fit the model obtained in Chapter 5 and evaluated in Chapter 6 (see Table 6.3). The results of fitting this model are presented in Table 7.13 using delayed entry as length of hospital stay. The results in the two tables are not identical, but the interpretations and conclusions we would reach are the same.

It is not our intention to reanalyze the WHAS500 data, but rather to illustrate how to use the proportional hazards model with left-truncated or delayed entry data that is also subject to right censoring. Once delayed entry is accounted for, there are no substantive changes in the methods used for model development, assessment, and interpretation.

In summary, the key elements defining a survival time with delayed entry are: (1) the observation must, by design of the study, exceed some minimum value, that may be the same or different for all subjects, and (2) the beginning or zero value of time must be known for each observation. Andersen, Borgan, Gill and Keiding (1993) present, in Chapter III, the mathematical details as well as insight-

Table 7.13 Estimated Coefficients, Standard Errors, z-Scores, Two-Tailed *p*-Values, and 95% Confidence Interval Estimates for the Final Proportional Hazards Model for the WHAS500 Data with Delayed Entry of Subjects, *n* = 459.

Variable	Coeff.	Std. Err.	z	$p>|z|$	95% CIE
bmifp1	−0.728	0.1933	−3.76	<0.001	−1.107, −0.349
bmifp2	0.155	0.0437	3.56	<0.001	0.070, 0.241
age	0.066	0.0093	7.12	<0.001	0.048, 0.084
hr	0.014	0.0033	4.29	<0.001	0.008, 0.020
diasbp	−0.012	0.0039	−3.13	0.002	−0.020, −0.005
gender	2.499	1.0608	2.36	0.018	0.420, 4.579
chf	0.901	0.1628	5.54	<0.001	0.582, 1.220
agexgender	−0.037	0.0134	−2.79	0.005	−0.064, −0.011

ful examples involving left truncation of survival time.

Left censoring of survival time is different from left truncation in that it occurs randomly at the individual subject level, while left truncation involves a selection process that applies to all subjects. A follow up time is left censored if we know that the event of interest took place at an unknown time prior to when the individual is first observed. Examples of left-censored data often involve age as the time variable and a life-course event. For example, in a study modeling the age at which "regular" smoking starts, the data may come from interviews of 12-year olds. A 12-year-old subject may report that he is a regular smoker but that he does not remember when he started smoking regularly. In this case, we know the observed time, 12, is larger than the time to event (i.e., the age when the subject became a regular smoker).

The defining characteristic of left-censored data is that the event is known to have occurred and the observed time is larger than the survival time. In a sense, left censoring is the opposite of right censoring, where we know that the event of interest has not occurred and that the observed time is less than the survival time.

Ware and DeMets (1976) proposed one solution for the analysis of left-censored data. They suggested turning the time scale around and treating the data as if they were right censored. This method works if the data are only subject to left censoring. In practice, however, if left censoring can occur, then right censoring is also likely to occur. In the example of age at first regular smoking, many study subjects will not be regular smokers at the time they are interviewed, and these observations of time are right censored. Alioum and Commenges (1996) present a method for fitting the proportional hazards model to arbitrarily censored and truncated data. We will not discuss their method because it is quite complex and requires computational skills greater than those assumed in the rest of this text. Klein and Moeschberger (2003) discuss general mechanisms for incomplete observation of survival time and necessary modifications in estimation methods. A somewhat simpler but less flexible approach is presented later in this section within the context of interval-censored data.

Right truncation occurs when, by study design, there is a selection process such that data are available only on subjects who have experienced the event. This typically occurs in settings where data come from a registry containing information on confirmed cases of a disease. For example, all subjects in a cancer registry, by definition, have cancer. Thus, any analysis of a time variable that uses confirmed diagnosis of cancer as the event of interest will involve right truncation. Extensions of the methods for left-truncated data or right-censored data for the analysis of right-truncated data are not especially straightforward. We will not consider analysis of right-truncated data further in this text. Instead we refer the reader to Klein and Moeschberger (2003) for a general discussion of likelihood construction and to Alioum and Commenges (1996) for methods using the proportional hazards model.

Another type of incomplete observation of time can occur if we do not know the zero value when we begin observing a subject. The observation may also be subject to right censoring. For example, in a study of survival time of patients with AIDS, suppose some subjects enter the study with active, confirmed disease, but no precise information can be obtained as to when they converted from HIV+ to AIDS. Thus, for these patients, the zero value of time, (when they actually developed AIDS) is unknown. Statistical methods have been developed to handle this setting (see DeGruttola and Lagakos (1989), Kim, DeGruttola and Lagakos (1993), Jewell (1994) and Klein and Moeschberger (2003) who describe this type of data as being doubly censored).

Interval-censored data is another form of incomplete observation of survival time that can involve left and right censoring as well as truncation. Interval censoring is used to describe a situation where a subject's survival time is known only to lie between two values. Data of this type typically arise in studies where follow up is done at fixed intervals. For example, in the WHAS, the aim is to model the survival time among patients admitted to a hospital for a myocardial infarction. Suppose that patients who were discharged alive from the hospital were contacted every 3 months to ascertain their vital status. Patients who die before the first contact at 3 months have survival times that are left censored at 3 months. We know the event took place prior to 3 months, yet we are unsure of the exact time. All that is known is that these survival times are at most 3 months. For subjects who die between two contacts, all that is known is that survival time is at least as long as the time of the earlier contact and is no longer than the time of the most recent contact (e.g., between 9 and 12 months). For subjects still alive at their last follow up, all we know is that their survival time is at least as long as the time associated with their last contact (e.g., alive at 18 months and then lost to follow up). These observations are right censored.

Lindsey and Ryan (1998), Carstensen (1996), and Farrington (1996) have considered regression models for arbitrarily interval-censored survival time that extend methods developed by Finkelstein (1986) specifically for the proportional hazards model as well as earlier developmental work by Prentice and Gloecker (1978). Carstensen and Farrington show how arbitrarily interval-censored data may be fit by considering the problem as a binary outcome regression problem. We illustrate this approach by modifying follow-up time in the GBCS data. Collett (2003) and Klein and Moeschberger (2003) present methods for interval-censored data similar to those presented here. Sun (2006) provides a more detailed and technical discussion of interval-censored failure time data.

Assume that all we know about the observed time for the ith subject is that it is bounded between two known values, denoted $a_i < T \leq b_i$. In addition, we know whether the event of interest occurred. The outcome is indicated by the usual censoring variable, $c_i = 1$ if the event occurred and $c_i = 0$ otherwise. Observations that are left censored have $a_i = 0$ and $c_i = 1$. Observations that are right censored have $b_i = \infty$ and $c_i = 0$.

Let the survival function at time t for a subject with covariate vector $\mathbf{x}_i$ and associated parameter vector $\boldsymbol{\beta}$ be denoted $S(t,\mathbf{x}_i,\boldsymbol{\beta})$. The probability of the observed interval for the ith subject is

$$\left[S(a_i,\mathbf{x}_i,\boldsymbol{\beta})\right]^{1-c_i}\left[S(a_i,\mathbf{x}_i,\boldsymbol{\beta})-S(b_i,\mathbf{x}_i,\boldsymbol{\beta})\right]^{c_i}. \tag{7.9}$$

The expression in (7.9) yields $\left[1-S(b_i,\mathbf{x}_i,\boldsymbol{\beta})\right]$ for left-censored observations, $\left[S(a_i,\mathbf{x}_i,\boldsymbol{\beta})-S(b_i,\mathbf{x}_i,\boldsymbol{\beta})\right]$ for non-censored observations, and $S(a_i,\mathbf{x}_i,\boldsymbol{\beta})$ for right-censored observations.

The first steps in obtaining estimators of parameters in a regression model are to construct the likelihood function and then to evaluate it with the chosen model. We will use the proportional hazards model, but the method is general enough that other models could be used, including the parametric models discussed in Chapter 8. The likelihood is the product of the terms obtained by evaluating (7.9) for each subject, namely

$$l(\boldsymbol{\beta})=\prod_{i=1}^{n}\left[S(a_i,\mathbf{x}_i,\boldsymbol{\beta})\right]^{1-c_i}\left[S(a_i,\mathbf{x}_i,\boldsymbol{\beta})-S(b_i,\mathbf{x}_i,\boldsymbol{\beta})\right]^{c_i}. \tag{7.10}$$

The computations and model fitting procedure are simplified if only a few values are possible for a and b. In this case, it is easier to refer to the interval-censored values by intervals on the time scale common to all subjects. Assume that we have $J+1$ such intervals denoted $\left(t_{j-1},t_j\right]$ for $j=1,2,\ldots,J+1$ with $t_0=0$ and $t_{J+1}=\infty$, and these intervals are the same for all subjects.

For ease of presentation, we let I_j denote the jth time interval $\left(t_{j-1},t_j\right]$. The binary variable indicating the specific time interval observed for the ith subject is defined as

$$y_{ij}=\begin{cases}1 & \text{if } \left(a_i,b_i\right]=I_j \\ 0 & \text{otherwise.}\end{cases}$$

In addition, we re-express the probability for the jth interval as

$$S\left(t_{j-1},\mathbf{x}_i,\boldsymbol{\beta}\right)-S\left(t_j,\mathbf{x}_i,\boldsymbol{\beta}\right)=S\left(t_{j-1},\mathbf{x}_i,\boldsymbol{\beta}\right)\left[1-\frac{S\left(t_j,\mathbf{x}_i,\boldsymbol{\beta}\right)}{S\left(t_{j-1},\mathbf{x}_i,\boldsymbol{\beta}\right)}\right]. \tag{7.11}$$

The right-most term in the square brackets in (7.11) is the conditional probability that the event occurs in the jth interval, given that the subject was alive at the end of interval $j-1$, $\Pr\left(t_{j-1} < T \le t_j \mid T > t_{j-1}\right)$. Under the proportional hazards model, the ratio of the survival function at successive interval endpoints can be simplified (algebraic steps not shown) to:

$$\frac{S\left(t_j, \mathbf{x}_i, \boldsymbol{\beta}\right)}{S\left(t_{j-1}, \mathbf{x}_i, \boldsymbol{\beta}\right)} = \exp\left[-\exp\left(\mathbf{x}_i'\boldsymbol{\beta} + \tau_j\right)\right], \qquad (7.12)$$

where

$$\tau_j = \ln\left\{-\ln\left[\frac{S_0\left(t_j\right)}{S_0\left(t_{j-1}\right)}\right]\right\}.$$

To further simplify the notation, let us denote the conditional probability in (7.11) as

$$\theta_{ij} = 1 - \exp\left[-\exp\left(\mathbf{x}_i'\boldsymbol{\beta} + \tau_j\right)\right]. \qquad (7.13)$$

Using the result in (7.13), it follows that the likelihood function in (7.10) may be expressed as follows:

$$l(\boldsymbol{\beta}) = \prod_{i=1}^{n}\prod_{j=1}^{J+1}\left\{\left[S\left(t_{j-1}, \mathbf{x}_i, \boldsymbol{\beta}\right)^{1-c_i}\right]\left[S\left(t_{j-1}, \mathbf{x}_i, \boldsymbol{\beta}\right) - S\left(t_j, \mathbf{x}_i, \boldsymbol{\beta}\right)\right]^{c_i}\right\}^{y_{ij}}$$

$$= \prod_{i=1}^{n}\prod_{j=1}^{J+1}\left\{\left[S\left(t_{j-1}, \mathbf{x}_i, \boldsymbol{\beta}\right)\right]\left[1 - \frac{S\left(t_j, \mathbf{x}_i, \boldsymbol{\beta}\right)}{S\left(t_{j-1}, \mathbf{x}_i, \boldsymbol{\beta}\right)}\right]^{c_i}\right\}^{y_{ij}} \qquad (7.14)$$

$$= \prod_{i=1}^{n}\prod_{j=1}^{J+1}\left\{S\left(t_{j-1}, \mathbf{x}_i, \boldsymbol{\beta}\right) \times \theta_{ij}^{c_i}\right\}^{y_{ij}}.$$

The next step involves expressing the survival function at an interval endpoint as a product of successive conditional survival probabilities, a process similar to the one used to develop the Kaplan–Meier estimator in Chapter 2, but using the expression in (7.13). The algebraic details are not shown, but the result is

$$S\left(t_{j-1}, \mathbf{x}_i, \boldsymbol{\beta}\right) = \prod_{l=1}^{j-1}\left(1 - \theta_{il}\right). \qquad (7.15)$$

Substituting the expression in (7.15) into the function in (7.14) results in the following likelihood function:

$$l(\boldsymbol{\beta}) = \prod_{i=1}^{n} \prod_{j=1}^{J+1} \left[\prod_{l=1}^{j-1} (1-\theta_{il}) \theta_{ij}^{c_i} \right]^{y_{ij}} . \tag{7.16}$$

Let the observed interval for the ith subject be denoted k_i, that is, $I_{k_i} = (a_i, b_i]$. The first thing to note in (7.16) is that the only time the terms in the product over j differ from 1 is when $j = k_i$. Thus the expression (7.16) simplifies to

$$l(\boldsymbol{\beta}) = \prod_{i=1}^{n} \theta_{ik_i}^{c_i} \prod_{j=1}^{k_i-1} (1-\theta_{ij}) . \tag{7.17}$$

The likelihood function in (7.17) can be made to look like the likelihood function for a binary regression model. We define a pseudo binary outcome variable as $z_{ij} = y_{ij} \times c_i$ and use it to re-express (7.17) as

$$l(\boldsymbol{\beta}) = \prod_{i=1}^{n} \prod_{j=1}^{k_i-1+c_i} (1-\theta_{ij})^{1-z_{ij}} \theta_{ij}^{z_{ij}} . \tag{7.18}$$

For each subject, i, (7.18) is the likelihood for $k_i - 1 + c_i$ independent binary observations with probabilities θ_{ij} and outcomes z_{ij}. This observation allows us to use standard statistical software to fit the interval-censored proportional hazards regression model.

Suppose that, in the GBCS, time to recurrence or censoring was not observed exactly, but instead only to within 12 month intervals. That is, the status of subjects was determined annually. To obtain data of this type, we form intervals by grouping follow up time in months $(12 \times days / 365.25)$ into seven intervals. The first six are of length 12 months and the last interval is for follow-up time exceeding 72 months:

$$\{(0,12],(12,24],(24,36],(36,48],(48,60],(60,72],(72,\infty]\} .$$

The results of cross tabulating the follow up times into seven intervals by the censoring indicator is shown in Table 7.13.

The first step in the model-fitting process is to expand the data for each subject $k_i - 1 + c_i$ times and create the values of j and z_{ij}. For example, in the GBCS, if a subject's recurrence time was in the third interval, between 24 and 36 months, then $k_i = 3$ and $c_i = 1$. This subject would contribute 3 lines to the expanded data

Table 7.13 Frequency Distribution of the Created Interval Censored Data in the GBCS by Censoring Status (n = 686)

Interval	Censoring Indicator		Total
	0	1	
$(0,12]$	28	56	84
$(12,24]$	35	109	144
$(24,36]$	68	59	127
$(36,48]$	64	39	103
$(48,60]$	85	22	107
$(60,72]$	74	11	85
$(72, \infty)$	33	3	36
Total	387	299	686

file. The covariates would be the same in each line; the interval indicator, j, would take on the values 1, 2, and 3; and the binary outcome variable, z, would be zero for the first 2 lines and 1 for the third line of data. If the follow up on the subject ended during the fifth interval, between 48 and 60 months without recurrence, then $k_i = 5$ and $c_i = 0$. This subject would contribute 5 lines of data, and the value of the binary outcome variable would be zero in all 5 lines. Similarly, if a subject's follow-up time exceeded 72 months without cancer recurrence, then $k_i = 7$ and $c_i = 0$. The subject would be represented with 7 lines of data, and the binary outcome variable would be zero for each line.

The binary regression model defined in (7.13) has as its link function, or linearizing transformation, the complementary log-log function, that is, $\ln\left[-\ln\left(1-\theta_{ij}\right)\right] = x_i'\beta + \tau_j$. The design variable, represented by τ_j in the model, is a 0/1 indicator variable for each time interval. All J of these variables are included in the model, which requires that we force the usual constant term to be zero.

An important point to keep firmly in mind is that the manipulations of the likelihood in (7.10)–(7.18) are designed to cast the interval-censored data problem in a form that would allow likelihood analysis by existing software. The problem is not a binary regression problem in the usual sense of the primary outcome variable being a 0/1 variable; however, we manipulated the problem to make it look like one.

The likelihood in (7.18) is identical to one that would be obtained using the general methods in Carstensen (1996) and Farrington (1996) under the restriction of a few intervals common to all subjects. If this assumption does not hold, then the more general method must be used. This method also yields a likelihood that may be analyzed using a binary regression model, but it requires a two-step fitting procedure. In addition, a second set of calculations is required to obtain standard errors of estimated model coefficients. For these reasons, we have chosen not to present the general regression method.

The creation of the expanded data set is more easily demonstrated using a few example subjects, shown in Table 7.14. The first line of data in this table is for a 46-year old subject who was followed for between 0 and 12 months and whose cancer had recurred some time during this interval. The second line of data is for a 65-year old subject who was followed for between 0 and 12 months and whose cancer had not recurred during this interval. These data are indicted by month = 12, interval = 1, censor = 1 or 0, and the binary outcome variable $z = 1$ or 0. The covariate chosen, for demonstration purposes only, is AGE.

The second block of four lines represents two subjects whose follow up time fell in the second interval. This is noted by month = 24. Subject 17's cancer recurred in this interval, while subject 321's did not recur. The first and third lines correspond to the fact that neither subject had a recurrence in the first year of follow up. For these lines the interval = 1 and $z = 0$. The second and fourth lines are for the second year of follow up, denoted by interval = 2. The recurrence for subject 17 is denoted by $z = 1$. The value of age is the same in both lines. Non-recurrence of the cancer for subject 321 is indicated by $z = 0$.

The third block of six lines represents two subjects (117 and 288): one whose cancer recurred in the third year of follow-up and one whose cancer did not recur. Both of these subjects contribute three lines of data, one for each of the three intervals. During the first two intervals of follow up, neither subject's cancer had recurred so, for each subject, $z = 0$. The value is changed to $z = 1$ in the third line for the subject whose cancer recurred and is kept at $z = 0$ for the one whose cancer did not recur while being followed.

The fourth block of five lines represents a subject (278) whose cancer recurred during the fifth year of follow up. Because the subject's cancer had not recurred during the first four intervals, $z = 0$ for these four lines and $z = 1$ for the fifth line. As in the previous examples, age remains constant at 70 in all five lines.

Data for subjects with their follow up time falling in other intervals would be expanded in a similar manner.

The technical details of expanding the data set will vary by software package, but most can perform the expansion without too much trouble. Analyses presented here were performed in STATA, where the data expansion is especially easy to perform.

To illustrate the model fitting, we fit a model containing age, hormone use, and tumor size. Table 7.15 presents the results of fitting the interval-censored proportional hazards model containing age, hormone use, and tumor size using the likelihood in (7.18) with the expanded data set. Even though age it is not significant, we have kept it in the model because it was useful in illustrating the expanded data and is clinically important.

Table 7.14 Examples of the Expanded Data Set Required to Fit the Binary Regression Model in Equation (7.18) for the GBCS

ID	Month	Interval	Censor	z	Age
230	12	1	1	1	46
621	12	1	0	0	65
17	24	1	1	0	62
17	24	2	1	1	62
321	24	1	0	0	49
321	24	2	0	0	49
117	36	1	1	0	65
117	36	2	1	0	65
117	36	3	1	1	65
288	36	1	0	0	57
288	36	2	0	0	57
288	36	3	0	0	57
278	60	1	0	0	70
278	60	2	0	0	70
278	60	3	0	0	70
278	60	4	0	0	70
278	60	5	1	1	70

The presentation and interpretation of the estimated coefficients for study covariates in Table 7.15 would proceed in exactly the same manner as illustrated in Chapter 6 for a fitted, non-interval-censored, proportional hazards model. In this regard, it is important to remember that, even though a binary regression program

Table 7.15 Estimated Coefficients, Standard Errors, z-Scores, Two-Tailed p-values, and 95% Confidence Intervals Estimates Based on the Interval Censored Proportional Hazards Model for the GBCS Data ($n = 686$)

Variable	Coeff.	Std. Err.	z	$p>|z|$	95% CIE
age	0.001	0.0061	0.22	0.823	−0.011, 0.013
hormon	−0.358	0.1283	−2.79	0.005	−0.609, −0.106
size	0.015	0.0036	4.10	<0.001	0.008, 0.022
int_1	−2.873	0.3712	−7.74	<0.001	−3.601, −2.146
int_2	−2.009	0.3595	−5.59	<0.001	−2.713, −1.304
int_3	−2.365	0.3695	−6.4	<0.001	−3.089, −1.640
int_4	−2.439	0.3780	−6.45	<0.001	−3.180, −1.698
int_5	−2.630	0.4023	−6.54	<0.001	−3.419, −1.842
int_6	−2.668	0.4525	−5.90	<0.001	−3.555, −1.781
Int_7	−2.764	0.6781	−4.08	<0.001	−4.093, −1.435

was used to obtain coefficient estimates, the model generating the likelihood is the proportional hazards model.

We can use the results of the fitted model and (7.15) to obtain estimates of the covariate–adjusted survival function. Because there are only seven time intervals, the survival function is not likely to be of great practical value. However, it might be of value in other settings with more intervals, so we present and illustrate the method. As in the non-interval censored setting, we begin by obtaining an estimator of the baseline survival function. In this case, the values are obtained at endpoints of each interval, using the interval-specific parameter estimates. It follows from the definition of τ_j, and the fact that $S_0(t_0 = 0) = 1$ that the estimator of the baseline survival function at the end of the first interval is

$$\hat{S}_0(t_1) = \exp\left[-\exp(\hat{\tau}_1)\right].$$

The estimator of the baseline survival function at the end of the second interval is

$$\hat{S}_0(t_2) = \hat{S}_0(t_1) \times \exp\left[-\exp(\hat{\tau}_2)\right].$$

In general, the estimator at the end of the jth interval, t_j, is

$$\hat{S}_0(t_j) = \hat{S}_0(t_{j-1}) \times \exp\left[-\exp(\hat{\tau}_j)\right], \tag{7.19}$$

for $j = 1, 2, \ldots, J$. As in the continuous time setting, the actual values of these estimators will not be particularly useful unless the data have been centered in such a way that having covariates equal to zero corresponds to a clinically plausible subject. We obtain the covariate-adjusted estimator of the survival function from the estimator of the baseline survival function in the same way as in the non interval-censored case, namely

$$\hat{S}(t_j, \mathbf{x}, \hat{\boldsymbol{\beta}}) = \left[\hat{S}_0(t_j)\right]^{\exp(\mathbf{x}'\hat{\boldsymbol{\beta}})}. \tag{7.20}$$

The covariate–adjusted survival function can also be used to provide a graphical, but model–based, comparison of survival experience in groups, such as those defined by hormone use. Because the model is not complicated, we do not need to use the modified risk score approach but, instead, compare the survival curves for the two hormone use groups at the median value of age, 53 years, and tumor size, 25 mm. In doing so, we must not perform the calculations in the expanded data set because it has more than one observation or data line per subject for those whose follow up goes beyond the first interval. We must either delete the extra lines from the expanded data set or return to the original data set to perform the calculations.

The first step is to calculate the two values of the risk score. This calculation uses the coefficients for age, hormone use, and tumor size from the model in Table 7.15. The covariate adjusted risk score for no hormone use is

$$\hat{r}_0 = 0.001 \times 53 + 0.015 \times 25$$
$$= 0.428$$

and the risk score for the hormone use group is

$$\hat{r}_1 = -0.358 + 0.001 \times 53 + 0.015 \times 25$$
$$= 0.070.$$

The estimated survival function for no hormone use is obtained by evaluating

$$\hat{S}(t_j, hormone = 0, age = 53, size = 25) = \left[\hat{S}_0(t_j)\right]^{\exp(0.428)}$$

for $j = 0,1,...,7$. The estimated survival function for hormone use is obtained by evaluating

$$\hat{S}(t_j, hormone = 1, age = 53, size = 25) = \left[\hat{S}_0(t_j)\right]^{\exp(0.070)}$$

for $j = 0,1,...,7$.

Figure 7.2 presents the graphs of the two estimated survival functions. The plotted points are connected by steps to emphasize that, in the interval-censored data setting, we have no information about the baseline survival function between interval endpoints and one must assume it is constant.

The graph itself is not particularly interesting in this example because only seven intervals were used. However, in an analysis with more intervals, it could be used to provide estimates of quantiles of survival time using the methods discussed in Chapter 4 and illustrated in Chapter 6.

In summary, the modeling paradigm for interval-censored survival data is essentially the same as for non-interval-censored data. Interpretation and presentation of the results of a fitted proportional hazards model is identical for the two types of data. However, model building with interval-censored data uses the binary regression likelihood in (7.18) if intervals are the same for all subjects. This implies that model building details, such as variable selection, identification of the scale of continuous covariates, and inclusion of interactions, use techniques based on binary regression modeling. These are discussed in detail for the logistic regression model in Hosmer and Lemeshow (2001) and may be used without modification for the complimentary log-log model. However, the methods for assess-

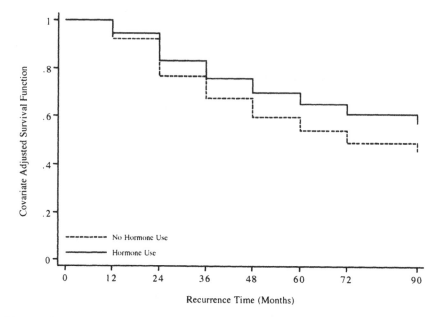

Figure 7.2 Graphs of the covariate adjusted risk-score-adjusted survival functions for the two hormone use groups based on the fitted model in Table 7.15 for the GBCS Data ($n = 686$).

ing model adequacy and fit discussed in Hosmer and Lemeshow (2001) are for use with the logistic regression model only. McCullagh and Nelder (1989, Chapter 12) discuss these methods for generalized linear models. We have not described details of how to obtain measures of leverage, residual, and influence, as well as overall goodness-of-fit from existing software packages for the complementary log-log link function.

It is possible that survival time could be thought of as being a discrete random variable. Kalbfleisch and Prentice (2002) discuss the discrete-time proportional hazards model and show that it may be obtained as a grouped–time version of the continuous-time proportional hazards model. The grouped-time model discussed by Kalbfleisch and Prentice is identical to the interval-censored model presented in this section, so analysis of a discrete-time proportional hazards model would use the methods described in this section.

EXERCISES

1. The model building example in Chapter 5 involved finding the best model in the WHAS500 data for lenfol (in years) as survival time and fstat as the censoring variable. The fit and adherence to model assumptions was assessed in Problem 5 in Chapter 6. In this problem and section, we call this model the "WHAS500 model."

   (a) Treating cohort year (variable: year) as a stratification variable, fit the WHAS500 model. Compare the estimated coefficients with those from the fit of the WHAS500 in Table 6.5. Are there any important differences (i.e., changes greater than 15 percent)?

   (b) Are there any significant interactions between the two-design variables for cohort year (use 1997 as the reference value) and the main effects in the WHAS500 model? In these models only interaction terms are included - not the main effects for the two design variables for cohort year. If there are any significant interactions, what are they and do they make clinical sense such that they should be kept in the model?

2. An alternative approach to the analysis of long-term survival in the WHAS500 data is to study the survival experience of patients post-hospital discharge using lenfol as survival time. Restrict the analysis to patients discharged alive (dstat = 0), but account for differing lengths of stay by defining los as the delayed entry time. Note that subjects with los = lenfol should be excluded, as 0 is not an allowable value for survival time in most software packages. Examine the effect on the WHAS500 model (see Table 6.5) of this alternative method of assessing long-term survival in the WHAS. Do any of the estimated coefficients change by more than 15 percent?

3. In the GBCS data, does hormone use improve survival after cancer recurrence, controlling for tumor grade and size?

4. Does revascularization improve survival experience when the analysis of the GRACE1000 data is restricted to the 695 patients who survived hospitalization (i.e., those patients with los < days)?

5. The survival time variable in the WHAS500 data, lenfol, is calculated as the days between the hospital admission date, admitdate, and the date of the last follow up, fdate. Follow up of patients is not done continuously but at various intervals. Thus, it is possible that a reported number of days of follow up could be inaccurate. To explore this, create a new variable monthfol = (12*lenfol/365.25). Use mnthfol to create discrete times, in multiples of 24

months (i.e., two-year intervals). For purposes of this problem, restrict analysis to the 496 subjects with, at most, 72 months of follow up.

(a) Use the method for fitting interval-censored data presented in Section 7.4, fit the WHAS500 model in Table 6.5. Compare the results of the two fitted models. Is this comparison helpful in evaluating the described grouping strategy as a method for dealing with imprecisely measured survival times?

(b) Use the fitted model in problem 3(a) and present covariate-adjusted survivorship functions comparing the survival experience of patients with and without congestive heart complications (chf).

(c) Describe a strategy for including cohort year (variable: year) as a stratification variable in the interval censored data analysis in problem 4(b). If possible, implement this strategy.

6. Data from the French Three Cities Study has been graciously provided to us by the 3C study investigators at Inserm Unit 708 in Paris, France. Data are available on approximately 8,500 subjects [see The 3C Study Group (2003)]. For the purposes of this problem we eliminated subjects with missing data and sampled censored subjects yielding a data set with 697 subjects and an event rate of 10 percent. Hence results from analyses in this problem do not apply to the main study. The data are available on the web sites as FRTCS.dat and are described in FRTCS.txt.

In this study the subject's age gender, systolic blood pressure, diastolic blood pressure and use of antihypertensive drugs are recorded at baseline. At two follow up visits the date of the visit and the measurements of systolic blood pressure, diastolic blood pressure and use of antihypertensive drugs are recorded. Hence these three covariates are examples of measured time varying covariates. The date of the event or end of follow up is recorded

(a) The first step in the analyses requires that the data for each subject be expanded from a single record to three records per subject, using the dates to create an entry time, exit time and covariate values for follow up from baseline to first follow up visit, from first follow up visit to second follow up visit and from second follow up visit to event or censoring. The single record data for the first subject are shown below: {id, age, sex (1 = male, 2 = female), age, date of baseline (ddmmmyy), systolic blood pressure (mmHg) at baseline, diastolic blood pressure (mmHg) at baseline, use of antihypertensive drugs (0 = no, 1 = yes) at baseline, similar data at follow up exams one and two, date of event or end of follow up and censor (1 = event, 0 = censor)}.

1, 65, 2, 25Feb99, 94, 63, 0, 27Jun01, 109, 59.5, 0, 02Jul03, 107.5, 56, 0, 25Feb04, 0

The expanded data for subject 1 are shown below. The time intervals (enter and exit) are defined as the number of days from baseline. For example, 1558 is the number of days from the baseline date of 25feb99 to the second exam date of 02Jul03. Because this subject did not experience an event, censor is equal to zero at the end of all three intervals. Subjects who have an event have a value of 1 at the end of the last interval.

id	age	sex	enter	exit	sbp	dbp	antihyp	censor
1	65	2	0	853	94	63	0	0
1	65	2	853	1588	109	59.5	0	0
1	65	2	1588	1826	107.5	56	0	0

(b) Following the creation of the expanded data set fit a proportional hazards model, using the counting process description of follow up, containing age, sex, systolic blood pressure, diastolic blood pressure and use of antihypertensive drugs.

(c) Estimate and interpret hazard ratios for each model covariate.

CHAPTER 8

Parametric Regression Models

8.1 INTRODUCTION

In the previous chapters, we focused on the use of either nonparametric or semiparametric models for the analysis of censored survival time data. The rationale for using these techniques, in particular the semiparametric proportional hazards regression model, was to avoid having to specify the hazard function completely. The utility of the proportional hazards model stems from the fact that a reduced set of assumptions is needed to provide hazard ratios that are easily interpreted and clinically meaningful. However, there may be settings in which the distribution of survival time, through previous research, has a known parametric form that justifies use of a fully parametric model to address the goals of the analysis better. A fully parametric model has some advantages: (1) full maximum likelihood may be used to estimate the parameters, (2) the estimated coefficients or transformations of them can provide clinically meaningful estimates of effect, (3) fitted values from the model can provide estimates of survival time, and (4) residuals can be computed as differences between observed and predicted values of time. An analysis of censored time-to-event data using a fully parametric model can almost have the look and feel of a normal-errors linear regression analysis.

In this chapter, we begin by considering a class of models called *accelerated failure time* models and discuss in detail three specific examples: the exponential, the Weibull, and the log-logistic regression models. We conclude the chapter with a few comments and observations on the use of parametric survival time models.

There are a number of texts that discuss parametric survival time-models (e.g., Cox and Oakes (1984), Crowder, Kimber, Smith and Sweeting (1991), Elandt-Johnson and Johnson (1980), Gross and Clark (1975), Lawless (2003), Lee and Wang (2003) and Nelson (1982, 1990)). Collett (2003) presents parametric models at a level comparable to the material in this chapter, while Klein and Moeschberger (2003) treat the topic at a slightly higher mathematical level. Andersen, Borgan, Gill and Keiding (1993) discuss theoretical aspects of parametric regression models.

A convenient and plausible way to characterize the distribution of time to event, denoted T, as a function of a single covariate is via the equation

$$T = e^{\beta_0 + \beta_1 x} \times \varepsilon. \tag{8.1}$$

Because time must be positive, we express it in (8.1) as the product of a strictly positive systematic component, $\exp(\beta_0 + \beta_1 x)$, and an error component, ε, that also must take on only positive values. A convenient choice is the exponential distribution, denoted $E(1)$. This is the distribution with survival function $S(t) = \exp(-t)$. This model can be "linearized" by taking the natural log of each side of the equation, yielding

$$\ln(T) = \beta_0 + \beta_1 x + \varepsilon^*, \tag{8.2}$$

where $\varepsilon^* = \ln(\varepsilon)$. If the error component, ε, follows the exponential distribution, then the error component ε^* follows the extreme minimum value distribution, denoted as $G(0,1)$. The model in (8.2) is called the *exponential regression model*. It can be generalized by allowing the shape parameter to be different from 1 by using the $G(0,\sigma)$ distribution, yielding model equation

$$\ln(T) = \beta_0 + \beta_1 x + \sigma \times \varepsilon^*. \tag{8.3}$$

The model in (8.3) is called the *Weibull regression model*.

Survival time models that can be linearized by taking logs are called *accelerated failure time* models. The reason for this terminology is that the effect of the covariate, as shown in (8.1), is multiplicative on the time scale. That is, the effect of the covariate is said to "accelerate" survival time. We have shown, in the previous chapters, that under the proportional hazards model, the effect of the covariates is multiplicative on the hazard scale. Another way to describe the distribution of the errors is the log-logistic distribution (i.e., log-survival time is logistic distributed) (8.3). Another popular distribution is the log-normal distribution (i.e., log-survival time is normally distributed). Because the logistic and normal distributions are similar and the logistic distribution can be expressed in closed form, we do not cover the log-normal accelerated failure-time model. The texts by Collett (2003) and Klein and Moeschberger (2003) discuss accelerated failure time models. Andersen, Borgan, Gill and Keiding (1993) discuss a model based on a general linearizing transformation.

Wei (1992) discusses semi-parametric approaches to fitting accelerated failure-time models. He suggests that, because the parameters in the accelerated failure-time models are interpreted as effects on the time scale, they may be more easily understood than hazard ratios by clinical investigators, especially those unfamiliar with survival time analyses. Fisher (1992), commenting on Wei's paper, notes that in his experience (and our as well) most research-oriented clinicians have little or no trouble understanding the proportional hazards model or the hazard ratio. To the contrary, they feel quite comfortable with it. As a result, the proportional hazards model is now accepted as the standard method for regression analysis of survival time in many applied settings. It is so deeply embedded in the statistical practice of some fields that it is unlikely that it will be replaced by another model in the foreseeable future. A parametric accelerated failure time regression model does have some appeal since it can, in some instances, provide a concise and easily interpreted analysis of censored survival time data.

8.2 THE EXPONENTIAL REGRESSION MODEL

We begin our detailed discussion of parametric regression models for time to-event-data with the single covariate model in (8.2), where the error distribution is log-exponential (i.e., the extreme minimum value distribution denoted $G(0,1)$). The survival function for this model is

$$S(t,x,\boldsymbol{\beta}) = \exp\left(-t/e^{\beta_0 + \beta_1 x}\right). \tag{8.4}$$

To obtain the median survival time, we set the right-hand side of (8.4) equal to 0.5 and solve the resulting equation. This yields an equation for the covariate specific median survival time of

$$t_{50}(x,\boldsymbol{\beta}) = -e^{\beta_0 + \beta_1 x} \times \ln(0.5). \tag{8.5}$$

When the covariate in (8.5) is dichotomous, coded 0 or 1, the ratio of the median survival time for the group with $x = 1$ to the group with $x = 0$ denoted, $\mathrm{TR}(x = 1, x = 0)$, is

$$\mathrm{TR}(x=1,x=0) = \frac{t_{50}(x=1,\boldsymbol{\beta})}{t_{50}(x=0,\boldsymbol{\beta})} = \frac{-e^{\beta_0 + \beta_1} \times \ln(0.5)}{-e^{\beta_0} \times \ln(0.5)} = e^{\beta_1}, \tag{8.6}$$

where TR denotes *time ratio*. Alternatively, the relationship between the two median times is

$$t_{50}(x=1,\boldsymbol{\beta}) = e^{\beta_1} t_{50}(x=0,\boldsymbol{\beta}). \tag{8.7}$$

If, for example, $\exp(\beta_1) = 2$, then the median survival time in the group with $x = 1$ is twice the median survival time in the group with $x = 0$. In a similar manner if $\exp(\beta_1) = 0.5$, then the median survival time in the group with $x = 1$ is one-half the median survival time in the group with $x = 0$. The multiplicative covariate effect on the time scale is clear and easy to understand. The result in (8.6) holds not only for the median but also for all percentiles. The quantity $\exp(\beta_1)$ is commonly referred to as the *acceleration factor*, even though its effect can be either to "accelerate" or "decelerate" survival time.

An alternative way to present the multiplicative effect is via the survival function. It follows from (8.4) that the relationship between the survival functions for the two groups is

$$S(t, x = 1, \beta) = S(te^{-\beta_1}, x = 0, \beta). \tag{8.8}$$

The interpretation of the result in (8.8) is that the value of the survival function at time t for the group with $x = 1$ may be obtained by evaluating the survival function for the group with $x = 0$ at time $t\exp(-\beta_1)$. The change in the sign of the coefficient is due to the fact that time percentiles and survival probabilities are inverse operations of one another.

The hazard function for the model in (8.4) is[1]

$$h(t, x, \beta) = e^{-(\beta_0 + \beta_1 x)}. \tag{8.9}$$

The hazard function in (8.9) depends only on the model coefficients and covariate values, hence is constant over time. This is both the exponential regression model's strength and weakness. The hazard function is simple, but may be too simple to provide a realistic description of the rate of event occurrence over time. We return to this point when we assess model fit.

The hazard ratio for a dichotomous covariate is

$$\text{HR}(x = 1, x = 0) = e^{-\beta_1}. \tag{8.10}$$

Thus, we see that the exponential regression model is an example of an accelerated failure time model with proportional hazards. Cox and Oakes (1984) show that the only accelerated failure time models that have proportional hazards are the exponential and Weibull regression models. If an exponential regression model fits the data, one may express the effect of covariates either as a time or as a hazard ratio.

---

[1] Here we use the fact that the hazard function is the ratio of the density function to the survival function and the equation for the density function is

$$f(t, x, \beta) = \{\exp[-(\beta_0 + \beta_1 x)]\} \exp[-t/\exp(\beta_0 + \beta_1 x)].$$

Some software packages, for example SAS, fit the linearized or log-time form of the model and provide estimates of the accelerated failure-time form of the coefficients. Other packages, for example STATA, provide a choice of expressing the results in terms of hazards or accelerated failure-time coefficients. One should always consult the software manual to confirm the form of the model fit and the scale (time or hazard) on which the results are displayed. With the exponential regression model, it is easy to switch between the two forms of the coefficients because each is simply the negative of the other. As we show in the next section, the Weibull model is bit more complicated in this respect.

In this chapter, we assume that observations are subject only to right censoring, but the analyses may be extended to other types of censoring and truncation using the methods discussed in Chapter 7 for the proportional hazards model.

We discussed using maximum likelihood estimation for time to event regression models with right censored data in Section 3.3 equations (3.14) – (3.16). Under the assumption that we have n independent observations of time, p covariates and a censoring indicator denoted $(t_i, \mathbf{x}_i, c_i)$, $i = 1, 2, \ldots, n$, the general equation for the log-likelihood function from (3.16) is

$$L(\boldsymbol{\beta}) = \sum_{i=1}^{n} \left\{ c_i \ln\left[f(t_i, \boldsymbol{\beta}, \mathbf{x}_i) \right] + (1 - c_i) \ln\left[S(t_i, \boldsymbol{\beta}, \mathbf{x}_i) \right] \right\}. \tag{8.11}$$

Under the assumption that the "errors," ε^*, are distributed as extreme minimum value $G(0,1)$ it follows that

$$f(y, \boldsymbol{\beta}, \mathbf{x}) = e^{\left[(y - \mathbf{x}'\boldsymbol{\beta}) - \exp(y - \mathbf{x}'\boldsymbol{\beta}) \right]}$$

and

$$S(y, \boldsymbol{\beta}, \mathbf{x}) = e^{-\exp(y - \mathbf{x}'\boldsymbol{\beta})},$$

where $y = \ln(t)$. Substituting these expressions into (8.11) and simplifying yields the log likelihood function

$$L(\boldsymbol{\beta}) = \sum_{i=1}^{n} c_i z_i - e^{z_i}, \tag{8.12}$$

where $z_i = y_i - \mathbf{x}_i'\boldsymbol{\beta}$, $y_i = \ln(t_i)$, $\mathbf{x}_i' = (x_{i0}, x_{i1}, \ldots, x_{ip})$ and $x_{i0} = 1$. We obtain the likelihood equations by differentiating the log-likelihood function with respect to the unknown parameters and setting the expressions equal to zero. This process yields the equation for the constant term of

$$\sum_{i=1}^{n}\left(c_i - e^{z_i}\right) = 0 \tag{8.13}$$

and equations for the non-constant covariates of

$$\sum_{i=1}^{n} x_{ij}\left(c_i - e^{z_i}\right) = 0, \tag{8.14}$$

for $j = 1, 2, \ldots, p$.   If we denote the solutions to (8.13) and (8.14) as $\hat{\boldsymbol{\beta}}' = \left(\hat{\beta}_0, \hat{\beta}_1, \ldots, \hat{\beta}_p\right)$, the model-based predicted or fitted values of time are computed as $\hat{t}_i = \exp\left(\mathbf{x}_i'\hat{\boldsymbol{\beta}}\right)$ for $i = 1, 2, \ldots, n$. In the usual linear regression model, the inclusion of the constant term in the model forces the mean of the observed and fitted values to be equal. However, in the exponential regression model, its effect is to force the sum of the ratio of observed to fitted values to be equal to the number of non-censored observations, that is,

$$\sum_{i=1}^{n} c_i = m = \sum_{i=1}^{n} \frac{t_i}{\hat{t}_i}. \tag{8.15}$$

The actual value of $\hat{\beta}_0$ depends, to a large extent, on m, the number of non-censored observations.   Thus, the fitted values are predictions of values from a censored exponential distribution — not the true mean survival time of a subject with covariate value $\mathbf{x}_i$.

We obtain the estimator of the variances and covariances of the estimator of the coefficients, using standard theory of maximum likelihood estimation, from the second partial derivatives of the log-likelihood function. The general form of the second partial derivative of the log-likelihood function in (8.12) is

$$\frac{\partial^2 L(\boldsymbol{\beta})}{\partial \beta_j \partial \beta_k} = -\sum_{i=1}^{n} x_{ij} x_{ik} e^{z_i}, \quad j, k = 0, 1, \ldots, p. \tag{8.16}$$

In this setting, estimators are based on the observed information matrix, denoted $\mathbf{I}(\hat{\boldsymbol{\beta}})$, which is the matrix with elements given by the negative of (8.16) evaluated at the estimator of the coefficients. The inverse of the observed information matrix provides the estimators of the variances and covariances, namely

$$\widehat{\text{Var}}\left(\hat{\boldsymbol{\beta}}\right) = \mathbf{I}(\hat{\boldsymbol{\beta}})^{-1}. \tag{8.17}$$

Table 8.1 Estimated Coefficients, Standard Errors, z-Scores, Two-Tailed p-values, and 95% Confidence Interval Estimates for the Exponential Regression Model in the WHAS100 data (n = 100)

Variable	Coeff.	Std. Err.	z	p > |z|	95% CIE
gender	−0.602	0.2814	−2.14	0.033	−1.153, −0.050
Constant	2.318	0.1890	12.26	< 0.001	1.947, 2.688

Typically, software packages provide estimates of the standard errors of each of the coefficients in the model that are the square roots of the elements on the main diagonal of the matrix in (8.17). Most packages provide an option for obtaining all the elements of (8.17). The endpoints of a $100(1-\alpha)$ percent Wald-statistic-based confidence interval for the jth coefficients are

$$\hat{\beta}_j \pm z_{1-\alpha/2}\hat{SE}\left(\hat{\beta}_j\right),\qquad\qquad(8.18)$$

where $z_{1-\alpha/2}$ is the upper $\alpha/2$ percentile of the standard normal distribution and $\hat{SE}\left(\hat{\beta}_j\right)$ denotes the estimator of the standard error of the estimator of the coefficient.

As a first example, we use the WHAS100 data and fit the exponential regresion model containing gender. The results of the fit are shown in Table 8.1.

The estimated coefficients shown in Table 8.1 are expressed on the log-time scale and, using (8.5), the estimated median time to death for males is

$$\hat{t}_{50}\left(gender=0\right)=-e^{2.318}\times\ln\left(0.5\right)=7.04$$

years, and the estimate for females is

$$\hat{t}_{50}\left(gender=1\right)=-e^{2.318-0.602}\times\ln\left(0.5\right)=3.86$$

months. The estimated time ratio, from (8.6), is

$$\hat{TR}\left(gender=1,gender=0\right)=e^{-0.602}=0.55.\qquad\qquad(8.19)$$

That is, the median time to death among females is estimated to be 0.55 times the median time to death among males.

The value of any estimated time percentile depends on the value of $\hat{\beta}_0=2.318$ which, in turn, depends on the observed number of actual survival times, m. Thus, the values of 7.04 years and 3.86 years are only useful for descriptive purposes in the 51 percent, $100 \times (51/100)$, of the data with observed survival times. Because the model is an accelerated failure-time model, the ratio of any time percentiles for females to males depends only on the coefficient for gender, $\hat{\beta}_1$. Hence, we feel that the ratio is a more useful summary measure of survival experience than are individual estimates of percentiles that depend on the proportion of observed non-censored survival times.

In particular, the interpretation of the estimated time ratio in (8.19) is that the survival time for females is estimated to be 55 percent of that of males. Another way to state the effect is that survival time among females is shortened by 45 percent. In a manner identical to that used in previous chapters for the hazard ratio, the confidence interval for the time ratio is obtained by exponentiating the endpoints of the confidence interval for the coefficient. In the example, the 95 percent confidence interval reported in Table 8.1 for $\hat{\beta}_1$ is obtained using (8.18). Thus, the 95 percent confidence interval for the time ratio is

$$\left(e^{-1.153} \leq TR \leq e^{-0.050} \right) = \left(0.32 \leq TR \leq 0.95 \right).$$

The interpretation of this confidence interval is that females have survival times estimated to be between 32 percent and 95 percent of males with 95 percent confidence. Alternatively, survival is shortened among females to between 5 percent and 68 percent of males.

Because the exponential regression model has proportional hazards, we can express the effect of covariates using hazard ratios. Using the negative of the coefficient for drug use from the results in Table 8.1 and (8.10), the estimated hazard ratio for female gender is

$$\hat{HR}\left(gender = 1, gender = 0 \right) = e^{0.602} = 1.83.$$

The endpoints of a 95 percent confidence interval are the inverse of those of the time ratio, namely

$$\left(e^{0.05} \leq HR \leq e^{1.153} \right) = \left(1.05 \leq HR \leq 3.17 \right).$$

These results show that females are dying at a rate estimated to be 1.83 times that of males, and it is consistent with the data that the hazard ratio could be as low as 1.05 or as high as 3.17.

The two descriptions of the effect are statistically equivalent, but one describes the effect on the time scale and the other with the hazard rate. For some investigators, time may be more easily understood than a rate expressed by the hazard function. For such an audience, results presented as time ratios are preferable to ones based on hazard ratios.

We emphasize that the dual interpretation of results discussed here is a consequence of the fact that the exponential regression model is both an accelerated failure-time model and a proportional hazards model. One should never automatically invert hazard ratios estimated from a fitted proportional hazards model and interpret them as estimated time ratios. Because there are many models with proportional hazards but only two of them are accelerated failure-time models.

The steps in building an exponential regression model are essentially identical to those described in detail in Chapter 5 for the proportional hazards model and, as such, are not repeated in this section. The only difference is that the log-likelihood function is used to compare models rather than the *partial* log-likelihood. Most software packages have routines for stepwise selection of covariates. As discussed in Chapter 5, issues of scale selection for continuous covariates, statistical adjustment, and selection of interactions are still vital steps in the model building process.

Because the model-building steps are the same as those presented in Chapter 5, we discuss only a few details. The techniques for checking the scale of all continuous covariates are similar to those illustrated in Chapter 5. Recall that possible methods include the use of design variables, smoothed residual plots, and fractional polynomials. Each of these methods may be used in the same way with an exponential regression model, with a few modifications. The smoothed residual plots discussed in Chapter 5 use the martingale residuals. The martingale residuals for a fitted exponential regression model are

$$\hat{M}_i = c_i - t_i e^{-x_i'\hat{\beta}} \tag{8.20}$$

and one may plot them using the method described for the proportional hazard model in Section 5.2. We remind the reader that application of the Grambsch, Therneau and Fleming (1995) plot assumes that the coefficients are on the log-hazard scale. If the model has been fit on the log-time scale, the sign of the coefficients has to be reversed before being added to the log of the ratio of smoothed values.

As an example of a more complicated model, we use the WHAS100 data and fit a model containing gender, age, their interaction and body mass index (bmi).

Table 8.2 Estimated Coefficients, Standard Errors, z-Scores, Two-Tailed p-values, and 95% Confidence Interval Estimates for the Preliminary Final Exponential Regression Model for the WHAS100 Data ($n = 100$)

Variable	Coeff.	Std. Err.	z	$p>|z|$	95% CIE
gender	−3.932	1.8098	−2.17	0.030	−7.480, −0.385
age	−0.053	0.0157	−3.39	0.001	−0.084, −0.022
gender × age	0.050	0.0241	2.06	0.039	0.002, 0.097
bmi	0.093	0.0376	2.49	0.013	0.020, 0.167
Constant	3.389	1.6200	2.09	0.036	0.214, 6.564

We regard the model in Table 8.2 as the preliminary final model until we check model adequacy and fit.

The methods and procedures for assessing the fit of an exponential regression model are nearly identical to those described in Chapter 6 for the proportional hazards model, with one exception. We check the hazard function for a specific parametric form rather than the more general proportional hazards assumption. The methods for identifying whether any subjects have an undue influence on the estimated parameters or are poorly fit use the same score function residuals used for the proportional hazards model. Not all software packages provide these score function residuals; however, they are not too difficult to calculate, as shown below.

Overall goodness of fit can be assessed using the test proposed by Grønnesby and Borgan (1996) and simplified by May and Hosmer (1998). This test was discussed in Section 6.5. The notes in Section 6.5 regarding its interpretation and the regularity conditions for the proofs given in Grønnesby and Borgan's paper also hold for the exponential regression model using right-censored data.

The score residuals are the basis for examining the influence of individual subjects on the values of the estimated parameters. These residuals are the individual contributions to score equations represented generally in (8.14). Specifically, the score residual for subject i on covariate j is the individual component of the derivative of the log-likelihood in equation (8.12), namely

$$\hat{L}_{ij} = x_{ij}\left(t_i e^{-x_i\beta} - c_i\right) = -x_{ij}\hat{M}_i \; . \qquad (8.21)$$

We denote the vector containing the score residuals for all the covariates as

$$\hat{\mathbf{L}}'_i = \left(\hat{L}_{i0}, \hat{L}_{i1}, \hat{L}_{i2}, \ldots, \hat{L}_{ip}\right). \qquad (8.22)$$

As was the case in (6.24) for the proportional hazards model and as described by Collett (2003, Section 7.4) for parametric regression models, the statistics for assessing the influence of the ith subject on the coefficients are the components of the vector

$$\Delta\hat{\boldsymbol{\beta}}_i = \hat{\mathrm{Var}}\left(\hat{\boldsymbol{\beta}}\right)\hat{\mathbf{L}}_i, \qquad (8.23)$$

which we refer to as scaled score residuals, where $\hat{\mathrm{Var}}\left(\hat{\boldsymbol{\beta}}\right)$ is the estimated covariance matrix of the estimated coefficients shown in (8.17). The covariate-specific score residuals in (8.21) and their respective individual components in (8.23) can be plotted against several measures. We feel that, when a diagnostic statistic relates to a specific covariate, using the values of that covariate leads to the most informative plot. With this plot, we are able to identify large values of the diagnostic statistic, and to determine at approximately which covariate values they occur. Figure 8.1 presents an example of such a plot.

A measure of the overall influence of a subject on the vector of coefficients, similar to the result in (6.25), is the statistic

$$ld_i = \hat{\mathbf{L}}_i' \widehat{\text{Var}}\left(\hat{\boldsymbol{\beta}}\right)\hat{\mathbf{L}}_i \, . \qquad (8.24)$$

This statistic was proposed by Hall, Rogers and Pregibon (1982) who suggested using a scaled version of it

$$\frac{ld_i}{\left(1 - ld_i\right)^2} \, . \qquad (8.25)$$

Either form, (8.24) or (8.25), could be used, but, to be in agreement with approaches described in Chapter 6, we use the unscaled form in (8.24). When referring to the statistic in (8.24), we use the same term(s) used in Chapter 6, namely likelihood displacement or Cook's distance statistic. The measure of overall influence depends on all covariates, so it makes sense to plot it against another summary statistic. We feel a plot using the martingale residuals with separate plotting symbols for censored and non-censored observations is most informative.

Unfortunately, most of the major software packages do not routinely calculate the values of the diagnostic statistics for parametric regression models, although this is likely to change in the future. At this time, only S-PLUS provides the diagnostic statistics. Users of other packages will need to write their own procedures to calculate the values of the diagnostic statistics. This requires some facility with creating matrices, performing matrix operations, and saving the results as new variables. Collett (2003) provides macros for use with SAS. The values of the diagnostic statistics for the model in Table 8.2 were calculated in STATA using a program we wrote.

As was the case in the proportional hazards model, there is no distribution theory to provide critical values for significance tests of the diagnostic statistics. The best approach is to plot them and look for values that seem too large. In Figure 8.1, we show the plots of the scaled score residuals from (8.23) for each of the four terms in the model. In Figure 8.1a, we see one residual that is large and negative for a female, id = 97. In figure 8.1b, we see one large positive and one large negative residual for two of the older subjects, id = 61 and 58, in the study. In Figure 8.1c, the scaled score residuals are plotted only for females, as their value is zero for males. In the figure, we see two large positive residuals for two of the younger females, id = 52 and 97. The scaled score residuals for body mass index in Figure 8.1d shows one large negative residual for a subject with a body mass index of about 36.5, id = 30.

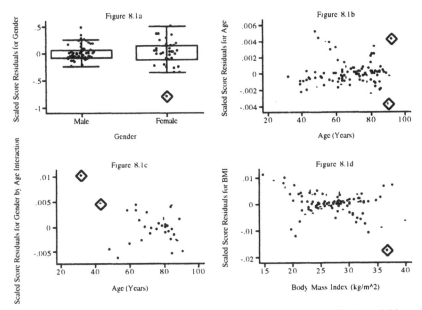

Figure 8.1 Graph of the scaled score residuals for the four terms in the fitted model in Table 8.2.

The graph of the overall likelihood displacement or Cook's distance is shown in Figure 8.2. The plot shows three subjects with large values of the statistic. Two of these subjects have positive martingale residuals, id = 30 and 97, indicating that the number of observed events, 1, was smaller than expected. The third point, id = 93, has a large negative martingale residual, indicating that the model expected this subject to have died before it was censored.

Using the plots of the diagnostic statistics, we have identified six subjects who could have a disproportionate influence on at least one of the estimated coefficients. The data for each subject and the coefficients(s) the subject appears to influence are shown in Table 8.3. The males are the oldest two males in the WHAS100 data and thus it is not surprising that they have a high influence on the main effect coefficient for age, which due to the interaction term in the model estimates of the effect of age among males. Subject 30 is an older female with among the highest values of BMI. Subjects 52 and 97 are the two youngest females and thus it is not surprising that they could influence the interaction coefficient, which adjusts the effect of age for females. Subject 97 is the youngest female and has the largest value of BMI in the WHAS100 data. We leave it as an exercise to demonstrate that deletion of these six subjects decreases the estimate of the coefficient for gender by 40 percent, decreases the interaction coefficient by 40

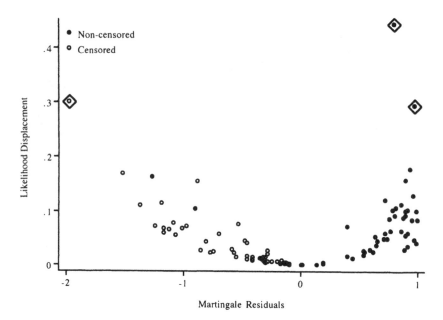

Figure 8.2 Graph of the likelihood displacement or Cook's distance statistic versus the martingale residuals from the model in Table 8.2.

percent and increases the coefficient for BMI by 30 percent. The coefficient for age only decreases by 3 percent. Other than for subjects 30 and 97, the data are clinically reasonable. As for subject 30, it is unusual to see an 85-year with a body mass index as high as 36. Unfortunately, with current levels of obesity in the US, it is not all that rare to have a 32-year-old female with a body mass index of nearly 40. In the end, the data for all six subjects is plausible enough that we cannot exclude any of them from the analysis.

Table 8.3 Six Subjects with High Influence for One or More Coefficients or Large Likelihood Displacement from the Fitted Model in Table 8.2

Study ID	Gender	Age	Body Mass Index	Influence On
30	Female	85	36.7	BMI
52	Female	43	25.3	Interaction
58	Male	92	24.4	Age
61	Male	90	24.8	Age
93	Female	80	20.6	Id
97	Female	32	39.9	Gender, Interaction and Id

The values of the diagnostic statistics depend on complicated relationships between the covariates, survival time, and censoring status. For this reason, it is not possible to provide specific cutpoints, which, when exceeded, indicate that an important change in a coefficient will occur. We think it is essential that one carefully examine the data for all subjects identified as being extreme in any diagnostic statistic and refit the model, deleting these subjects. Clinical criteria should always be used to make the final decisions about the continuing role of such subjects in the analysis.

We discussed methods for assessing the assumption of proportional hazards in Chapter 6. With a fully parametric model, this analysis step is replaced with one that determines whether the data support the particular parametric form of the hazard function. The most frequently employed method uses the model-based estimate of the cumulative hazard function to form the Cox–Snell residuals (see Cox and Snell (1968)). They noted that the values of the estimated cumulative hazard function may be thought of as observations from a censored sample from an exponential distribution with parameter equal to one. The diagnostic plot compares the model-based cumulative hazard to one obtained from a nonparametric (Kaplan–Meier or Nelson–Aalen) estimator. The nonparametric estimator uses the model-based estimates of the cumulative hazard at each observed time as the time variable and the censoring indicator from the original survival time variable as the censoring variable. If the parametric model is correct, this plot should follow a line through the origin with slope equal to one.

The estimator of the Cox–Snell residuals from an exponential regression model is obtained by exponentiating the additive residuals on the log-time scale. Specifically,

$$\hat{H}\left(t_i, \mathbf{x}_i, \hat{\boldsymbol{\beta}}\right) = \exp\left(y_i - \mathbf{x}_i'\hat{\boldsymbol{\beta}}\right) = t_i e^{-\mathbf{x}_i'\hat{\boldsymbol{\beta}}}, \tag{8.26}$$

for $i = 1, 2, \ldots, n$. The estimates for the current fitted model are obtained using the coefficients in Table 8.2. The pairs $\left(\hat{H}\left(t_i, \mathbf{x}_i, \hat{\boldsymbol{\beta}}\right), c_i\right)$, $i = 1, 2, \ldots, n$, are used to compute the Kaplan–Meier estimator shown in (2.1) or the Nelson–Aalen cumulative hazard estimator in (2.35). That is, the values of $\hat{H}\left(t_i, \mathbf{x}_i, \hat{\boldsymbol{\beta}}\right)$ define time and the values of c_i define the events. We denote this estimator as $\hat{H}_{\text{km},i}$. Figure 8.3 presents a plot of the pairs, $\left[\hat{H}\left(t_i, \mathbf{x}_i, \hat{\boldsymbol{\beta}}\right), \hat{H}_{\text{km},i}\right]$, for $i = 1, 2, \ldots, 100$, along with the referent straight line.

In this figure, the plotted pairs of points initially fall on the referent line and then fall mostly below the line. This provides some evidence that an assumption of a constant baseline hazard function based on the fitted exponential regression model may not be appropriate for these data.

We complete our assessment of fit with the Grønnesby-Borgan test described in Section 6.5. The risk score in this setting is based on the coefficients in Table

8.2, and it refers to risk on the time scale rather than on the hazard scale. We suggested that the number of groups be chosen such that G = integer of {maximum of [2 and minimum of (10 and the number of events divided by 40)]}. In the WHAS100 data, there are 51 deaths, which, when divided by 40, is 1.275. Thus, the number of groups is $2 = \max\left[2, \min\left(10, 1.275\right)\right]$. We can use the score, likelihood ratio, or Wald test for the significance of adding the design variables to the model. When we perform the overall goodness-of-fit test with two groups, the value of the likelihood ratio test for the inclusion of the single design variable is 0.54, which, with 1 degree of freedom, has a p-value of 0.464, which is not statistically significant. A summary of the observed and estimated expected number of events within each of the two groups is presented in Table 8.4. The individual p-values are not significant, and the overall test supports model fit. We note that, if we use 5 or more groups, the goodness-of-fit test rejects model fit. This is one of the disadvantages of a test where the choice of the number of groups can influence the test statistic value. We recommend that one look at the goodness of fit of a model with more than one test or graph. If at least one indicates some clear evidence of problems with the fit, the model and associated assumptions should be investigated further. In our example, the graph seemed to indicate that the exponential model fit might be problematic. Using two groups, the overall test does

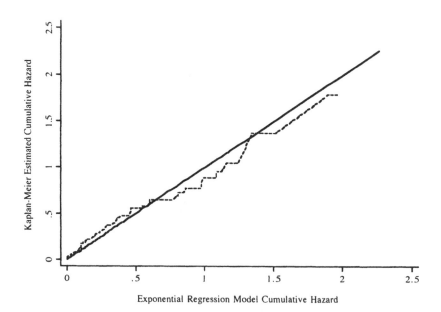

Figure 8.3 Graph of the Kaplan–Meier estimate of the cumulative hazard versus the exponential regression model estimate of the cumulative hazard from the model in Table 8.2. The solid line is the referent line with slope = 1.0 and intercept = 0.

Table 8.4 Observed Number of Events, Estimated Number of Events, z-Score, and Two-Tailed p-value within Each Decile of Risk Based on the Model in Table 8.2

Decile of Risk	Observed Number of Events	Estimated Number of Events	z	p - value
1	34	35.28	–0.22	0.83
2	17	15.72	0.32	0.75
Total	51	51		

not provide evidence of a problematic fit. As May and Hosmer (2004) show, if too many groups are used for data sets with a small to medium number of events, this test tends to reject the null hypothesis of adequate fit more often than it should. On the other hand, with only two groups, the test does not have much power to detect model violations. As a result, this overall goodness-of-fit test can only be expected to detect gross model violations for data sets with a small number of events.

At this point we have two choices: We can take the view that the departure from model fit seen in Figure 8.3 is not significant and proceed with model interpretation, or we can see whether an alternative parametric model provides a better fit than the exponential regression model. We comment on the first choice before proceeding with the details of the second in the next section.

The methods for providing an interpretation of a fitted exponential accelerated failure time regression model follow the same procedures used in Section 6.6 for the proportional hazards model. The only difference is that exponentiated coefficients provide estimates of the multiplicative effect on the time rather than estimating the hazard rate. As in Section 6.6, the key step is to specify the values of the covariates yielding a clinically interesting comparison. The time ratio is the exponentiation of the difference in the linear part of the model. That is, the time ratio comparing two levels of the covariates in the model is, in general,

$$\hat{TR}\left(\mathbf{x}=\mathbf{x}_1,\mathbf{x}=\mathbf{x}_0\right)=\exp\left[\left(\mathbf{x}_1-\mathbf{x}_0\right)'\hat{\boldsymbol{\beta}}\right]. \tag{8.27}$$

The model in Table 8.2 contains an interaction between gender and age. Following the approach used in Section 6.6, see (6.27) – (6.29), the estimated time ratio for females versus males age 60 is

$$\hat{TR}\left(gender=1,gender=0|age=60,bmi\right)=\exp\left(-3.932+0.05\times60\right)=0.39,$$

and the endpoints of the 95 percent Wald-based confidence interval are $(0.16, 0.92)$. The interpretation is that survival times for 60-year-old females are 0.39 times those of 60-year-old males. The confidence interval suggests that they could be between 0.16 to and 0.95 times the survival times of 60-year-old males. Similar calculations would be used to estimate female gender effect for other ages.

As another example, the estimated time ratio comparing subjects who differ by 5 kg/m^2 in body mass index is

$$\hat{TR}\left(bmi = b + 5, bmi = b \mid gender, age\right) = \exp\left[5 \times 0.093\right] = 1.59 \,.$$

The endpoints of the Wald-based confidence interval are $\left(1.10, \ 2.31\right)$. Thus, after controlling for gender and age, the survival times for subjects with a 5 kg/m^2 larger body mass index are 59 percent longer than those of subjects with the smaller body mass index. The confidence interval suggests that the estimate could be between 10 and 131 percent longer[2].

Again we refer the reader to Section 6.6 for formulae, computational details, and examples. There, the results deal with hazard ratios rather than time ratios, but the functions of the estimated coefficients are identical.

Before we conclude that the model in Table 8.2 is our final model, we examine other possible parametric models. Two other models that are a natural extension of the exponential model are the piecewise exponential model and the Weibull model. The piecewise exponential model assumes that the exponential model holds for segments of the time interval while allowing different levels of hazard for the different segments. The interested reader is referred to Zhou (2001) and Allison (1995) for a less technical discussion and Anderson, Borgan, Gill and Keiding (1993) for a more mathematical discussion of piecewise exponential models. We discuss the Weibull model in the next section.

8.3 THE WEIBULL REGRESSION MODEL

The basic form of a Weibull accelerated failure-time regression model was presented in (8.3). The main difference between it and the exponential regression model discussed in the previous section is that the parameter σ in the distribution of the "error" term of the accelerated failure-time form of the model can be different from 1.0. The inclusion of this parameter in the model leads to a slightly more complicated hazard function and related regression model parameters. For this reason, we begin our discussion of the Weibull model in the single covariate setting to compare and contrast it with the exponential regression model.

The hazard function for the single covariate Weibull regression model is

---

[2] We found, when modeling the WHAS500 data in Chapter 5, that body mass index was not linear in the log hazard function. This is also the case in the WHAS100 data, and we address this issue in the exercises.

$$h(t,x,\boldsymbol{\beta},\lambda) = \frac{\lambda t^{\lambda-1}}{\left(e^{\beta_0+\beta_1 x}\right)^{\lambda}}, \tag{8.28}$$

where, for convenience, we use $\lambda = 1/\sigma$. This hazard function can be expressed in either proportional hazards or accelerated failure-time form. The proportional hazards form of the function is obtained as follows:

$$h(t,x,\boldsymbol{\beta},\lambda) = \lambda t^{\lambda-1} e^{-\lambda(\beta_0+\beta_1 x)}$$
$$= \lambda t^{\lambda-1} e^{-\lambda\beta_0} e^{-\lambda\beta_1 x}$$

so

$$h(t,x,\boldsymbol{\beta},\lambda) = \lambda\gamma t^{\lambda-1} e^{-\lambda\beta_1 x}$$
$$= h_0(t) e^{\theta_1 x}, \tag{8.29}$$

where $\gamma = \exp(-\beta_0/\sigma) = \exp(\theta_0)$, $\theta_1 = -\beta_1/\sigma$ and the baseline hazard function is $h_0(t) = \lambda\gamma t^{\lambda-1}$. Although the parameter σ is a variance-like parameter on the log-time scale, $\lambda = 1/\sigma$ is commonly called the *shape parameter*. In the remainder of this chapter, we will refer to σ as the shape parameter. The parameter γ is called a *scale parameter*. The expression for the hazard function in (8.29) leads to a hazard ratio interpretation of the parameter θ_1.

The accelerated failure-time form of the hazard function is obtained by expressing (8.28) as follows:

$$h(t,x,\boldsymbol{\beta},\lambda) = \lambda t^{\lambda-1} e^{-\lambda(\beta_0+\beta_1 x)}$$
$$= \lambda\gamma \left(te^{-\beta_1 x}\right)^{\lambda-1} e^{-\beta_1 x}. \tag{8.30}$$

The rationale for presenting both forms of the hazard function is that different software packages use different parameterizations when fitting a model. For example, SAS uses the accelerated failure-time model parameterization in (8.30) and reports estimates of the $\boldsymbol{\beta}$ form of the coefficients and σ. STATA offers the option of providing estimates of either parameterization. If the accelerated failure-time (or log-time) form is chosen, estimates of $\boldsymbol{\beta}$ and σ are provided. If the proportional hazards (or log-hazards) form is chosen, estimates of $\boldsymbol{\theta}$ and σ are provided. The relationship between the two sets of coefficients is $\boldsymbol{\theta} = -\boldsymbol{\beta}/\sigma$. In the remainder of this section, we use the accelerated failure time formulation of the model.

The survival function corresponding to the accelerated failure-time form of the hazard function in (8.30) is

$$S(t,x,\boldsymbol{\beta},\sigma)=\exp\left\{-t^{\lambda}\exp\left[(-1/\sigma)(\beta_0+\beta_1 x)\right]\right\}. \tag{8.31}$$

We obtain the equation for the median survival time by setting the survival function equal to 0.5 and solving for time, yielding

$$t_{50}(x,\boldsymbol{\beta},\sigma)=\left[-\ln(0.5)\right]^{\sigma}e^{\beta_0+\beta_1 x}. \tag{8.32}$$

For example, if the covariate is dichotomous and coded 0/1, the time ratio at the median survival time is

$$\mathrm{TR}(x=1,x=0)=\frac{t_{50}(x=1,\boldsymbol{\beta},\sigma)}{t_{50}(x=0,\boldsymbol{\beta},\sigma)}=\frac{\left[-\ln(0.5)\right]^{\sigma}e^{\beta_0+\beta_1}}{\left[-\ln(0.5)\right]^{\sigma}e^{\beta_0}}=e^{\beta_1}. \tag{8.33}$$

A similar result is obtained for other percentiles of survival time. Thus, we see that the interpretation of the $\boldsymbol{\beta}$ form of the coefficients is the same as in the exponential regression model.

Rather than providing the details of parameter estimation for both the univariable and multivariable models as was done with the exponential regression model, we present only the general multivariable model. The equation for the log-likelihood function for a sample possibly containing right-censored data is obtained using

$$z_i = \frac{y_i - \mathbf{x}_i'\boldsymbol{\beta}}{\sigma},$$

which yields the log-likelihood function

$$L(\boldsymbol{\beta},\sigma)=\sum_{i=1}^{n}c_i\left(-\ln(\sigma)+z_i\right)-e^{z_i}. \tag{8.34}$$

The score equation for the jth regression coefficient is obtained by taking the derivative of (8.34) with respect to β_j and setting it equal to zero, yielding

$$\frac{\partial L(\boldsymbol{\beta},\sigma)}{\partial \beta_j}=\sum_{i=1}^{n}\frac{-x_{ij}}{\sigma}\left(c_i-e^{z_i}\right)=0, \quad j=0,1,2,\ldots,p. \tag{8.35}$$

The score equation for the shape parameter, σ, is

$$\frac{\partial L(\boldsymbol{\beta},\sigma)}{\partial \sigma}=\frac{-m}{\sigma}+\sum_{i=1}^{n}\frac{-z_i}{\sigma}\left(c_i-e^{z_i}\right)=0. \tag{8.36}$$

Some software packages (e.g., STATA) parameterize the log-likelihood function in terms of $-\ln(\sigma)$ because this makes the score equation easier to solve from a computational point of view. Regardless of the form used, all packages report an estimate of σ. The solutions to (8.35) and (8.36) are denoted as $\hat{\boldsymbol{\beta}}$ and $\hat{\sigma}$, respectively.

As is the case in any application of maximum likelihood, the estimator of the covariance matrix of the parameter estimator is obtained from the observed information matrix. The individual elements of this matrix to be evaluated are

$$-\frac{\partial^2 L(\boldsymbol{\beta},\sigma)}{\partial \beta_j \, \partial \beta_k} = \frac{1}{\sigma^2} \sum_{i=1}^{n} x_{ij} x_{ik} e^{\hat{z}_i} \,,$$

$$-\frac{\partial^2 L(\boldsymbol{\beta},\sigma)}{\partial \beta_j \, \partial \sigma} = \frac{1}{\sigma^2} \sum_{i=1}^{n} x_{ij} z_i e^{\hat{z}_i} \,,$$

and

$$-\frac{\partial^2 L(\boldsymbol{\beta},\sigma)}{\partial \sigma \, \partial \sigma} = \frac{m}{\sigma^2} + \frac{1}{\sigma^2} \sum_{i=1}^{n} z_i^2 e^{\hat{z}_i} \,.$$

When evaluated as the solution to the likelihood equations, the information matrix may be expressed as

$$\mathbf{I}\left(\hat{\boldsymbol{\beta}},\hat{\sigma}\right) = \frac{1}{\hat{\sigma}^2} \begin{bmatrix} \mathbf{X}'\hat{\mathbf{V}}\mathbf{X} & \mathbf{X}'\hat{\mathbf{V}}\hat{\mathbf{z}} \\ \hat{\mathbf{z}}'\hat{\mathbf{V}}\mathbf{X} & \hat{\mathbf{z}}'\hat{\mathbf{V}}\hat{\mathbf{z}} + m \end{bmatrix}, \tag{8.37}$$

where $\mathbf{X}$ is an n by $p+1$ matrix containing the values of the covariates, $\hat{\mathbf{V}} = \mathrm{diag}\left(e^{\hat{z}_i}\right)$, an n by n diagonal matrix, and $\hat{\mathbf{z}}' = \left(\hat{z}_1, \hat{z}_2, \ldots, \hat{z}_n\right)$, with

$$\hat{z}_i = \frac{y_i - \mathbf{x}_i'\hat{\boldsymbol{\beta}}}{\hat{\sigma}} \,.$$

The estimator of the covariance matrix of the estimators of the parameters is

$$\hat{\mathrm{Var}}\left(\hat{\boldsymbol{\beta}},\hat{\sigma}\right) = \left[\mathbf{I}\left(\hat{\boldsymbol{\beta}},\hat{\sigma}\right)\right]^{-1}. \tag{8.38}$$

The details of the model-building process for the Weibull regression model are the same as those presented in the previous section for the exponential regression model. The martingale residuals used in the Grambsch, Therneau and Fleming (1995) plots for checking the scale of continuous covariates and for model assessment are

$$\hat{M}_i = c_i - \exp(\hat{z}_i)$$
$$= c_i - t_i^{\hat{\lambda}} \exp\left(-\hat{\lambda} \mathbf{x}_i \hat{\boldsymbol{\beta}}\right) , \tag{8.39}$$

where $\hat{\lambda} = 1/\hat{\sigma}$.

We illustrate the Weibull model by fitting the same covariates as used in the exponential regression model shown in Table 8.2. Table 8.5 presents the results of this Weibull fit.

A related model development issue is whether the Weibull model, with its additional parameter, offers an improvement over the simpler exponential model for a given set of covariates. One step in this evaluation is a test of the hypothesis that $\sigma = 1$. This hypothesis may be tested using a Wald test or the confidence interval formed from its estimate and associated standard error. Shown at the bottom of Table 8.5 is a Wald test and confidence interval for the log form of the parameter σ, as estimated in STATA, and similar statistics for the parameter estimate itself. The confidence interval for σ was formed from the endpoints of the interval for $-\ln(\sigma)$. The Wald test for σ is not reported because, based on properties of other similarly bounded parameters such as the odds ratio, one would expect tests and estimates based on the log form to have better statistical properties. The confidence interval for $-\ln(\sigma)$ does contain zero, and the p-value for the Wald test is 0.070. This indicates that the Weibull regression model presented in Table 8.5 may provide some, $0.05 < p < 0.10$, improvement over the exponential model presented in Table 8.2.

Table 8.5 Estimated Coefficients, Standard Errors, z-Scores, Two-Tailed p-values, and 95% Confidence Interval Estimates for the Weibull Regression Model for the WHAS100 data ($n = 100$)

Variable	Coeff.	Std. Err.	z	$p > |z|$	95% CIE
gender	−4.689	2.2848	−2.05	0.040	−9.168, −0.211
age	−0.064	0.0206	−3.10	0.002	−0.104, −0.024
gender × age	0.059	0.0304	1.94	0.052	−0.000, 0.119
bmi	0.106	0.0465	2.27	0.023	0.014, 0.197
Constant	3.972	2.0470	1.94	0.052	−0.040, 7.984
−ln(Sigma)	−0.225	0.1242	−1.81	0.070	−0.469, 0.018
Sigma	1.253	0.1556			0.982, 1.598

Other packages report only the parameter estimate of σ and its estimated standard error. In SAS, the test of the hypothesis that $\sigma = 1$ is performed when one fits the exponential model and it is based on the score test for the addition of σ to the model.

As noted above, the Weibull model may provide a better fit to the data than does the exponential regression model. To confirm this, we need to use the same diagnostic statistics, plots and tests that are used to assess the fit of the exponential regression model.

The value of the score residuals for the ith subject on the jth regression coefficient is obtained by evaluating the individual terms in (8.35) at the estimator, namely

$$\hat{L}_{ij} = -\frac{x_{ij}}{\hat{\sigma}}\left(c_i - e^{\hat{z}_i}\right). \tag{8.40}$$

The score residuals for the shape parameter are obtained from (8.36) in a similar manner, and are

$$\hat{L}_{ip+1} = -\frac{c_i}{\hat{\sigma}} - \frac{\hat{z}_i}{\hat{\sigma}}\left(c_i - e^{\hat{z}_i}\right). \tag{8.41}$$

If we parameterize the model in terms of $-\ln(\sigma)$ then the score residuals are

$$\hat{L}_{ip+1} = c_i + \hat{z}_i\left(c_i - e^{\hat{z}_i}\right). \tag{8.42}$$

The vector of $p+2$ score residuals is

$$\hat{\mathbf{L}}_i' = \left(\hat{L}_{i0}, \hat{L}_{i1}, \ldots, \hat{L}_{ip}, \hat{L}_{ip+1}\right).$$

As is the case with the exponential regression model, the scaled score residuals that provide estimates of the effect that each subject has on individual parameter estimates are obtained by extending (8.22) to the current model using the expression for $\widehat{\text{Var}}\left(\hat{\boldsymbol{\beta}}, \hat{\sigma}\right)$ in (8.38), namely

$$\Delta\left(\hat{\boldsymbol{\beta}}, \hat{\sigma}\right)_i = \widehat{\text{Var}}\left(\hat{\boldsymbol{\beta}}, \hat{\sigma}\right)\hat{\mathbf{L}}_i. \tag{8.43}$$

The likelihood displacement or Cook's-distance-type measure of overall effect is, by extension of (8.23),

$$ld_i = \mathbf{L}_i'\widehat{\text{Var}}\left(\hat{\boldsymbol{\beta}}, \hat{\sigma}\right)\hat{\mathbf{L}}_i. \tag{8.44}$$

As in the previous section, we plot the individual scaled score residuals for the four terms in the model in Figures 8.4a to 8.4d. Because the transformed shape parameter, $-\ln(\sigma)$, is not a function of model covariates, we show a box plot of its scaled score residuals in Figure 8.5. The likelihood displacement or Cook's distance measure is plotted against the estimated martingale residuals in (8.39), shown in Figure 8.6.

The plots in Figure 8.4 and 8.6 identify the same six subjects as those flagged for further study in Figure 8.1 and Figure 8.2, namely subjects 30, 52, 58, 61, 93, and 97. Two additional subjects, 1 and 31, have large negative values for the influence diagnostic for the shape parameter in Figure 8.5. The data for these eight subjects are listed in Table 8.6.

We leave it as an exercise to demonstrate that deletion of these eight subjects decreases the estimate of the coefficient for gender by 38 percent, decreases the interaction coefficient by 40 percent and increases the coefficient for BMI by 40 percent. The coefficient for age decreases by a relatively modest 13 percent. The same comments apply to the influence and clinical plausibility of the data for subjects 30, 52, 58, 61, 93, and 97 and, as such, we cannot exclude any of them from the analysis. An interesting result is that, when the eight subjects are deleted, the modeled shape parameter, $-\ln(\sigma)$, is no longer borderline significant with $p = 0.61$. Investigating further, we find that when we delete only subjects 1

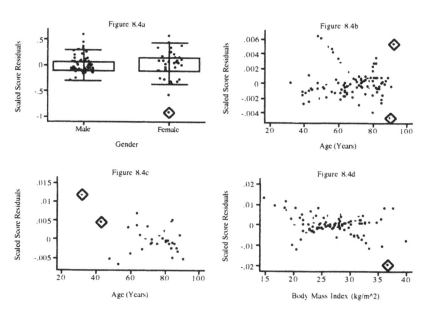

Figure 8.4 Graph of the scaled score residuals for the four covariates in the fitted Weibull regression model in Table 8.5.

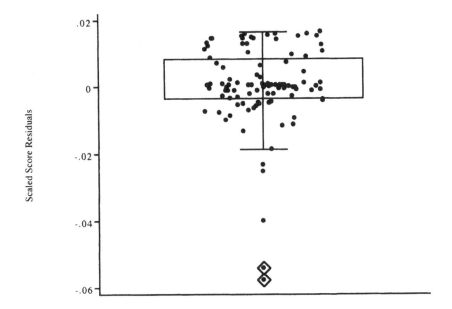

Figure 8.5 Box plot of the scaled score residuals for the transformed shape parameter, $-\ln(\sigma)$ from the Weibull regression model in Table 8.5.

and 31, the subjects seen as having large negative scaled score residuals in Figure 8.5, the shape parameter is also not significant with $p = 0.41$. The data for these two subjects is not particularly unusual but each died after six days of follow-

Table 8.6 Subjects with High Influence for One or More of the Model Parameters or Large Likelihood Displacement from the Fitted Model in Table 8.5

Study ID	Gender	Age	Body Mass Index	Influence On
1	Male	65	31.4	sigma
30	Female	85	36.7	BMI
31	Male	72	28.0	sigma
52	Female	43	25.3	Interaction
58	Male	92	24.4	Age
61	Male	90	24.8	Age
93	Female	80	20.6	ld
97	Female	32	39.9	Gender, Interaction and ld

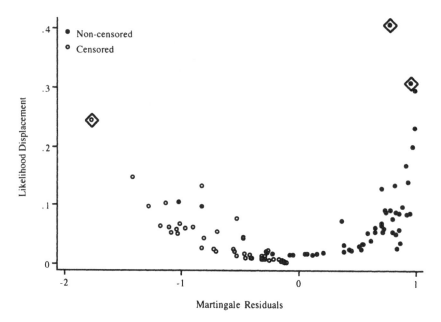

Figure 8.6 Graph of the likelihood displacement or Cook's distance statistic versus the martingale residuals from the model in Table 8.5.

up; this represents the shortest two survival times in the WHAS100 data. Hence, it appears that these relatively short follow-up times affect the departure from constant hazard. While interesting from a statistical view point, there is no real clinical reason to exclude the two subjects. Therefore, it appears that the Weibull may provide a better fit than the exponential regression model.

The next step in the assessment of model fit is to plot the Kaplan-Meier estimator against its Cox–Snell residuals (i.e., the regression-model based estimated cumulative hazard function) in the same manner as shown in Figure 8.3 for the exponential regression model. The estimator of the cumulative hazard function for the Weibull regression model is

$$\hat{H}\left(t_i, \mathbf{x}_i, \hat{\boldsymbol{\beta}}, \hat{\sigma}\right) = \exp\left[\left(y_i - \mathbf{x}_i'\hat{\boldsymbol{\beta}}\right)/\hat{\sigma}\right]$$
$$= \exp\left(\hat{z}_i\right),$$

so

$$\hat{H}\left(t_i, \mathbf{x}_i, \hat{\boldsymbol{\beta}}, \hat{\sigma}\right) = \left(t_i e^{-\mathbf{x}_i'\hat{\boldsymbol{\beta}}}\right)^{\hat{\lambda}},$$

for $i = 1, 2, \ldots, n$. Alternatively, one may calculate the values from the martingale residuals as

$$\hat{H}\left(t_i, \mathbf{x}_i, \hat{\boldsymbol{\beta}}, \hat{\sigma}\right) = c_i - \hat{M}_i .$$

Figure 8.7 presents the Cox–Snell residual diagnostic plot. When we compare the plot in Figure 8.3 with the one in Figure 8.7, we see that the estimated cumulative hazard for the Weibull regression model falls closer to the referent line, indicating better adherence to the parametric assumptions. The likelihood ratio form of the Grønnesby–Borgan test has a value of $G = 4.70$ which, with 1 degree of freedom, yields $p = 0.030$. This does not seem to support overall model fit. A summary of the observed and estimated expected number of events within each of the two groups is presented in Table 8.7. Here we see that the p-values for the two risk groups are not significant, which supports model fit. Recall that in Section 8.2, we mentioned that we have not checked the scale of age or bmi and, when done in the exercises, it may change the model covariates and subsequent fit. Regardless, the results shown here are typical of those often encountered in practice where some analyses support model fit while others do not. At this point, we favor the Weibull model because its shape parameter is modestly significant.

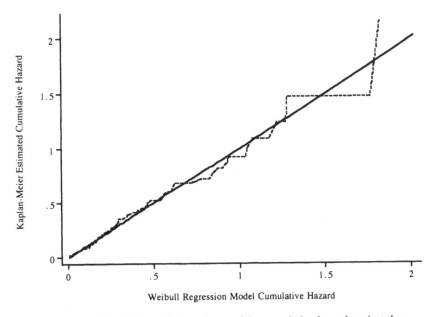

Figure 8.7 Graph of the Kaplan–Meier estimate of the cumulative hazard against the Weibull regression model estimate of the cumulative hazard based on the model in Table 8.5. The solid line is the referent line with slope = 1.0 and intercept = 0.

Table 8.7 Observed Number of Events, Estimated Number of Events, z-Score, and Two-Tailed p-value within Each Risk Group Based on the Fitted Weibull Model in Table 8.5

Risk Group	Observed Number of Events	Estimated Number of Events	z	p - value
1	33	36.97	−0.65	0.52
2	18	14.03	1.05	0.29
Total	51	51		

Estimates of time ratios from a fitted Weibull model are obtained by exponentiating the product of a coefficient and the stated differences in the covariate. The process is the same as that used for the exponential regression model in Section 8.2. Because the estimates of the coefficients for the model covariates in Table 8.5 are similar to those in Table 8.2, we leave as an exercise the actual calculation of the time ratios with confidence intervals.

In this particular example, it is constructive to examine the estimated baseline hazard functions for the fitted exponential and Weibull regression models. The estimator of the baseline hazard for the exponential model is obtained from (8.9) and is

$$h_{0e}\left(t, \hat{\boldsymbol{\beta}}\right) = \exp\left(-\hat{\beta}_0\right). \tag{8.45}$$

The estimator of the baseline hazard for the Weibull model is obtained from (8.29) and is

$$h_{0w}\left(t, \hat{\boldsymbol{\beta}}, \hat{\sigma}\right) = \frac{1}{\hat{\sigma}} \exp\left(-\hat{\beta}_0 / \hat{\sigma}\right) t^{((1/\hat{\sigma})-1)}. \tag{8.46}$$

The text symbols "e" and "w" in the subscripts of (8.45) and (8.46) refer to exponential and Weibull, respectively. As in the case of the proportional hazards model, for the value of the baseline hazard function to be clinically meaningful, we must define the covariate value of zero to be meaningful. To do this, we refit the model in Tables 8.2 and 8.5, centering age at 70 years and bmi at 27 kg/m^2 and compute the interaction using gender and age centered. Hence, a subject with covariates equal to zero corresponds to a 70-year old male subject with body mass index 27 kg/m^2. Plots of the two estimated baseline hazard functions are shown in Figure 8.8.

This figure illustrates the difference in the shapes of the two estimated baseline hazard functions. The estimated baseline hazard function of the exponential model, by definition, has a constant value of 0.111. The Weibull model, on the other hand, has a baseline hazard that begins at a higher value than the exponential baseline hazard, drops sharply and then continues to fall gradually to its minimum of 0.08. The average baseline hazard for the Weibull is 0.105. Hence, the two models have nearly the same average baseline hazard rate, but the Weibull model is much more specific. For these data, the pattern of a progressive decrease in risk over time is quite reasonable because the risk of dying from a myocardial infarction is greatest in the time immediately after it occurs. The parameter controlling whether the baseline hazard decreases or increases is the shape parameter σ. If the shape parameter is greater than 1.0 then the hazard decreases because the power t in (8.46) is raised to a term that is less than 1.0, $\left[(1/\sigma)-1\right]<1$. The reverse occurs if the shape parameter is less than 1.0. The multiplier, $(1/\sigma)\exp(-\beta_0/\sigma)$, determines the scale of the descent or ascent in the baseline hazard function.

In this example, when all aspects of the two models are considered, we continue to favor the Weibull model. It fits the data better and has the more clinically plausible hazard function.

This comparative analysis is only possible because both the exponential and Weibull models are also proportional hazards models. This type of model comparison could not be done using the accelerated failure time hazard functions because the function for the Weibull model in (8.30) depends on both covariate val-

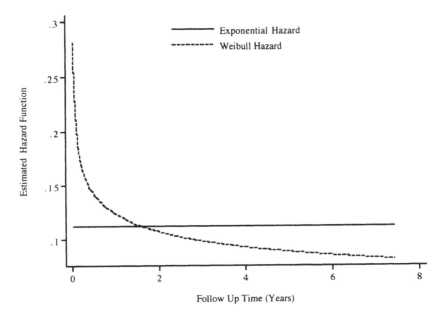

Figure 8.8 Plots of the estimated baseline hazard function for the exponential regression model in Table 8.2 and the Weibull regression model in Table 8.5, with age centered at 70 years and body mass index centered at 27 kg/m².

ues and coefficients in such a way as to prevent a baseline hazard function from being independent of covariates.

It is also possible to graph estimated covariate-adjusted survival functions using fitted parametric regression models. To illustrate this, we show (in Figure 8.9) the estimated survival functions for 70-year-old males and females with a body mass index of 27 kg/m^2. Using the results of the fitted model in Table 8.5 and the equation for the survival function in (8.31), the estimated survival function for males is

$$\hat{S}\left(t, gender = 0, age = 70, bmi = 27, \hat{\boldsymbol{\beta}}, \hat{\sigma}\right) = \exp\left\{-t^{\left(\frac{1}{1.253}\right)} \exp\left(-\frac{\hat{r}_m}{1.253}\right)\right\},$$

where $\hat{r}_m = 3.972 - 4.689 \times 0 - 0.064 \times 70 + 0.059 \times 0 \times 70 + 0.106 \times 27$. The estimate survival function for females is

$$\hat{S}\left(t, gender = 1, age = 70, bmi = 27, \hat{\boldsymbol{\beta}}, \hat{\sigma}\right) = \exp\left\{-t^{\left(\frac{1}{1.253}\right)} \exp\left(-\frac{\hat{r}_f}{1.253}\right)\right\},$$

where $\hat{r}_f = 3.972 - 4.689 \times 1 - 0.064 \times 70 + 0.059 \times 1 \times 70 + 0.106 \times 27$.

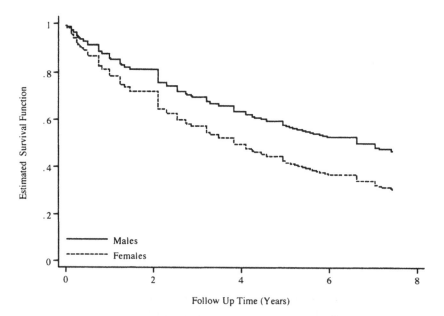

Figure 8.9 Plots of the estimated survival functions for 70-year-old males and females with body mass index 27 kg/m^2 using the fitted Weibull regression model in Table 8.5.

The covariate-adjusted survival functions, plots, or lists, may be used to estimate median survival times and/or five-year survival probabilities. Using a list of the estimated functions in Figure 8.9, the estimated median survival time for males is 7.2 years and, for females, the estimate is 3.8 years, while the estimated five-year survival probabilities are 0.58 for males and 0.43 for females. Both estimates, median survival time and five-year survival probability, point to a poorer survival experience for females. Again, we remind the reader that these data are a specially selected sample from the main Worcester Heart Attack Study data and thus, the results do not apply to the main study.

Modeling survival time data via accelerated failure time models is different from normal-errors linear regression modeling in that one has the choice of several possible "error" distributions. So far, we have considered two of them, the exponential and Weibull distributions. In the next section we consider another popular and useful model: the log-logistic accelerated failure time model.

8.4 THE LOG-LOGISTIC REGRESSION MODEL

The single covariate log-logistic accelerated failure time model may be expressed as

$$\ln(T) = \beta_0 + \beta_1 x + \sigma\varepsilon, \tag{8.47}$$

where the error term, ε, follows the standard logistic distribution, which we will discuss in more detail later in this section. The appealing feature of the log-logistic model is that the slope coefficient can be expressed in such a way that it can be interpreted as an odds-ratio.

To develop the odds-ratio interpretation, we begin by expressing the survival function for the model in (8.47) as

$$S(t, x, \boldsymbol{\beta}, \sigma) = \left[1 + \exp(z)\right]^{-1}, \tag{8.48}$$

where z, as before, is the standardized log-time outcome variable, i.e., $z = (y - \beta_0 - \beta_1 x)/\sigma$ and $y = \ln(t)$. The odds of a survival time of at least t is

$$\frac{S(t, x, \boldsymbol{\beta}, \sigma)}{1 - S(t, x, \boldsymbol{\beta}, \sigma)} = \exp(-z). \tag{8.49}$$

As an example, assume that the covariate is dichotomous and coded 0/1. The odds-ratio at time t, formed from the ratio of the odds in (8.49) evaluated at $x = 1$ and $x = 0$, is

$$OR(t, x = 1, x = 0) = \frac{\exp\left[\dfrac{-(y - \beta_0 - \beta_1 \times 1)}{\sigma}\right]}{\exp\left[\dfrac{-(y - \beta_0 - \beta_1 \times 0)}{\sigma}\right]} = \exp(\beta_1/\sigma). \qquad (8.50)$$

Note that the ratio in (8.50) is independent of time. If the odds-ratio in (8.50) were 2.0, the interpretation would be that the odds of survival beyond time t among subjects with $x = 1$ is twice that of subjects with $x = 0$, and this holds for all t.

An alternative interpretation is obtained when we express the median survival time as a function of the regression coefficients. Setting the survival function in (8.48) equal to 0.5 and solving for t, we obtain an equation for the median survival time of

$$t_{50}(x, \boldsymbol{\beta}, \sigma) = \exp(\beta_0 + \beta_1 x), \qquad (8.51)$$

and the time ratio at the median is

$$TR(t_{50}, x = 1, x = 0) = \exp(\beta_1). \qquad (8.52)$$

As expected with an accelerated failure-time model, the exponentiated coefficient provides the acceleration factor on the time scale. In particular, if the time ratio in (8.52) is 2.0, the median survival time in the group with $x = 1$ is twice that of the group with $x = 0$. Because the percentiles of the survival time distribution in (8.48) are of the form

$$t_p(x, \boldsymbol{\beta}, \sigma) = \left[(1 - p)/p\right]^\sigma \exp(\beta_0 + \beta_1 x),$$

the result in (8.52) holds at all values of time. Cox and Oakes (1984) show that the log-logistic model is the only accelerated failure time model with the proportional odds property in (8.49).

As was the case with the exponential and Weibull models, maximum likelihood is the method usually employed to fit a log-logistic model to a set of data subject to right censoring. It follows from results for the standard logistic distribution [see Evans, Hastings and Peacock (1993) or Klein and Moeschberger (2003)] that the contribution of a non-censored time to the likelihood is

$$(1/\sigma)\exp(z)/\left[1 + \exp(z)\right]^2,$$

and that of a censored time is

$$\left[1+\exp(z)\right]^{-1},$$

where, for a multivariable model, $z = (y - \mathbf{x}'\boldsymbol{\beta})/\sigma$. It follows that the log-likelihood function for a sample of n independent observations of time, covariates and censoring indicator, denoted $(t_i, \mathbf{x}_i, c_i)$, $i = 1, 2, \ldots, n$, is

$$L(\boldsymbol{\beta}, \sigma) = \sum_{i=1}^{n} c_i \left\{ -\ln(\sigma) + z_i - 2\ln\left[1 + \exp(z_i)\right] \right\} - (1 - c_i)\ln\left[1 + \exp(z_i)\right]$$

$$= -m \times \ln(\sigma) + \sum_{i=1}^{n} c_i \left\{ z_i - \ln\left[1 + \exp(z_i)\right] \right\} - \ln\left[1 + \exp(z_i)\right], \tag{8.53}$$

where m is the number of non-censored observations. The score equation for the jth regression coefficient is obtained by taking the derivative of the log-likelihood in (8.53) with respect to β_j and, setting this equal to 0, yields

$$\frac{\partial L(\boldsymbol{\beta}, \sigma)}{\partial \beta_j} = \sum_{i=1}^{n} \frac{-x_{ij}}{\sigma} \left[c_i - (1 + c_i) \frac{e^{z_i}}{1 + e^{z_i}} \right] = 0, \quad j = 0, 1, 2, \ldots, p. \tag{8.54}$$

The score equation for σ is

$$\frac{\partial L(\boldsymbol{\beta}, \sigma)}{\partial \sigma} = \frac{-m}{\sigma} + \sum_{i=1}^{n} \frac{-z_i}{\sigma} \left(c_i - (1 + c_i) \frac{e^{z_i}}{1 + e^{z_i}} \right) = 0. \tag{8.55}$$

Some packages, for example STATA, estimate $\ln(\sigma)$ and report the values of $\widehat{\ln(\sigma)}$ and $\hat{\sigma} = \exp\left[\widehat{\ln(\sigma)}\right]$.

As is the case in any application of maximum likelihood, the estimator of the covariance matrix of the parameter estimator is obtained from the observed information matrix. The individual elements of this matrix to be evaluated are

$$-\frac{\partial^2 L(\boldsymbol{\beta}, \sigma)}{\partial \beta_j\, \partial \beta_k} = \frac{1}{\sigma^2} \sum_{i=1}^{n} x_{ij} x_{ik} (1 + c_i) \frac{e^{z_i}}{\left(1 + e^{z_i}\right)^2},$$

$$-\frac{\partial^2 L(\boldsymbol{\beta}, \sigma)}{\partial \beta_j\, \partial \sigma} = \frac{1}{\sigma^2} \sum_{i=1}^{n} x_{ij} z_i (1 + c_i) \frac{e^{z_i}}{\left(1 + e^{z_i}\right)^2} - \frac{1}{\sigma^2} \sum_{i=1}^{n} \left[c_i - (1 + c_i) \frac{e^{z_i}}{\left(1 + e^{z_i}\right)} \right],$$

and

$$-\frac{\partial^2 L(\boldsymbol{\beta},\sigma)}{\partial\sigma\,\partial\sigma} = \frac{m}{\sigma^2} + \frac{1}{\sigma^2}\sum_{i=1}^{n} z_i^2\left(1+c_i\right)\frac{e^{z_i}}{\left(1+e^{z_i}\right)^2} + \frac{1}{\sigma^2}\sum_{i=1}^{n} z_i\left[c_i - \left(1+c_i\right)\frac{e^{z_i}}{\left(1+e^{z_i}\right)}\right].$$

Because the score equations sum to zero when evaluated at their solution, it follows that

$$\frac{1}{\hat{\sigma}^2}\sum_{i=1}^{n}\left[c_i - \left(1+c_i\right)\frac{e^{\hat{z}_i}}{\left(1+e^{\hat{z}_i}\right)}\right] = 0$$

and

$$\frac{m}{\hat{\sigma}^2} + \frac{1}{\hat{\sigma}^2}\sum_{i=1}^{n}\hat{z}_i\left[c_i - \left(1+c_i\right)\frac{e^{\hat{z}_i}}{\left(1+e^{\hat{z}_i}\right)}\right] = 0.$$

Hence, the information matrix may be expressed as

$$\mathbf{I}(\hat{\boldsymbol{\beta}},\hat{\sigma}) = \frac{1}{\hat{\sigma}^2}\begin{bmatrix} \mathbf{X}'\hat{\mathbf{V}}\mathbf{X} & \mathbf{X}'\hat{\mathbf{V}}\hat{\mathbf{z}} \\ \hat{\mathbf{z}}'\hat{\mathbf{V}}\mathbf{X} & \hat{\mathbf{z}}'\hat{\mathbf{V}}\hat{\mathbf{z}} \end{bmatrix}, \tag{8.56}$$

where $\mathbf{X}$ is an n by $p+1$ matrix containing the values of the covariates, $\hat{z}_i = \left(y_i - \mathbf{x}_i\hat{\boldsymbol{\beta}}\right)/\hat{\sigma}$, $\hat{\mathbf{z}}' = \left(\hat{z}_1,\hat{z}_2,\dots,\hat{z}_n\right)$ and $\hat{\mathbf{V}}$ is an n by n diagonal matrix with general element

$$\hat{\mathbf{V}} = \text{diag}\left[\left(1+c_i\right)\frac{e^{\hat{z}_i}}{\left(1+e^{\hat{z}_i}\right)^2}\right].$$

The estimator of the covariance matrix of the estimators of the parameters is

$$\hat{\text{Var}}\left(\hat{\boldsymbol{\beta}},\hat{\sigma}\right) = \left[\mathbf{I}(\hat{\boldsymbol{\beta}},\hat{\sigma})\right]^{-1}. \tag{8.57}$$

Following the results in Collett (2003, Section 7.4) the score equations and the estimator of the covariance matrix may be used to generate score residuals, scaled score residuals and the likelihood displacement statistic in the same manner as for the exponential and Weibull regression models. Following the approach used in

(8.20) and (8.39) to calculate the estimated martingale residuals, it follows from (8.48) that

$$
\begin{aligned}
\hat{M}_i &= c_i - \left\{ -\ln\left[\hat{S}\left(t_i, \mathbf{x}_i, \hat{\boldsymbol{\beta}}, \hat{\sigma}\right) \right] \right\} \\
&= c_i - \ln\left[1 + e^{\hat{z}_i} \right].
\end{aligned}
\tag{8.58}
$$

While the result in (8.58) looks like a martingale residual, it does not satisfy the property that they sum to zero. This is not a problem when they are used in plots but does have implications if we use them to assess goodness of fit with the Grønnesby–Borgan test. We return to this point later in this section.

We conclude this section with an example, fitting the same model to the WHAS100 data used in the previous two sections. The results of the fit are shown in Table 8.8.

The first thing we note is that the estimator of the shape parameter is not significantly different from 1.0 with $p = 0.734$. Unfortunately, the log-logistic model does not simplify to another model when the shape parameter is equal to 1. The equation describing the hazard as a function of follow-up time is

$$
h(t, \mathbf{x}, \boldsymbol{\beta}, \sigma) = \frac{1}{\sigma} \times \frac{1}{t} \times \frac{e^{\hat{z}}}{1 + e^{\hat{z}}}.
\tag{8.59}
$$

The hazard function for this model is monotonic, decreasing for $\sigma \geq 1$ and it increases and then decreases for $\sigma < 1$. To see this more clearly, Figure 8.10 shows the plot of the estimated log-logistic hazard function from the model fit in Table 8.8 but using age centered at 70 years, bmi centered at 27 kg/m^2, and the gender-by-age interaction computed using centered values of age. Hence, it is the hazard function for 70 year old males with a body mass index of 27 kg/m^2. The estimate

Table 8.8 Estimated Coefficients, Standard Errors, z-Scores, Two-Tailed p-values, and 95% Confidence Interval Estimates for the Log-Logistic Regression Model for the WHAS100 data ($n = 100$)

Variable	Coeff.	Std. Err.	z	$p > |z|$	95% CIE
gender	−4.695	2.2916	−2.05	0.040	−9.186, −0.204
age	−0.065	0.0210	−3.10	0.002	−0.106, −0.024
gender × age	0.059	0.0313	1.88	0.061	−0.003, 0.120
bmi	0.110	0.0458	2.40	0.016	0.020, 0.200
Constant	3.468	2.0260	1.71	0.087	−0.503, 7.439
ln(Sigma)	0.041	0.1210	0.34	0.734	−0.196, 0.278
Sigma	1.042	0.1261			0.822, 1.321

of the intercept in this model is $\hat{\beta}_0 = 1.883$, and the estimate of the shape parameter, $\hat{\sigma}$, is as shown in Table 8.8. The other three hazard functions plotted in Figure 8.10 use the same value for $\hat{\beta}_0$ and $\sigma = 1.25, 0.5, 0.25$.

Increasing sigma to 1.25 will sharpen the initial drop in the hazard. When sigma is equal to 0.5, the hazard rises gradually and begins to decline at about 6 years. The hazard for sigma equal to 0.25 rises in an almost "S" shaped manner and, while not shown, begins to decrease at about 9 years. Hence, the log-logistic model has a hazard function that provides more flexibility than the Weibull model, whose hazard only increases or decreases monotonically, but it is perhaps best suited for settings where the hazard rises and then falls.

The hazard for the fitted log-logistic model in Figure 8.10 looks similar to the hazard function for the Weibull model in Figure 8.8 for survival time greater than one year. For the first year of follow up, the Weibull hazard in Figure 8.8 begins at a higher value and then drops more rapidly. We consider an approach to choosing between two or more unrelated parametric models later in this section.

The estimated coefficients for the covariates in Table 8.8 are nearly identical to those of the fitted Weibull regression model in Table 8.5 and are reasonably close to those from the fitted exponential regression model in Table 8.2. Hence, estimates of time ratios and their interpretation from the fitted log-logistic model

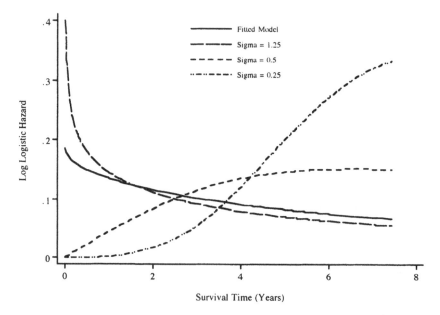

Figure 8.10 Plots of hazard functions from the fitted log-logistic model with $\hat{\beta}_0 = 1.883$ and $\hat{\sigma} = 1.04, 1.25, 0.5, 0.25$.

would not differ substantially from the results presented for the exponential regression model in Section 8.2. As such, we do not present them here and leave verification as an exercise.

The next step in the analysis is to examine plots of the scaled score residuals and likelihood displacement statistic for highly influential subjects. These are presented in Figure 8.11 for the model covariates, in Figure 8.12 for the shape parameter, and in Figure 8.13 for the likelihood displacement. Of interest is that the subjects who influenced the fit of the Weibull regression model are also influential for the fit of the log-logistic model. A total of six subjects have values that stand out in one or more of the plots: 1, 30, 31, 56, 67, and 97. These subjects' data and the parameter(s) they influence are listed in Table 8.9. Of these subjects, 1, 30, 31, and 97 were also influential in the fit of the Weibull regression model.

When we fit the model deleting the six subjects in Table 8.9, the estimate of the coefficient for gender decreases by 20 percent, the coefficient for age decreases by 3 percent, the coefficient for interaction decreases by 17 percent, and the coefficient for body mass index increases by 39 percent. We discussed the data and their effects on parameter estimates for subjects 1, 30, 31, and 97 in Section 8.3. As shown in Table 8.9, the data for subjects 56 and 67 are not especially unusual. Hence, it is a little puzzling why these two subjects seem to exert any influence and, in particular, on the gender coefficient. In fact, when we delete just

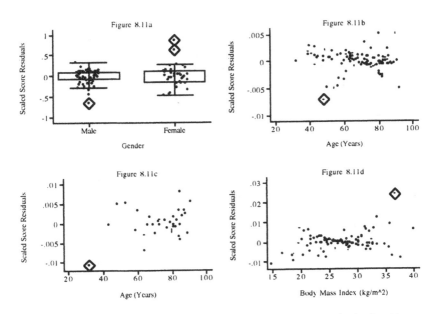

Figure 8.11 Graph of the scaled score residuals for the four covariates in the fitted log-logistic regression model in Table 8.8.

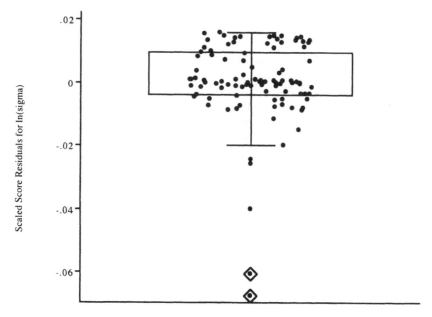

Figure 8.12 Box plot of the scaled score residuals for the transformed shape parameter, $\ln(\sigma)$, from the log-logistic regression model in Table 8.8.

these two subjects, the coefficient for gender changes by just 1 percent. We think this provides an excellent example of the importance of deleting the subjects identified as having large scaled-score residuals and refitting the model. There are no critical values for these diagnostic statistics, and we identify subjects as ones whose values seem large relative to the other subjects. While they may appear to have influence, one can only tell for sure by deleting the subjects and refitting the model. As was the case in the previous section, the data for all

Table 8.9 Subjects with High Influence for One or More of the Model Parameters or Large Likelihood Displacement from the Fitted Log-Logistic Model in Table 8.8

Study ID	Gender	Age	Body Mass Index	Influence On
1	Male	65	31.4	sigma
30	Female	85	36.7	BMI and ld
31	Male	72	28.0	sigma
56	Female	64	24.4	Gender
67	Male	48	31.6	Gender and Age
97	Female	32	39.9	Gender, Interaction and ld

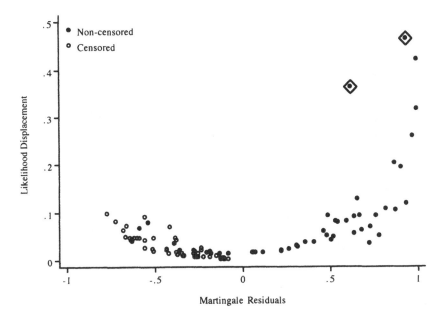

Figure 8.13 Graph of the likelihood displacement or Cook's distance statistic versus the martingale residuals from the log-logistic model in Table 8.8.

subjects are clinically plausible and hence they should not be excluded from the analysis.

The estimator of the Cox Snell residuals, the log-cumulative hazard, is obtained from the estimator of the multivariable form of the survival function in (8.48) and, for the ith subject, it is

$$\hat{H}\left(t_i, \hat{\boldsymbol{\beta}}, \hat{\sigma}\right) = \ln\left[1 + \exp\left(\hat{z}_i\right)\right]. \tag{8.60}$$

Figure 8.14 shows the plot of the Kaplan–Meier estimator against these residuals.

For the most part, the plotted points follow the referent line. There is slightly more departure from the line at larger values of the cumulative hazard than was seen in the corresponding plot for the Weibull model shown in Figure 8.8. Based on this plot, it would appear that the log-logistic model provides a reasonable fit to the data.

We noted that, in the case of a fitted log-logistic regression model, it is not necessarily true that the sum of the 0-1 censoring variable and the estimated cumulative hazard function are equal. Hence, it is not clear that the theory behind the Grønnesby–Borgan test would hold in this setting.

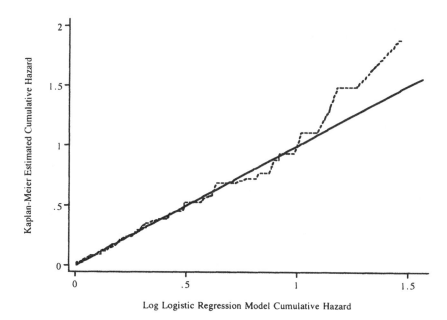

Figure 8.14 Graph of the Kaplan–Meier estimate against the log-logistic regression model estimate of the cumulative hazard based on the fitted model in Table 8.8. The solid line is the referent line with slope = 1.0 and intercept = 0.

The three models fit to the data from the WHAS100 study are not directly comparable. Akaike (1974) proposed an information criterion (AIC) statistic to compare different models and/or models with different numbers of parameters. For each model the value is computed as

$$\text{AIC} = -2 \times (\text{log-likelihood}) + 2(p+1+s), \qquad (8.61)$$

where p denotes the number of covariates in the model (not including the constant term), $s = 0$ for the exponential model and $s = 1$ for the Weibull and log-logistic models. The values of AIC are 276.42 for the exponential model in Table 8.2, 274.82 for the Weibull model in Table 8.5, and 277.76 for log-logistic model in Table 8.8. These three values are quite similar and reflect what was seen in the analysis. There are no large differences in the fit or the inferences from the three models. Each offers an accelerated failure time interpretation, and the estimates of effect are not very different. The Weibull model, with the smallest value of AIC, seems to be the best fitting of the three.

8.5 OTHER PARAMETRIC REGRESSION MODELS

There is an extensive literature on parametric models to analyze survival time data. A number of texts that present a significant amount of material on parametric analysis of survival time data are listed at the end of Section 8.1. Delving much further into this topic would take us beyond the scope of this text, and we conclude this chapter with a few observations and comments on parametric survival time models.

The principal benefit of any parametric model is the specificity it provides for modeling the data, especially the hazard function's description of the underlying aging process. Parametric models offer a wide variety of possible shapes for the hazard function, ranging from a simple constant hazard to complex "bathtub" shaped functions that might be appropriate for modeling human life over a long time span. In general, these models are most effectively used when the investigator has considerable knowledge of the aging process in the subjects being studied. Clinical plausibility is a vital aspect of any choice of hazard function.

One should not use a complicated parametric model without prior knowledge that the hazard function is plausible for the problem at hand. In the vast majority of current applications of survival time data analysis that follow humans over time, this prior knowledge is not available. Therefore, use of the semi-parametric models discussed in the previous chapters provides a safe and proven method for analysis. This is not to say that parametric models should be avoided, but rather they should be used with caution and with a keen eye to the plausibility of the parametric form of the hazard.

EXERCISES

1. A model containing gender, age, their interaction, and body mass index is used in Sections 8.2, 8.3, and 8.4 to illustrate the exponential, Weibull, and log-logistic regression models. In those sections, we used scaled score residuals and the likelihood displacement statistic to identify subjects who seemed to have an influence on parameter estimates. Results were reported in these sections on the effect deleting these subjects has on parameter estimates, percentage change in the estimates of the coefficients. Verify that the reported results are correct.

2. The fitted exponential model in Table 8.2 was used in Section 8.2 to estimate time ratios for the model covariates. Estimate these same time ratios using the fitted Weibull model in Table 8.5 and the fitted log-logistic model in Table 8.8.

3. We noted in Sections 8.2 – 8.4 that we had not checked the scale of the covariates age and body mass index.

   (a) Is there evidence of non-linearity in any of the three models for either continuous covariate?

   (b) If there is evidence (hint: consider the variable bmi), does modeling it as non-linear change any or all of the three fitted models, (exponential, Weibull, or log-logistic)? If so, then fit the new model and estimate the time ratios for the model covariates.

4. Fit an exponential regression model containing Treatment (tx) and CD4 count (cd4) using the ACTG320 data.

   (a) Using the fitted model,, compute point and 95 percent confidence interval estimates of the time ratio for treatment and for an increase of 50 in CD4. Interpret these estimates within the context of the study.

   (b) Using the fitted model, compute point and 95 percent confidence interval estimates of the hazard for treatment and for an increase of 50 in CD4. Interpret these estimates within the context of the study.

   (c) Compare the time ratio and hazard ratio estimates computed in problems 4(a) and 4(b). In particular, which estimate time or hazard ratio do you think would be more easily understood by non-statistically trained clinicians?

   (d) Why can the fitted exponential regression model be used to compute both time and hazard ratio estimates?

5. Repeat problem 4 using the Weibull regression model.

6. Repeat problem 4 part (a) using the log-logistic regression model.

7. Which of the three models, the exponential, Weibull, or log-logistic regression model, fit in problems 4-6 is the best fitting model? Justify your response using plots, statistical tests, and AIC.

8. Fit an exponential regression model to the WHAS500 data using the covariates in the main effects proportional hazards model shown in Table 5.6.

   (a) Assess the scale of age, heart rate, diastolic blood pressure and body mass index. Are the results the same or different from those obtained for the proportional hazards model in Chapter 5?

   (b) Using the correctly scaled model from problem 8(a), assess the need for interactions in the exponential regression model. Are the interactions the same or different from those selected in Chapter 5 for the proportional hazards model?

(c) Compute the diagnostic statistics to assess the model obtained in problem 8(b). Explore the effect on the estimates of the coefficients of any influential subjects identified through use of the diagnostic statistics.

(d) Assess the overall fit of the model from problem 8(c) via the Grønnesby-Borgan test.

(e) Assess the adherence of the fitted model to the exponential errors assumption via the plot of the Cox–Snell residuals.

(f) Describe the estimates of effect of the covariates in the final exponential regression model using time ratios, with 95 percent confidence intervals.

9. Fit a Weibull regression model containing the covariates in the final exponential regression model from problem 8. Repeat problem 8(f) for the Weibull model.

10. Fit a log-logistic regression model containing the covariates in the final Weibull regression model from problem 8. Repeat problem 8(f) for the log-logistic model.

11. Which of the models fit in problems 8, 9 and 10 best fits these data?

CHAPTER 9

Other Models and Topics

9.1 INTRODUCTION

The central theme of the previous eight chapters is modeling survival time when there is a single event of interest that terminates observation. This situation, in which each subject may experience the event of interest only once, describes the majority of applied settings when follow-up time is observed. There are situations, however, when the event of interest may occur more than one time for each subject. Another is a setting in which the disease process progresses through several stages, each with its own event time. For example, a subject's cancer may be treated and then recur some time later with treatment and recurrence happening several times. The follow up may ultimately end due to death. We discuss several approaches to modeling recurrent event data in Section 9.2.

Another extension of the standard modeling situation occurs when subgroups of responses are correlated due to study design. This lack of independence of response can occur in any setting in which survival time is influenced by unmeasured factors that are the same within groups of subjects and are thought to have significant group-to-group variability. When these factors are present in the usual normal errors linear model setting, they are called *random effects*. Survival analysis models incorporating such factors are called *frailty models*. These models have also been suggested for use in the recurrent event setting. We discuss frailty survival-time models in Section 9.3.

Investigators employing statistical methods often have less data than they would like to have. Sample sizes tend to be limited by cost and time constraints. Alternatively, there are situations when follow-up time is available in such a large cohort that it is impractical to use all the data. When this happens, nested case-control studies have been suggested as a way to model a covariate's effect at a considerably reduced cost. We discuss this approach to modeling survival time data in Section 9.4.

In previous chapters, we used regression models in which the covariate's effect on the hazard rate was multiplicative. Models of this type yield hazard rate

286

ratio estimates of effect that are meaningful and easily interpreted. We have largely ignored additive models, as they are not as easy to fit or interpret. We discuss a few additive models in Section 9.5. One of the additive models we discuss is based on coefficients whose values depend on time, e.g. $\beta(t)$. We explore, in Section 9.5, how information from the fit of this additive model can shed light on time-dependent effects for the proportional hazards model. We then illustrate how to fit a proportional hazards model with a discrete time-dependent effect.

In Section 9.6, we discuss a few methods to select sample size for a typical time-to-event study. We also discuss missing values and strategies for handling this nettlesome but commonly occurring problem.

9.2 RECURRENT EVENT MODELS

The idea that an event can occur multiple times in the course of the subject's follow-up is a conceptually easy extension of the single-event model. We often encounter things that break, are repaired, and then break again. Cancer is a good example. Following treatment, the cancer may go into remission but, may recur later. The process of treatment and recurrence may be repeated multiple times in a subject. The defining characteristic of a recurrent event is that we observe the same event in a single subject multiple times during the follow-up period. A specific example is basal cell carcinoma, a type of skin cancer, that may occur multiple times and at many different sites during a subject's lifetime. Other types of multiple observations per subject can occur when the subject is simultaneously at risk for more than one event. In some diseases, a subject may progress over time into different manifestations of the disease (e.g., some may be physical and others may be biochemical and each has a time to event). In this section we do not discuss this latter type of data.

Modeling of recurrent event data is not typically addressed in a text of this level. Therneau and Grambsch (2000) present a more mathematical and computationally detailed discussion of recurrent event data, with examples, than we present in this section. Clayton (1994) discusses recurrent events and compares them to generalized linear models, such as Poisson and logistic regression. Hougaard (2000) considers a number of methods for recurrent events within the context of multivariate survival data and illustrates them with examples. Kalbfleisch and Prentice (2002) treat it at a fairly theoretical level using the counting process approach. Kelly and Lim (2000) study via simulation all of the methods we discuss here and make specific recommendations. Cain and Cole (2005) perform additional simulations and use these to sharpen the focus of the recommendations of Kelly and Lim.

A number of proportional hazards-type models have been proposed for use with recurrent event data. The easiest way to explain the similarities and differences in the models is by describing how we handle the data for two hypothetical subjects using each model. Suppose we have n independent subjects in our study. One of these subjects experienced the event of interest at 9, 13, and 28 months of follow-up, and was followed for another 3 months with no additional events before the study ended. The second subject experienced the event at 10 and 15 months, and follow-up ended at the second event. We also assume that a sufficient number of subjects had four recurrent events to allow modeling this number of recurrent events.

The simplest modeling approach is to use the counting process formulation described in detail in Andersen, Borgan, Gill and Keiding (1993). In this formulation, follow-up time is broken into segments defined by the events. The data for our hypothetical subjects under the counting process model are shown in the panel labeled "AG" for Andersen and Gill (1982) in Table 9.1. We describe the data using time intervals, event indicators, and strata. The purpose of the stratum variable will become clear when we describe the other modeling approaches. In the counting process model, the events are assumed to be independent, and a subject contributes to the risk set for a specific event time as long as the subject is under observation at the time the event occurs. The first hypothetical subject will be in the risk set for any event occurring between 0 and 31 months. Under an assumption of no tied event times, this subject contributes the events defining the risk sets at 9, 13, and 28 months. The second subject will be in the risk sets for any events occurring between 0 and 15 months. This subject contributes the events defining the risk sets at 10 and 15 months. The data for the first subject could be described as data for four different subjects: the first begins follow-up at time 0 and has the event at 9 months, the second has delayed entry at 9 months and is followed until 13 months, when the event occurs, the third has delayed entry at 13 months and is followed until 28, months when the event occurs, and the fourth has delayed entry at 28 months, is followed until 31 months, and is censored at that time. Data for our second hypothetical subject may be described in a similar manner.

We see from the data construction that the model treats the events as being independent and does not differentiate a first event from a second or third, and so on. This model can include time-varying covariates of any type.

In theory, we could model the data in this setting using any hazard function, but we will use the proportional hazards function. It follows that the partial likelihood is identical to the standard proportional hazards partial likelihood [see (3.17)]. If we denote the number of recurrent events for the ith subject as m_i then the total number of events modeled is $m = \Sigma m_i$. The correlation from observing multiple events within the same subject is accounted for by adjusting the estimates of the standard errors using a method that we describe after discussing the data layout for each model.

The counting process model is particularly easy to fit, as many software packages allow follow up time to be described by a time defining the beginning of an interval and a time defining the end of an interval where the subject was either lost to follow up or experienced the event. For example SAS, STATA and S-PLUS allow this type of data input.

Table 9.1 Data Layout under Four Recurrent Event Models for Two Hypothetical Subjects

Model	Subject 1			Subject 2		
	Time Interval	Event	Stratum	Time Interval	Event	Stratum
AG	(0, 9]	1	1	(0, 10]	1	1
	(9, 13]	1	1	(10, 15]	1	1
	(13, 28]	1	1			
	(28, 31]	0	1			
PWP-CP	(0, 9]	1	1	(0, 10]	1	1
	(9, 13]	1	2	(10, 15]	1	2
	(13, 28]	1	3			
	(28, 31]	0	4			
PWP-GT	(0, 9]	1	1	(0, 10]	1	1
	(0, 4]	1	2	(0, 5]	1	2
	(0, 15]	1	3			
	(0 , 3]	0	4			
WLW	(0, 9]	1	1	(0, 10]	1	1
	(0, 13]	1	2	(0, 15]	1	2
	(0, 28]	1	3	(0, 15]	0	3
	(0, 31]	0	4	(0, 15]	0	4
TT-R	(0, 9]	1	1	(0, 10]	1	1
	(0, 13]	1	2	(0, 15]	1	2
	(0, 28]	1	3			
	(0, 31]	0	4			

Two conditional models for recurrent event data have been suggested in Prentice, Williams and Peterson (1981). The models are conditional in the sense that a subject is assumed not to be at risk for a subsequent event until a prior event has occurred. For example, hypothetical subject 1 is assumed not to be at risk for a third event until the second event occurred and is not at risk for a fourth event until the third event occurs. A stratum variable is used to keep track of the event number.

The difference between the two conditional models is the time scale used. One model uses time defined by the beginning of the study while the second uses time since the previous event. The data layouts for the two models are labeled "PWP-CP" and "PWP-GT," respectively, in Table 9.1. The follow up time for the two hypothetical subjects under the CP (conditional probability) model is handled via the same type of time intervals and event indicators used in the counting process model. The stratum variable indicates the specific event number for which the subject is at risk. In the GT (gap time) model, follow-up time begins at zero for each event and ends at the length of time until the next event, the gap time.

Under the assumption that all the covariates are fixed at the beginning of the study, the proportional hazards function for the sth event under conditional model PWP-CP is

$$h_s(t, \mathbf{x}, \boldsymbol{\beta}_s) = h_{0s}(t) \exp(\mathbf{x}' \boldsymbol{\beta}_s) \qquad (9.1)$$

and, under conditional model PWP-GT, it is

$$h_s(t, \mathbf{x}, \boldsymbol{\beta}_s) = h_{0s}(t - t_{s-1}) \exp(\mathbf{x}' \boldsymbol{\beta}_s), \qquad (9.2)$$

where t_{s-1} denotes the time at which the previous event occurred. Parameter estimates for either model may be obtained by using the stratified partial likelihood in (7.2) and (7.3), with data as shown in Table 9.1. Event-specific parameter estimates are obtained by including stratum by covariate interactions in the model. Time-varying covariates can also be incorporated. The risk sets used in the partial likelihood are composed of subjects at risk for a specific event at time t. These sets will be completely different under the two models, because each uses a different time scale. Thus, we expect the two models to yield different values for the estimate of the effect of the same covariate. We consider this point in more detail in the example below.

Wei, Lin and Weissfeld (1989) proposed a marginal event-specific model for the analysis of recurrent event data. The model is marginal in the sense that each event is considered as a separate process. Under this model, time for each event starts at the beginning of follow-up for each subject. All subjects are considered at risk for all events, regardless of how many events they actually experience. The data layout for the two hypothetical subjects is shown in the panel labeled "WLW" in Table 9.1. Recall that in this study we are modeling up to four recurrent events. Our hypothetical subject 1 had three events, and the first three intervals record the total length of time to each event, the event indicator variable is equal to 1, and the stratum variable records the specific event. Note that this subject has an additional fourth interval that records the total length of follow up, has event indicator variable equal to 0 and stratum variable equal to 4. This interval records the "marginal" time the subject was at risk for the fourth event. The data for our second hypothetical subject follow this same pattern. This subject had two events, and the first two intervals denote the total follow-up time until each event. The third interval records the marginal follow-up time to the third event, and, because the event was not observed, the event indicator variable is equal to zero. The marginal follow up time for the fourth event is the same and is repeated with stratum variable equal to 4. All subjects in the study contribute follow up times to all possible recurrent events, whether they experienced that particular recurrence or not.

Under the assumption that all covariates are fixed, the proportional hazards function for the sth event is of the same form as the one in (9.1), and parameter estimates can be obtained using the stratified partial likelihood in (7.2) and (7.3).

Stratum-specific parameter estimates are obtained by including stratum-by-covariate interactions in the model. This model will also accommodate time-varying covariates.

Kelly and Lim (2000) consider a model similar to the WLW model called Total Time-Restricted (TT-R). This model uses the same intervals as WLW, but deletes those that correspond with strata for which no additional follow up time is added. For example, in Table 9.1 the intervals for strata 3 and 4 for the second subject are deleted as this subject has two events and was not observed after the second event.

From a purely computational point of view, once the data for each subject has been put into the specific form shown in Table 9.1, we can use existing software to fit any of the models. SAS users can consult the help features of PROC PHREG version 9 and higher for examples on how to set up their data and fit each of the models in Table 9.1. STATA users should go to the following link for similar information, http://www.stata.com/support/faqs/stat/stmfail.html .

Before considering an example, we discuss a method for adjusting the estimates of the variance of the coefficients to account for the correlation among the observations on an individual subject. Lin and Wei (1989) proposed an extension of White's (1980, 1982) robust variance estimator to the proportional hazards model setting. The extension is similar to the "information sandwich" estimator proposed by Liang and Zeger (1986a, 1986b) for use with correlated data in generalized linear models. Lin and Wei proposed that the estimator be based on the vector of changes in the estimate when the ith subject is deleted. This is the influence diagnostic defined in (6.23). The Lin and Wei robust estimator for the usual single-event proportional hazards model is

$$\hat{R}(\hat{\beta}) = \hat{Var}(\hat{\beta})[\hat{L}'\hat{L}]\hat{Var}(\hat{\beta}), \qquad (9.3)$$

where $\hat{Var}(\hat{\beta})$ is the information-matrix-based estimator in (3.26), and $\hat{L}$ is the n by p matrix whose rows contain the vector of score residuals, $\hat{L}_i$, defined in (6.17).

In the recurrent event setting, subjects may contribute more than one score residual. The actual number will depend on which of the four models is fit. The robust estimator is still based on (9.3), but it uses a value of $\hat{L}_i$ obtained by summing over all the score residuals contributed by the ith subject. This estimator is available as an option in many software packages, including SAS, S-PLUS and STATA. We do not discuss the robust estimator further, but refer the reader to Lin and Wei (1989) for details. In the examples, we use only the robust information-estimator because it is vital to correct the estimator for the correlation between the multiple event or censored times observed for each subject.

The model building details involved in fitting any of the four models are the same as those discussed in Chapter 5, namely checking the scale of continuous covariates, dealing with issues of adjustment or confounding, and assessing the inclusion of interactions. Because all four models are fit using conventional software for a one-event proportional hazards model, the methods are identical to those discussed and illustrated in Chapter 5. Model fit can be assessed using the same residual and influence measures discussed in Chapter 6.

The May and Hosmer (1998) approach to calculating the Grønnesby-Borgan goodness-of-fit test may be used with the counting process model, because this model treats each event as if it were a first event. The other four models make an explicit differentiation between events. The extension of the goodness-of-fit test to the setting of multiple events has not been studied.

To illustrate the use of recurrent event models, we use data from a study in which successive endpoints occur, but the event defining the endpoints is a landmark in the course of disease remission of psoriasis. The data are from a recent study of the influence of a mindfulness-based stress reduction intervention in the treatment of psoriasis. Kabat–Zinn et al. (1998) report the details of the study's design and implementation and the results of an analysis aimed at a general medical audience. Patients in the study had severe psoriasis and were beginning a treatment program prescribed by their physician. The treatment (LIGHT) was either phototherapy (LIGHT = 0) or photochemotherapy (LIGHT = 1). A portion of the intervention consisted of listening to a tape of soothing music while undergoing treatment. Patients within each light group were randomized to one of two tape groups (TAPE). One tape group (TAPE = 1) received instruction on the use of mindfulness-based stress reduction techniques and employed these during the treatment sessions. The other tape group (TAPE = 0) did not receive any aspect of the mindfulness-based intervention.

Four possible successive endpoints were observed. The first endpoint was the number of days until study personnel noted a *first response* to treatment. The second endpoint was the number of days until a specific major lesion showed evidence of the effect of treatment, called the *turning point*. The third endpoint was the number of days until this key lesion was half-cleared, the *halfway point*. The fourth and final endpoint was the number of days until the key lesion cleared completely, the *clearing point*.

Our goal in this example is not to provide a definitive analysis of the data from the Kabat–Zinn study, but rather to illustrate the use of the recurrent event models. One covariate that affected the response to treatment was the number of years the patient had psoriasis (YRSPSOR), and it is included in all of our models.

Table 9.2 presents the results of fitting the CP, PWP-CP, PWP-GT, WLW, and TT-R models to the psoriasis data. Results from partial likelihood ratio tests (not shown) indicate that the stratum by covariate interaction terms required by the PPWP-CP, PWP-GT, WLW, and TT-R models to obtain event-specific coefficient estimates, are not significant. The results of checking the scale of years with psoriasis support treating this covariate as linear in the log-hazard function. In addition, the interaction between LIGHT and TAPE is not significant in any of the models. The results in Table 9.2 are obtained by defining event type as a stratification variable.

Because the primary purpose of the example is to compare the four models, we focus this discussion on the estimated coefficients for TAPE. The coefficient for TAPE is significant in all four models, but it varies in magnitude. Even though the rank order of the p-values is the same for all three variables in Table 9.2, it is not possible to conclude that the observed order holds in all cases.

The counting process (CP) model uses time defined from the beginning of the study, treats all events as if they were the same type of event, and assumes all events are independent. In the psoriasis study, the follow-up times for the 32 subjects, when expanded into time intervals using the method shown in Table 9.1, created 110 intervals of which 96 ended in an event. The counting process model uses a partial likelihood based on the observed survival times of the 96 events. Anyone under observation at the particular time is in the risk set for that event. For example, if a subject experienced his/her second event at 34 days, the risk set would contain all subjects who were still being followed (under treatment in our example) at 34 days regardless of how many events they may have already experienced. This implies that the risk set could contain a subject who had not yet had his/her first event as well as a subject who had experienced 3 events. This property of not taking into account the order or type of event makes the counting process model simple but unrealistic in many settings. For this reason, we feel it is not a useful model for the psoriasis data, in which there is a clear time sequence in the events. Having said this, we interpret the coefficient for TAPE as if the model did make sense for illustrative purposes only. We obtain estimates of hazard ratios, as

Table 9.2 Coefficient Estimates, Robust Standard Errors, Robust z-Scores, and Two-Tailed p-Values for Five Recurrent Event Models Fit to the Psoriasis Data ($n = 32$)

Model	Var.	Coeff.	Robust Std. Err.	Robust z	$p > |z|$
	TAPE	0.390	0.126	3.09	0.002
AG	LIGHT	0.401	0.123	3.26	0.001
	YRSPSOR	0.009	0.006	1.59	0.113
	TAPE	0.838	0.254	3.30	0.001
PWP-CP	LIGHT	1.118	0.272	4.10	<0.001
	YRSPSOR	0.021	0.014	1.52	0.130
	TAPE	0.616	0.249	2.48	0.013
PWP-GT	LIGHT	0.811	0.227	3.57	<0.001
	YRSPSOR	0.016	0.013	1.26	0.207
	TAPE	1.030	0.325	3.17	0.002
WLW	LIGHT	1.540	0.312	4.94	<0.001
	YRSPSOR	0.028	0.019	1.47	0.143
	TAPE	0.955	0.320	2.99	0.003
TT-R	LIGHT	1.448	0.304	4.76	<0.001
	YRSPSOR	0.026	0.018	1.42	0.156

before, by exponentiating estimated coefficients. The estimated hazard ratio for the effect of the mindfulness intervention (TAPE) is 1.48. This is interpreted to mean that subjects having the mindfulness therapy are estimated to be experiencing events at a rate that is 48% higher than subjects not having this treatment adjunct. Estimated hazard ratios could be computed and interpreted in a similar manner for the other covariates. As is the case with all models, estimated hazard ratios for any continuous covariate should be based on a meaningful change in the covariate. In summary, the counting process model is perhaps the simplest of the four models to fit and interpret. Its simplicity is both its major strength and weakness when applied to recurrent event data.

The two conditional models take the specific order of events into account, but define time in different ways. The PWP-CP model uses time defined from the beginning of the study, while the PWP-GT model "resets the clock" after an event is observed, and thus the risk sets are different for the two models. For example, consider the time to the second event for the two subjects in Table 9.1. Under the PWP-GT model, both subjects are in the risk set for the second event from time 0 to 4 months. Under the PWP-CP model, the first subject enters the risk set for the second event at 9 months and leaves at 13 months, while the second subject does not enter the risk set for the second event until 10 months and leaves at 15 months. Not only are the times of entry and removal from the risk sets different under the two models, but the lengths of time the subjects are in the risk sets are different.

The PWP-CP model is the logical choice if one is interested in obtaining event specific estimates of effect modeled over the full time course of the recurrent event process. The PWP-GT model should be used when the goal of the analysis is to obtain event specific estimates of effect and time is modeled using gap time between events. Of these two approaches, we think that the logical choice for the psoriasis data is the PWP-CP because the goal is to document the full time course of the therapy.

Estimated hazard ratios are computed and interpreted in the standard manner. Under the PWP-CP model, the estimated hazard ratio for the effect of the addition of the mindfulness therapy is 1.85. We interpret this to mean that the rate of attainment of the endpoints is 85 percent higher in the group receiving the mindfulness adjunct to therapy. Estimated hazard ratios could be computed and interpreted in a similar manner for the other variables in the model. As was recommended for the counting process model for recurrent events, confidence interval estimates and Wald-type tests should use the robust standard error. In summary, the two conditional approaches provide models that allow one to take into account both the occurrence of multiple events and the time order of the events.

The WLW model takes a different approach to the multiple event process. Under this model, the total time to each of the possible recurrent events is modeled. Each subject contributes to the risk set for each event as long as he/she is still being followed at the time that is defining the risk set. For example, consider the time to the third event for the two subjects in Table 9.1. The first subject experienced a third event at 28 months and is in the risk set for the third event from time 0 to 28 months. The second subject experienced two events, yet under time 0 to 28 months. The second subject experienced two events, yet under the marginal model is considered to be at risk for the third (and fourth for that matter) from time 0 to 15 months. In a sense, the marginal model looks at each event separately and models all of the available data for that event. In many settings, this would be a completely unrealistic model because it may be clinically impossible to observe, say, the third event if the first and second had not yet occurred. In addition, Kelly and Lim (2000) demonstrate that, when a treatment administered at the start of follow up is only effective on the first event, there is a strong carry-over effect in the WLW model and effects for later events might be observed, even if they do not exist.

Estimated hazard ratios and confidence intervals are computed in the usual manner. The estimated hazard ratio for the effect of the mindfulness therapy is 2.80. The interpretation is similar to the other models, but the rate of attainment of the endpoints is 180 percent greater in the group receiving the mindfulness adjunct to therapy. Hazard ratios for the other covariates in the model could be computed and interpreted in a similar manner.

The TT-R model considers follow up time in the same way as the WLW model, but does not include stratum for which no follow up time is added, such as the third stratum when there is no follow up beyond the second event. Based on their simulations, Kelly and Lim (2000) recommend its use when event-specific estimates of effect are desired and one wishes to model effect over the full study time. In a sense, it is similar to the PWP-CP model, but with fewer restrictions on the risk sets. The estimated hazard ratio for TAPE is 2.6 under this model, which is interpreted to mean that subjects receiving the mindfulness adjunct to therapy are experiencing events at a rate that is 2.6 times greater than subjects not on this therapy.

The results in Table 9.2 are consistent across the models in that the rank order of the magnitude of the estimates for all three covariates is: AG, PWP-GT, PWP-CP, TT-R, and then WLW. It would be helpful if this were always the case; but we are aware of no published work that supports the consistency of these relationships. The estimated models presented in Table 9.2 are somewhat simpler than one might encounter in other examples or settings because none of the stratum-by-covariate interaction terms were significant. The effect of each covariate could be described by a single coefficient. In settings where the interactions are significant, stratum- or event-specific estimates of the effect must be computed. Depending on how the design variables for the interaction are created, the estimate of the effect of the covariates may involve coefficients for main effects as well as interaction coefficients. The method for estimating and interpreting a hazard ratio in this case is the same as that discussed and illustrated in Section 6.6.

Unlike other settings in this book where we considered a single model, we have shown in this section that, for recurrent event data, there are five possible proportional hazards-based models, and even more if one delves more deeply into the literature. Hence we conclude with a few summary recommendations, which draw heavily on the results in Kelly and Lim (2000) and Cain and Cole (2005) for choosing a model. First the AG model, with its assumption of independence of and order of events, seems unrealistically simple for most settings. We do not recommended the WLW model because of its unrealistic inclusion of dummy records for unobserved events and observed treatment carry-over effect in the simulations. We recommend that you use the PWP-GT model when you are interested in modeling time from last event. We feel the PWP-CP and TT-R models are both appropriate when the goal is modeling over the full time course. They model the same effect, but subjects contribute to the risk sets in slightly different ways. For example, subject 2 in Table 9.1 contributes 5 "months" to the risk sets under the PWP-CP model and "15" months under the TT-R model. While Kelly and Lim recommend TT-R we feel more comfortable with PWP-CP as it forms its risk sets in a more natural way over the time course (i.e., beginning after an event is observed). All of the above recommendations have to be tempered by the results in Cain and Cole (2005) that suggest that when the data arise from a subject specific random effects model of the type described in the next section the parameters being estimated by these marginal or population average models are, in fact, closer to the null than their subject counterparts. Hence the interpretation applies to groups or "averages" of subjects. Regardless of which model is used one should always employ the robust estimator of the variances and covariances of estimated parameters.

As with any fitted statistical model, it is important to assess its adequacy and fit before using the estimated coefficients for inferential purposes. Furthermore, it is important to evaluate how well the fitted proportional hazards model adheres to the proportional hazards assumption. Because each of the models is fit using standard proportional hazards software, the methods for carrying out this step are the same as those described in Chapter 6 for the single event setting.

9.3 FRAILTY MODELS

Up to this point, all of the statistical models we have used to describe the distribution of survival time have assumed that the hazard function is completely specified, given the baseline hazard function and the values of the covariates (i.e., there are no other factors influencing survival). For example, in a study comparing two forms of treatment for a particular type of cancer, we might, in addition to treatment, include age, and gender in the model and assume that the proportional hazards model is correct. In this case, all subjects of the same treatment, age, and gender are assumed to have the same underlying distribution of survival time. This is not to say that all observed subjects of the same treatment, age and gender will have the same observed survival time. Rather, we assume that, if there is no censoring, the observed survival times are independent observations from a distribution with the same parameters. In some studies, particularly those involving human subjects, there may be factors other than the measured covariates that could significantly affect the distribution of survival time. This condition is often referred to as heterogeneity of the subjects. Among the early papers on this subject is the work by Vaupel, Manton and Stallard (1979), who used the concept of frailty to describe differences in survival time among apparently similar individuals. Considerable work has been done in this area, but much of it is beyond the mathematical level assumed for this text. In this section, we therefore present an introductory overview of frailty models. Hougaard (1995, 2000) presents an excellent overview of the models proposed for use in this area. Aalen (1994) provides a relatively non-technical summary with some examples, with a focus on fully parametric models. Klein and Moeschberger (2003) present methods based on incorporating frailty in a proportional hazards model and discuss some of the technical and computational details. Therneau and Grambsch (2000) also provide a more technical and computationally oriented discussion of frailty models including examples. Nielsen, Gill, Andersen and Sørensen (1992) present a more theoretical treatment based on the counting process approach. Andersen, Borgan, Gill and Keiding (1993) discuss frailty models from the counting process perspective and illustrate the use of these models with examples.

At the individual subject level, the basic idea of a frailty model is to incorporate an unmeasured "random" effect into the hazard function to account for heterogeneity among the subjects. When the observed data consist of triples $(t_i, \mathbf{x}_i, c_i)$, $i = 1, 2, \ldots, n$ denoting the observed follow-up times, the vector of p covariates and a right censoring indicator variable, the hazard function at time t for the ith subject is, under the proportional hazards model,

$$h(t, \mathbf{x}_i, \beta) = h_0(t) \exp(\mathbf{x}_i' \boldsymbol{\beta}). \tag{9.4}$$

A frailty model includes, in the hazard function, the value of an additional unmeasured covariate, the frailty, denoted z_i, yielding a hazard function

$$h_f(t, \mathbf{x}_i, \boldsymbol{\beta}) = z_i h(t, \mathbf{x}_i, \boldsymbol{\beta}). \tag{9.5}$$

This idea extends to models with time-varying covariates, with the usual change in notation. We use the subscript f in (9.5) to represent a hazard function that has been modified by the inclusion of a frailty. An important statistical assumption is that the frailty is independent of any censoring that may take place. Much of the work in this area [see Hougaard (2000), Aalen (1994) and Klein and Moeschberger (2003)] has dealt with the appropriate choice of statistical distribution for the frailty. Because the hazard cannot be negative, distributions must have only positive values. This and other technical issues have led, most frequently, to the use of the Gamma distribution (i.e., a model that assumes that the frailties represent a sample from a Gamma distribution with mean equal to 1 and variance parameter θ). If the value of the frailty, z_i in (9.5) is greater than 1, the subject has a larger-than-average hazard and is said to be more "frail." On the other hand, if the value of the frailty is less than 1, the subject is less "frail" than an average subject. Aalen (1994) points out that there are advantages to using a fully parametric model, such as the Weibull regression model, with a frailty. Not only is estimation easier, it is also possible to describe explicitly the effect that frailties have on hazard ratios over time. In particular, due to the fact the "most" frail individuals tend to fail early in the follow-up, the average hazard ratio tends to decrease over time |see Aalen (1994) for an example and Hougaard (2000) for additional discussion of this point|. Because the major thrust of this text is modeling with the proportional hazards model, we do not consider parametric models with frailties in any more detail. We note that the parametric models considered in Chapter 8 may be fit with a frailty in STATA However, we do not illustrate this situation with examples in this section.

Frailty models have often been used to model dependency in the responses among groups of subjects. In these settings, if the value of the frailty is assumed to be constant within groups, the models are called *shared frailty models*. Suppose that we have $i = 1, 2, \ldots, g$ groups and $j = 1, 2, \ldots, n_i$ subjects in the ith group. In this case we denote the data as $\left(t_{ij}, \mathbf{x}_{ij}, c_{ij} \right)$. The hazard function for ij^{th} subject under the shared frailty model is

$$h_f \left(t, \mathbf{x}_{ij}, \boldsymbol{\beta} \right) = z_i h \left(t, \mathbf{x}_{ij}, \boldsymbol{\beta} \right), \tag{9.6}$$

where some of the covariates in $\mathbf{x}_{ij}$ may be at a group level and are constant over subjects within each group. For example, in an animal carcinogenicity study, the responses of members of the same litter are not likely to be independent. Another example occurs when multiple events have been observed on the same subject, as discussed in the previous section. Liang, Self, Bandeen–Roche and Zeger (1995) discuss the use of frailty models with multivariate failure time data. The shared frailty model has been extended by Pickels et al. (1994) and Yashin, Vaupel and Jachine (1995) to allow different but correlated frailties among observations within a group.

The idea of using an unmeasured covariate or random effect to account for heterogeneity or dependence of responses among groups of subjects is not new or unique to survival time models. This idea has been proposed for use in many generalized linear models. Clayton (1994) and Neuhaus (1992) provide broad overviews of the topic. Collett (2002) and Hosmer and Lemeshow (2000) each discuss random effects logistic regression models.

One problem is that software that fits the proportional hazards model may not have an option to include a frailty in the hazard. Klein and Moeschberger (2003) provide SAS macros that fit the Gamma frailty proportional hazards model at their web site. STATA and S-Plus have the capability to include a frailty.

Several different methods have been proposed to fit frailty models. One method involves an application of the Estimation-Maximization (EM) algorithm.[1] A detailed discussion of the implementation of the EM algorithm may be found in Klein and Moeschberger (2003). They suggest that a simpler implementation proposed by Nielsen, Gill, Andersen and Sørensen (1992) could also be used. We describe the application of the EM algorithm below.

The frailty models in this section were fit in STATA, which uses an approach described by Therneau and Grambsch (2000). This method approaches the problem by considering the frailties as being like design variables. As a result, STATA's implementation requires that a matrix be inverted that is of the order: number of frailties plus model parameters. For example, for the individual frailty model in (9.5), the matrix is of dimension $n + p$, which can be nearly as time consuming to invert in the iterative calculations as the notoriously slow EM-algorithm takes to converge. In addition, STATA uses numerical differentiation, which has caused numerical problems in some of our example data sets when we attempt to fit the individual frailty model. (This was the case, for example, in the final model in Table 6.5 for the WHAS500 data.)

O'Quigley and Stare (2002) consider modeling and computational aspects of fitting frailty models. They use the term *frailty model* to describe the individual frailty model in (9.5) and the term *random effects model* to describe the shared frailty model in (9.6). Their results and simulations show that simply having a model covariate that is nonproportional in the hazard can lead us to incorrectly conclude from the fit of the frailty model that there is unaccounted heterogeneity between the subjects. Thus, they feel that there is little is to be gained from a fit of the frailty model. Based on this, we feel it would be much better to use methods that focus on specific model departures such as those described in Chapter 6 to assess proportional hazards. This is good news for the practitioner because the frailty model can be tricky to fit, as noted above. In addition, O'Quigley and Stare point out that the random effects/shared frailty model in (9.6) is a more restrictive version of the stratified proportional hazards model considered in Section 7.2. The hazard function in (9.6) can be expressed as a stratified model as follows

$$
\begin{aligned}
h_f\left(t, \mathbf{x}_{ij}, \boldsymbol{\beta}\right) &= z_i h\left(t, \mathbf{x}_{ij}, \boldsymbol{\beta}\right) \\
&= h_0\left(t\right) z_i e^{\mathbf{x}_{ij}'\boldsymbol{\beta}} \\
&= h_{0i}\left(t\right) e^{\mathbf{x}_{ij}'\boldsymbol{\beta}},
\end{aligned}
\tag{9.7}
$$

where $h_{0i}\left(t\right) = h_0\left(t\right) z_i$ is the stratum-specific baseline hazard function under the random effects / shared frailty model. The hazard function in (9.7) is of the same

---

[1] The EM algorithm has been used in many settings since it was first described by Dempster, Laird and Rubin (1977). This algorithm and its application in medical settings are discussed in a series of papers in *Statistical Methods in Medical Research* **6**(1) 1997.

form as the general stratified proportional hazards model in (7.1), only more restrictive in that, rather than being completely unspecified, it involves the strong parametric assumption that z_i is a Gamma-distributed random variable with mean 1 and variance θ. The fact that the model in (9.7) is a stratified model led O'Quigley and Stare (2002) to compare, via simulations, fitting the model as a random effects model and as a stratified model when the data are generated from the random effects model. Both methods yield consistent estimates of the coefficients in the model, but the estimated variances from the random effects model are expected to be smaller because that fit is based on the correct model. Based on the simulations, they conclude that if the group size is 5 or larger, there is little practical difference between the two estimation approaches. Thus, they recommend using the stratified model, because it is immensely simpler to fit. For group size 2, for example twin studies, the gain in efficiency (i.e., smaller variances) of the random effects model is considerable and thus they recommend using it. For group sizes 3 or 4, the random effects model is more efficient but not dramatically so. In this case, all things being equal, we would prefer to fit the random effects model.

The practical difficulty in these recommendations is that the random effects model is best in settings when it might be most difficult to fit. If you encounter numerical problems, then you could try the slow but steady EM method, which we describe next (see Klein and Moeschberger (2003) for more detail).

The EM algorithm estimates the regression parameters for each of a fixed set of values of the variance parameter, θ, of the Gamma frailty distribution. The solution is the one yielding the largest value of a "profile" log-likelihood, whose equation is shown below in (9.13). The specific steps are as follows:

Step 1: Fit the proportional hazards model (without frailty) containing the covariates of interest. Following the fit, obtain the estimate of the baseline cumulative hazard function for each subject, $\hat{H}_0(t_i)$, discussed in Section 3.5. Use this to obtain the estimate of the cumulative hazard for each subject,

$$\hat{H}\left(t_i, \mathbf{x}_i, \hat{\boldsymbol{\beta}}\right) = \hat{H}_0\left(t_i\right) \exp\left(\mathbf{x}_i'\hat{\boldsymbol{\beta}}\right).$$

Step 2: Create a set of possible values for the variance parameter θ. Typically, this set is constructed by beginning with a small value, for example, 0.25, and increasing by 0.25 until reaching some maximum value, for example, 4 or 5. For each of the values of θ in this set, steps 3, 4 and 5 are followed.

Step 3: The estimation step (E) consists of computing, for each subject, an estimate of the value of their frailty as

$$\hat{z}_i = \frac{1 + \theta \times c_i}{1 + \theta \times \hat{H}\left(t_i, \mathbf{x}_i, \hat{\boldsymbol{\beta}}\right)}. \tag{9.8}$$

Step 4: The maximization step (M) consists of fitting the proportional hazards model with the same covariates, but including $\hat{z}_i$ in the hazard function, as follows

$$
\begin{aligned}
h_f\left(t, \hat{z}_i, \mathbf{x}_i, \boldsymbol{\beta}\right) &= h_0(t)\hat{z}_i \exp\left(\mathbf{x}_i'\boldsymbol{\beta}\right) \\
&= h_0(t)\exp\left[\mathbf{x}_i'\boldsymbol{\beta} + \ln\left(\hat{z}_i\right)\right].
\end{aligned}
\tag{9.9}
$$

As shown, one may include $\ln\left(\hat{z}_i\right)$ as a model covariate with a coefficient fixed and equal to 1.0. Including a term in a model with a fixed coefficient equal to 1.0 is common in applications of Poisson regression, and occasionally logistic regression, where it is called an *offset*. Some software packages, for example STATA, allow the user to specify an offset when fitting a proportional hazards model.

Following the fit of the model in (9.9), we must estimate the baseline hazard that now includes the estimated frailty term

$$
\hat{h}_{f0}\left(t_i\right) = \frac{c_j}{\displaystyle\sum_{l \in R\left(t_j\right)} \hat{z}_i \exp\left(\mathbf{x}_i'\hat{\boldsymbol{\beta}}\right)},
\tag{9.10}
$$

the cumulative baseline hazard function

$$
\hat{H}_{f0}\left(t_i\right) = \sum_{t_j \le t_i} \hat{h}_{f0}\left(t_j\right),
\tag{9.11}
$$

and the cumulative hazard containing the frailty, namely

$$
\hat{H}_f\left(t_i, \mathbf{x}_i, \hat{\boldsymbol{\beta}}\right) = \hat{H}_{f0}\left(t_i\right)\exp\left(\mathbf{x}_i'\hat{\boldsymbol{\beta}}\right).
\tag{9.12}
$$

The E- and M-steps are repeated until convergence is achieved. We note that, in the second and subsequent applications of the E-step, one uses the cumulative hazard containing the frailty, (9.12), computed in the previous M-step.

Step 5: Evaluate the profile log-likelihood in (9.13) using the specified value of θ and the results from the fit in the M-step at convergence. Let $m_i = \sum_{j=1}^{n_i} c_{ij}$ denote the number of observed events in the ith group. The equation for the profile log-likelihood, from Klein and Moeschberger [2003, equation (13.3.2)] is

$$L\left(\theta,\hat{\boldsymbol{\beta}}\right) = \sum_{i=1}^{g} m_i \ln(\theta) - \ln\left[\Gamma\left(\frac{1}{\theta}\right)\right] + \ln\left[\Gamma\left(\frac{1}{\theta} + m_i\right)\right]$$

$$+ \sum_{j=1}^{n_i} c_{ij} \left\{ \mathbf{x}'_{ij}\hat{\boldsymbol{\beta}} + \ln\left[h_{f0}\left(t_{ij}\right)\right] \right\} \qquad (9.13)$$

$$- \left(\frac{1}{\theta} + m_i\right)\ln\left[1 + \theta\sum_{j=1}^{n_i} \ln\left[1 + \theta\hat{H}_f\left(t_{ij}, \mathbf{x}_{ij}, \hat{\boldsymbol{\beta}}\right)\right]\right].$$

Note that the value of the middle term in (9.13) is the log-likelihood for the model fit in the M-step.

Steps 1 to 5 are performed for all chosen values of θ. The maximum likelihood estimate of θ is the value maximizing (9.13). Nielsen, Gill, Andersen and Sørensen (1992) describe an easily employed method for using the calculated values of (9.13) to obtain an empirical estimate of the MLE, $\hat{\theta}$. Significance tests for model coefficients may be performed either using Wald tests or a profile likelihood ratio test. The Wald test uses estimated standard errors from a covariance matrix obtained from the negative of the inverse of the matrix of second derivatives of the profile log-likelihood. Klein and Moeschberger (2003) provide equations for the elements of a matrix given in by Andersen, Klein, Knudsen and Tabanera y Placios (1997) that correct for an underestimation in the variance of the estimate of the MLE of the Gamma-variance parameter. Nielsen, Gill, Andersen and Sørensen (1992) suggest using a profile likelihood ratio test where one compares twice the difference in profile log-likelihood of the fitted model and the one obtained from fitting the model deleting the covariate but using the same value of $\hat{\theta}$.

A significance test for the variance parameter, θ, can also be performed in one of two ways. Commenges and Andersen (1995) proposed a score test described in some detail in Klein and Moeschberger (2003). A more easily performed test is to use the likelihood ratio test suggested by Nielsen, Gill, Andersen and Sørensen (1992). Under the hypothesis that $\theta = 0$, the random effects model reduces to the standard proportional hazards model and the value of the profile log-likelihood in (9.13) is the usual partial log-likelihood from fitting the proportional hazards model minus the number of non-censored follow-up times. That is,

$$L\left(\theta = 0, \hat{\boldsymbol{\beta}}\right) = \sum_{i=1}^{g}\sum_{j=1}^{n_i} c_{ij}\left\{\mathbf{x}'_{ij}\hat{\boldsymbol{\beta}} + \ln\left[h_0\left(t_{ij}\right)\right]\right\} - \sum_{i=1}^{g} m_i . \qquad (9.14)$$

The first term in (9.14) is simply the partial log-likelihood from the model fit in step 1 of the EM procedure, and the second term is the number of events. The likelihood ratio test statistic is

$$G = 2\left[L\left(\hat{\theta},\hat{\boldsymbol{\beta}}\right) - L\left(0,\hat{\boldsymbol{\beta}}\right) \right], \qquad (9.15)$$

with a p-value computed using a mixture of a chi-square distribution with one degree of freedom and a distribution with point mass 1.0 at the value $\theta = 0$. STATA implements this test by returning a p-value of 1.0 if the estimate of θ is close to zero and returns $p = 0.5 \times \Pr\left[\chi^2(1) > G\right]$ if the estimate is not zero (see Gutierrez, Carter and Drukker (2001)).

The complicated nature of these calcualtions is one of the motivating factors why Aalens (1994) favor the use of a fully parametric model. In the parametric model, the actual values of the unobserved frailties can be "averaged" out of the model in the way they are handled in random effects logistic regression. Andersen, Klein, Knudsen and Tabanera y Placios (1997) also suggest that one consider the use of parametric models rather than the proportional hazards models.

To provide an example, we use the WHAS500 data and fit models containing body mass index, heart rate, diastolic blood pressure, and congestive heart complications. To illustrate the random effects/shared frailty setting, we formed groups based on age. We sorted on age and then formed 250 groups of size 2, 100 groups of size 5 and 50 groups of size 10. In each of these cases, we fit both the random effects (shared frailty) model and the stratified model. We also fit the (individual) frailty model (i.e., 500 groups of size 1) and the usual proportional hazards model. The results are presented in Table 9.3. Note that the fitted random effects model excludes age, which is known from analyses in earlier chapters to be significant. Thus, there should be some heterogeneity displayed in the fit of the random effects models for which we have not accounted

The results presented in Table 9.3 are in basic agreement with the simulations in O'Quigley and Stare (2002). The efficiency of the stratified model relative to the random effects model increases as the group size increases. For the continuous covariates, the differences between the random effects estimates of the coefficients and the stratified estimates is of the general magnitude seen in Figure 4 of O'Quigley and Stare (2002). They did not simulate any dichotomous covariates, so we do not know if the increase in the difference between the estimates of the coefficient for chf from group size 5 to 10 is important or merely random. In summary, the results in Table 9.3 do support the recommendation that little is to be gained by using the more complicated random effects model when the group size is 5 or larger. Having said this, we feel that, rather than adopt an all or nothing approach, we would prefer to use the frailty model when it may be conveniently and easily estimated and to use the stratified model when the sample size is so large that the frailty model's computations are prohibitively slow and difficult.

We know from the model building in Chapter 5 that a fitted model containing body mass index, heart rate, diastolic blood pressure and congestive heart complications is not the best model for the WHAS500 data. However, it is adequately complex for the purposes of illustrating estimation and interpretation of covariate effects and other post-fit descriptors of survival experience following the fit of a random effects model. In this regard, we consider the model in Table 9.3 a fit with 250 groups of size 2. In this case, the estimate of the random effect variance parameter is $\hat{\theta} = 0.245$ with $p = 0.045$, indicating significant heterogeneity. All estimated standard errors of estimated coefficients are conditional on this value. Estimates of hazard ratios are conditional on having the same value of the shared random effect. For example, the estimated hazard ratio for congestive heart complications is $\hat{HR} = \exp(1.006) = 2.7$. The interpretation is that among subjects with the same value of the random effect or frailty, those with congestive heart complications are dying at a rate that is 2.7 times greater than those without congestive heart complications. The estimated hazard ratio for a 5 kg/m^2 increase in body mass index is $\hat{HR} = \exp(5 \times -0.083) = 0.66$. Thus, among subjects with the same value of the random effect or frailty, an increase of 5 kg/m is associated with a 34 percent decrease in the rate of dying. Computation and interpretation is similar for the hazard ratios for the other model covariates.

Most packages that fit the frailty / random effects model have the capability to compute and save estimates of the shared or individual frailties as well as save estimates of the baseline hazard and cumulative hazard in (9.10) and (9.11) for the "baseline" random effect of $z_i = 1$ as well as the corresponding estimated baseline survival function. To illustrate how the inclusion of random effects can change the estimated survival function, we refit the 250-by-2 model in Table 9.3, centering body mass index at 26, heart rate at 85, and diastolic blood pressure at 79, which are approximately the respective median values. Hence, the estimated baseline survival function, denoted $\hat{S}_{0f}(t)$, estimates the survival experience among subjects with these three covariate values and no congestive heart complications, $chf = 0$, and random effect $z_i = 1$ or $w_i = \ln(z_i) = 0$. The estimated survival function for subjects with congestive heart complications, $chf = 1$, is

$$\hat{S}_{1f}(t) = \left[\hat{S}_{0f}(t)\right]^{\exp(0.994)},$$

where 0.994 is the value of the estimated coefficient for congestive heart complications for the 250-by-2 case in Table 9.3.

To illustrate the effect that the random effects can have on the estimated survival function, we saved the individually estimated shared random effects and found that the minimum value on the log scale was –0.800 and the maximum value was 0.379. We use these values to obtain "high" and "low" survival functions as follows

$$\hat{S}_{0fh}(t) = \left[\hat{S}_{0f}(t)\right]^{\exp(-0.8)},$$

Table 9.3 Fit of the Proportional Hazards Model, Frailty Model, Random Effects Models, and Stratified Models with Estimated Coefficients, Standard Errors, Estimated Gamma Variance with LR Test p-value, Percent Difference of Coefficient from the Frailty Model and Relative Efficiency of the Standard / Stratified to the Frailty / Random Effects Model

Variable	Frailty Model		Standard PH Model		Diff. in Coeff.[#]	Percent Relative Efficiency[&]
	500 Groups of Size 1					
	Coeff.	S.E.	Coeff.	S.E.		
bmi	−0.083	0.0158	−0.081	0.0153	−0.003	94.3
hr	0.013	0.0030	0.012	0.0029	0.000	93.0
diasbp	−0.016	0.0036	−0.016	0.0035	−0.001	93.8
chf	0.994	0.1497	0.953	0.1445	0.040	93.1
Theta	0.094	0.2420				
LR Test p value	0.344					
	Random Effects		Stratified Model			
	250 Groups of Size 2		250 Strata of Size 2			
Variable	Coeff.	S.E.	Coeff.	S.E.		
bmi	−0.082	0.0163	−0.034	0.0253	−0.099	41.8
hr	0.013	0.0031	0.016	0.0058	0.010	29.3
diasbp	−0.017	0.0037	−0.006	0.0061	−0.021	36.8
chf	0.994	0.1555	0.440	0.2534	0.838	37.6
Theta	0.209	0.1594				
LR Test p value	0.073					
	100 Groups of Size 5		100 Strata of Size 5			
Variable	Coeff.	SE.	Coeff.	SE.		
bmi	−0.071	0.0162	−0.050	0.0196	−0.087	68.5
hr	0.013	0.0032	0.011	0.0038	0.009	67.8
diasbp	−0.016	0.0037	−0.008	0.0046	−0.019	66.0
chf	0.965	0.1562	0.931	0.1943	0.808	64.6
Theta	0.311	0.1383				
LR Test p value	0.001					
	50 Groups of Size 10		50 Strata of Size 10			
Variable	Coeff.	S.E.	Coeff.	S.E.		
bmi	−0.062	0.0162	−0.040	0.0177	−0.022	84.1
hr	0.011	0.0031	0.010	0.0033	0.001	87.2
diasbp	−0.014	0.0037	−0.011	0.0040	−0.003	84.2
chf	0.884	0.1536	0.829	0.1672	0.054	84.4
Theta	0.352	0.1401				
LR Test p value	<0.001					

#: $\hat{\beta}_f - \hat{\beta}_s$, &: $100 \times \left[\widehat{SE}_t^2 / \widehat{SE}_s^2 \right]$

$$\hat{S}_{0fl}(t) = \left[\hat{S}_{0f}(t)\right]^{\exp(0.379)},$$

$$\hat{S}_{1fh}(t) = \left[\hat{S}_{1f}(t)\right]^{\exp(-0.8)},$$

and

$$\hat{S}_{1fl}(t) = \left[\hat{S}_{1f}(t)\right]^{\exp(0.379)}.$$

These six estimated survival functions are plotted in Figure 9.1, where they appear as two groups of three curves. The estimated baseline survival function for $chf = 0$ is the solid line step function second from the top. Its "high" and "low" functions are plotted with short dashed lines (first and third from the top). The estimated baseline survival function for $chf = 1$ is the step function with plotting pattern " $- \cdot -$ " (second from the bottom). Its "high" and "low" functions are plotted with long dashed lines (first and third from the bottom). Note that the function $\hat{S}_{1fh}(t)$ falls quite close to the function $\hat{S}_{0fl}(t)$. Hence, subjects with congestive heart complications and a "small" random effect have a survival experience similar to subjects without congestive heart complications, thus describing the essence of how inclusion of random effects can allow for between-subject variability in response. The coefficient for chf in Table 9.3 is significant, based on a Wald test with $p < 0.001$. This implies that the two "baseline" survival functions, $\hat{S}_{0f}(t)$ and $\hat{S}_{1f}(t)$, are significantly different from each other. Because we do not have an estimate of the variance of the individually estimated random effects, we cannot determine, using a statistical test, whether the estimated survival curves at the "high" and "low" values differ from each other or the baseline survival curves.

Because the model was fit with 250 groups of size 2, there are 250 values of the estimated random effects. So in essence, there are 250 possible estimated survival curves with $chf = 0$ and another 250 with $chf = 1$, each computed in the same manner as the functions plotted in Figure 9.1. To further explore the variability in the estimated survival curves, we plot 42 of the 500 possible curves in Figure 9.2. There are 21 with $chf = 0$ evaluated at the $1, 13, 25, 37, \ldots, 229, 241^{st}$ largest values of z_i and another 21 with $chf = 1$ at the same 21 values of z_i. The estimated curves in Figure 9.2 fall into two clusters, with some overlap. The upper group contains the 21 with $chf = 0$ and the lower 21 have $chf = 1$. The spread within group clearly illustrates the variability in response from the random effect. The curves are all of the same basic form, which is a result of the model in (9.6) and the assumption that the random effects come from a Gamma distribution with mean 1 and estimated variance of 0.245.

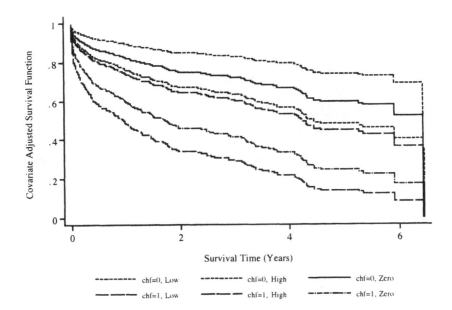

Figure 9.1 Plots of the covariate-adjusted survival functions for the absence or presence of congestive heart complications (chf = 0 or 1) at three levels (low, high and zero) of the estimated random effect.

To compare and contrast the covariate adjusted survival functions from the fit of the random effects and stratified models in Table 9.1, we would have to plot 42 estimated survival curves from the fitted stratified model for the same 21 strata / groups used in Figure 9.2. The difficulty is that, when the software saves the estimated baseline survival functions from the stratified fit, there are only two values per stratum; hence the plots are not useful.

In summary, frailty or random effects models can provide a useful, though computationally challenging, way to account for correlation among responses and is recommended when the group size is less than 5. In settings when the number of subjects "sharing" the same frailty is 5 or more one may obtain similar, though slightly less efficient, estimates from a fit of stratified proportional hazards model. However, in this case one may not have sufficient within stratum data to obtain meaningful estimates of the covariate adjusted survival function.

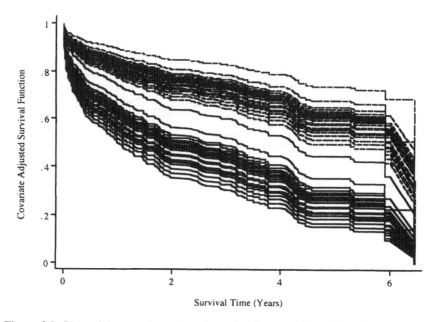

Figure 9.2 Plots of the covariate adjusted survival functions for chf = 0 (dashed lines) and chf = 1 (solid lines) at the same 20 estimated values of the random effect.

9.4 NESTED CASE-CONTROL STUDIES

In some situations, such as large epidemiologic studies with time-varying covariates, the data may be so extensive that it would be impractical to fit survival time models using the entire cohort of subjects. In other cases, new research may indicate that data on an additional covariate should have been collected, but the process of collecting new information on all subjects would be too extensive to be feasible. In studies of this type, one may choose to use what is known as a *nested case-control study*.[2]

In a nested case-control study, one may estimate the regression parameters in the proportional hazards model with risk sets that contain a reduced number of subjects. Briefly, the data are obtained by selecting a sample (without replacement) of a fixed number of subjects who did not fail from the risk set at each observed survival time. These subjects become the controls for the case whose survival time defines the risk set. This design is discussed from an epidemiologic perspective in Clayton and Hills (1993). Construction of the partial likelihood was first considered by Oakes (1981). A series of papers by Borgan and Langholz

---

[2] Those readers who are unfamiliar with the case-control study may wish to consult Rothman and Greenland (1998).

(1993), Langholz and Borgan (1995) and Borgan, Goldstein and Langholz (1995) reviews the construction of the partial likelihood, derives score equations for estimation, presents methods for inference, and provides examples.

Methods for implementing the design assume there are no tied survival times, so we must decide how to handle ties that might exist in the data. Borgan and Langholz (1993) suggest that tied survival times be broken randomly and that the random order be used as if it were the real order in the survival times. We illustrate one method of breaking ties in the example.

The number of control subjects selected will affect the efficiency of the nested case-control analysis relative to an analysis based on the complete risk set at each survival time. Clayton and Hills (1993) point out that the ratio of the standard errors of coefficient estimates from the two methods of analysis is approximately

$$\frac{\text{SE}\left(\hat{\beta}\middle|\text{case-control}\right)}{\text{SE}\left(\hat{\beta}\middle|\text{full cohort}\right)} \approx \sqrt{1+\frac{1}{n_c}},$$

where n_c is the number of controls selected from each risk set. This expression suggests that little would be gained from using more than five controls.

Once the number of controls to be selected is determined, the sampling of controls from each risk set must be done independently of all other study factors. Eligible subjects may be selected as controls in more than one risk set. To simplify the notation somewhat, we denote the $n_c + 1$ subjects, consisting of the n_c controls and one case, in the nested case control study risk set at survival time t_i as $\tilde{R}(t_i)$. If we assume there are no time-varying covariates among the p covariates in the model, the partial likelihood is

$$l_{\text{ncc}}(\boldsymbol{\beta}) = \prod_{i=1}^{n_c} \frac{e^{x_i'\boldsymbol{\beta}}}{\sum\limits_{j \in \tilde{R}(t_i)} e^{x_j'\boldsymbol{\beta}}}. \tag{9.16}$$

The subscript "ncc" in (9.16) is used to differentiate this partial likelihood from the one in (3.19) for the full cohort. The distinction between the two partial likelihoods goes well beyond a subscript because the model in (9.16) cannot be fit using a proportional hazards regression program. The risk sets for the partial likelihood for the full cohort analysis are nested. That is, subjects in a risk set at time t are contained in all risk sets at time less than t, but that is not true of the risk sets in (9.16). The likelihood in (9.16) is identical to that of a matched case control study, with one case and n_c controls per matched set, with survival times defining the matched sets [see Hosmer and Lemeshow (2000, Chapter 7)]. Thus, the regression coefficients from the nested case-control study may be obtained by using any matched logistic regression routine that can handle multiple controls per case.

From a practical point of view, the only impediment to using a nested case control design is the actual selection of the sample of controls from the risk set. STATA has eased the burden by providing a command, sttocc, that executes the sampling and creates an output data set containing all the information needed to fit the model in (9.16) using the conditional logistic regression program. Users of other packages are encouraged to check their favorite package's web site and/or make an inquiry to its user group list server.

Time-varying covariates can be included in the partial likelihood in (9.16) simply by letting the covariate values depend on time, for example, by using $x(t_i)$ in place of x. In practice this means that fewer calculations of the values of the time-varying covariates are necessary because one needs only the values of the covariates at the times that define the case control sets, and only for those subjects in the set.

The ACTG320 study provides a good data set to illustrate the nested case-control study because it is a large study with few events. The sampling was performed using STATA. The software automatically breaks tied survival times randomly, but we performed this step manually (prior to sampling) to have better control of the analysis. For tied event times, we subtract an independently generated

Table 9.4 Key Variables from Creation of the Nested Case Control Study from the ACTG320 Study, for the First Three Risk Sets

Set	Case Control Indicator	Study ID	Case Time	Follow-up Time
1	0	525	0.639	133
1	0	213	0.639	161
1	0	861	0.639	329
1	0	631	0.639	300
1	0	1136	0.639	102
1	1	486	0.639	0.639
2	0	1019	1.749	263
2	0	965	1.749	280
2	0	267	1.749	248
2	0	1017	1.749	216
2	0	45	1.749	291
2	1	788	1.749	1.749
3	0	759	6.517	187
3	0	578	6.517	117
3	0	971	6.517	280
3	0	120	6.517	291
3	0	145	6.517	287
3	1	823	6.517	6.517

observation from the $U(0,0.5)$ distribution from observed follow-up times. This process broke all the tied survival times but left any ties among the censored observations intact.

Among the 1151 subjects with complete data, there were 96 uncensored follow-up times, and application of the sampling procedure produced a new data set with $576 = 6 \times 96$ data records. Key data for the first 3 sets of one case and 5 sampled controls is shown in Table 9.4. Selecting 5 controls per case was possible because the minimum number in any risk set was 312. While not a problem in the ACTG320 example, to have the sampling be fully independent, survival times with fewer than n_c non-failing subjects would not be used.

The study ID numbers for the subjects selected are shown in the third column of Table 9.4, and the survival times for cases are shown in the fourth column. Follow-up time for each subject is shown in the last column. We note that these times are both non-integer and integer valued. The integer-valued times correspond to subjects whose observed time is censored, while non-integer times correspond to subjects who died (i.e., the observed follow-up time minus a $U(0,0.5)$ random number). We note that in each set, follow-up time is longer for the controls than for the case, as expected. An analysis of the selected controls (not shown) indicated that a few subjects appeared in multiple sets, but no subject appears more than four times. Subjects appear in multiple sets because the number in the full cohort risk sets becomes increasingly smaller as follow-up time increases, thus increasing the chance that a subject will be selected as a control in later sets. We also note that subjects who eventually define case control sets as the case could have been selected as a control at an earlier follow-up time. In fact this occurs in 17 of the 96 sets of observations.

Conditional logistic regression was used to fit a model containing treatment (tx), age and CD4 count (cd4) with outcome variable case control status and stratifying on set. The first two columns of Table 9.5 present the results of this fit. The next two columns contain the estimated coefficients and standard errors from the fit of the model to the full ACTG320 data set with $n = 1151$ subjects. The last column contains the ratio of estimated standard errors of the coefficients.

Table 9.5 Estimated Coefficients, Standard Errors, and the Ratio of the Estimated Standard Errors Comparing the Fit in the Nested Case Control Sample to the Full Data Set for the Final Model for the UIS Study

Variable	Nested Case Control		Full Data Set		Ratio
	Coeff.	Std. Err.	Coeff.	Std. Err.	
tx	−0.701	0.2474	−0.659	0.2150	1.15
age	0.021	0.0134	0.028	0.0111	1.20
cd4	−0.017	0.0027	−0.017	0.0025	1.08

The results in Table 9.5 indicate that the coefficient estimates obtained from the nested case control study are close to those obtained from the full data set. In addition, the ratios of the estimated standard errors are each close to the theoretical ratio of $1.095 = \sqrt{1 + 1/5}$. The conclusions about the significance of treatment and estimated hazard ratios for all three covariates would certainly be the same for both analyses. In particular, the methods used in Chapter 6 to provide estimates and confidence intervals for hazard ratios may be used with the results of a nested case control analysis.

Borgan, Goldstein and Langholz (1995) derive the estimator of the baseline survival function. We can use this estimator in a manner identical to that shown in Chapter 6 to provide estimates and graphs of covariate-adjusted survival probabilities. The estimator of the baseline survival for the nested case control study is similar in format to the one used for the frailty models in the previous section in that it includes a specific weighting factor for each risk set. The estimator of the baseline hazard at the ith observed survival time is given by the equation

$$\hat{h}_{0\text{ncc}}\left(t_i\right) = \frac{1}{\displaystyle\sum_{j \in \tilde{R}(t_i)} w_i e^{x_j' \hat{\beta}}}, \tag{9.17}$$

where the value of the weight is $w_i = n(t_i)/(n_c + 1)$ and $n(t_i)$ denotes the number of subjects in the risk set at time t_i in the original cohort. The estimator of the cumulative baseline hazard function at time t is

$$\hat{H}_{0\text{ncc}}\left(t\right) = \sum_{t_i \le t} \hat{h}_{0\text{ncc}}\left(t_i\right), \tag{9.18}$$

and the estimator of the cumulative hazard function for the ith subject at time t is

$$\hat{H}_{\text{ncc}}\left(t, \mathbf{x}_i, \hat{\boldsymbol{\beta}}\right) = \hat{H}_{0\text{ncc}}\left(t\right) \exp\left(\mathbf{x}_i' \hat{\boldsymbol{\beta}}\right). \tag{9.19}$$

The estimator of the survival function is of the same form as the estimator when the full cohort is analyzed using the proportional hazards model, namely

$$
\begin{aligned}
\hat{S}_{\text{ncc}}\left(t, \mathbf{x}_i, \hat{\boldsymbol{\beta}}\right) &= \exp\left[-\hat{H}_{\text{ncc}}\left(t, \mathbf{x}_i, \hat{\boldsymbol{\beta}}\right)\right] \\
&= \left[\hat{S}_{0\text{ncc}}\left(t\right)\right]^{\exp\left(\mathbf{x}_i' \hat{\boldsymbol{\beta}}\right)},
\end{aligned} \tag{9.20}
$$

where the estimator of the baseline survival function is

$$\hat{S}_{0ncc}(t) = \exp\left[-\hat{H}_{0ncc}(t)\right]. \tag{9.21}$$

Note that we again use the subscript "ncc" in (9.17)–(9.21) to emphasize that these estimators are obtained from a nested case control study.

As an example of the use of the estimator of the survival function, we calculate the estimated covariate-adjusted survival functions for the two levels of treatment, fixing age at its median, 38 years, and CD4 count at its median 68. Using the estimated coefficients in Table 9.5, the two estimated survival functions are

$$\hat{S}_{ncc}(t, tx = 0, age = 38, cd4 = 68) = \left[\hat{S}_{0ncc}(t)\right]^{\exp(0.021 \times 38 - 0.017 \times 68)} \tag{9.22}$$

and

$$\hat{S}_{ncc}(t, tx = 1, age = 38, cd4 = 68) = \left[\hat{S}_{0ncc}(t)\right]^{\exp(-0.701 + 0.021 \times 38 - 0.017 \times 68)}. \tag{9.23}$$

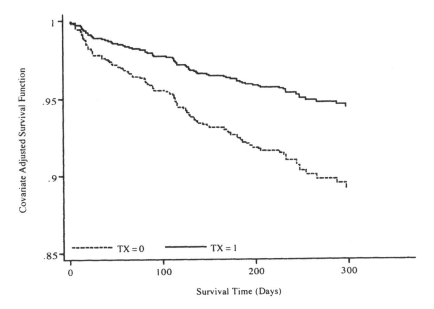

Figure 9.3 Graph of the covariate-adjusted survival functions for the two treatments in the ACTG320 nested case control analysis.

Figure 9.3 presents graphs of the estimated survival functions in (9.22) and (9.23), plotted at the 96 observed survival times in the nested case control study. The estimated survival functions may be used to estimate quantiles of the survival distribution in the same manner as described in Chapter 2 as well as illustrated for a covariate-adjusted survival function in Chapter 6.

Because a random process is used to select the control subjects, it would be impossible for you to reproduce the results shown in Table 9.5 and Figure 9.3. Each time a new nested case control data set is created, the composition of the control group will change. However, the results from any new sample should not differ appreciably from those reported here.

In summary, the nested case-control study offers the possibility of fitting data from a follow-up study using information on fewer subjects than the total number of subjects in the complete cohort. If an adequate number of controls are used, the results from the nested study should agree with those that would have been obtained had the entire cohort been used.

9.5 ADDITIVE MODELS

Up to this point, we have focused on *multiplicative* regression models for the analysis of survival-time data. In these models, the combined effect of the covariates is obtained by multiplying their separate effects. For example, in a proportional hazards model containing sex and age, the multiplicative nature of the hazard function is seen if we rearrange the terms as follows:

$$
\begin{aligned}
h(t, \mathbf{x}, \boldsymbol{\beta}) &= h_0(t) \times (\text{effect of sex}) \times (\text{effect of age}) \\
&= h_0(t)\left(e^{\beta_1 \text{SEX}}\right) \times \left(e^{\beta_2 \text{AGE}}\right) \\
&= h_0(t) e^{\beta_1 \text{SEX} + \beta_2 \text{AGE}}.
\end{aligned}
\tag{9.24}
$$

In a similar manner, the fully parametric models presented in Chapter 8 can also be shown to be multiplicative.

As we showed in detail in previous chapters, multiplicative models are extremely useful in practice because either the estimated coefficients themselves or simple functions of them can be used to provide estimates of hazard ratios. In addition, statistical software is readily available and easy to use to fit models, check model assumptions, and assess model fit. The widespread use of multiplicative models, particularly the proportional hazards model, in applied settings is largely due to these factors.

However, there may be times when a measure of the additive effect of a covariate is preferred over a relative measure. There are several different forms of additive models, including the *additive relative hazard model* mentioned in Section 3.2. If we use a hypothetical model containing sex and age, the additive relative hazard function is

$$h(t,\mathbf{x},\boldsymbol{\beta}) = h_0(t) \times (1 + \text{effect of sex} + \text{effect of age})$$
$$= h_0(t)(1 + \beta_1 \text{SEX} + \beta_2 \text{AGE}). \tag{9.25}$$

If we code $\text{SEX} = 1$ for male and $\text{SEX} = 0$ for female then, under the model in (9.25), the hazard ratio for male versus female at $\text{AGE} = a$ is

$$\text{HR}(\text{SEX} = 1, \text{SEX} = 0, \text{AGE} = a) = \frac{(1 + \beta_1 + \beta_2 a)}{(1 + \beta_2 a)},$$

which is not a simple function of the coefficient for sex. The coefficient for sex, β_1, is the additive increase or decrease in the hazard ratio from male gender. One rather obvious problem with this model is that, if inferences are based on hazard ratios, it is impossible, except in a univariate model, to isolate the effect of a single covariate. Under this model, the difference in the hazard for males and females, at $\text{AGE} = a$, is

$$h(t, \text{SEX} = 1, \text{AGE} = a, \boldsymbol{\beta}) - h(t, \text{SEX} = 0, \text{AGE} = a, \boldsymbol{\beta}) = h_0(t)\beta_1,$$

which depends on both the coefficient for sex and the unspecified baseline hazard function.

Two other forms of the additive relative hazard model that have been suggested, expressed in terms of the two variable example, are

$$h(t,\mathbf{x},\boldsymbol{\beta}) = h_0(t)\left(1 + e^{\beta_1 \text{SEX}} + e^{\beta_2 \text{AGE}}\right) \tag{9.26}$$

and

$$h(t,\mathbf{x},\boldsymbol{\beta}) = h_0(t)\left(1 + e^{\beta_1 \text{SEX} + \beta_2 \text{AGE}}\right). \tag{9.27}$$

In theory, the additive relative hazard models may be easily expanded to include interactions between covariates, nonlinear terms for continuous covariates, time-varying covariates and stratification variables. Thus, fitting the models should be no more difficult than fitting the proportional hazards model. The EGRET software package (EGRET for Windows, (1999)) offers the option to fit the additive relative hazard models shown in (9.25) and (9.26). However, one may have trouble fitting these models containing more than just a few dichotomous covariates because the range of allowable values for the coefficients, those yielding a positive hazard function, is tightly constrained by the additive form of the model. Despite the possible clinical appeal of additive relative hazard models, they are not practical, which may be why they have not been used more frequently in applied research.

Two fully additive models have received attention in the statistical literature. One of these is a semi-parametric model (see Breslow and Day, 1987) where, for the hypothetical two-variable model, the hazard function is

$$
\begin{aligned}
h(t, \mathbf{x}, \boldsymbol{\beta}) &= h_0(t) + \text{effect of sex} + \text{effect of age} \\
&= h_0(t) + \beta_1 \text{SEX} + \beta_2 \text{AGE}.
\end{aligned} \tag{9.28}
$$

Under this model, the difference in the hazard rate for males and females of a common age is

$$
h(t, \text{SEX} = 1, \text{AGE} = a, \boldsymbol{\beta}) - h(t, \text{SEX} = 0, \text{AGE} = a, \boldsymbol{\beta}) = \beta_1 .
$$

The regression coefficient, β_1, is the additive change from the baseline hazard function for males, holding age fixed. Similarly, the quantity β_2 is the additive change in hazard rate for a 1-year increase in age, holding sex fixed at either male or female. The model in (9.28) can easily be expanded to include nonlinear terms for continuous covariates, interactions, time-varying covariates and stratification variables.

Lin and Ying (1994) derive an estimator of the regression coefficients from models of the form shown in (9.28) that does not require iterative calculations. They prove that their estimator has a large-sample normal distribution, with mean equal to the true coefficients, and they derive an estimator of the covariance matrix of the estimator of the coefficients. One can use these estimators, with the standard normal distribution or chi-square distribution, for hypothesis tests and confidence intervals. They also derive an estimator of the baseline cumulative hazard function that can, when combined with the estimates of the coefficients and a vector of covariate values, be used to estimate the covariate-adjusted survivorship function. One potential problem with their estimator of the coefficients is that it can yield an estimate of the baseline cumulative hazard function that is a non-monotonic increasing function of time. In addition, the estimate can be negative, leading to estimated survival probabilities greater than one. They suggest that we work around these problems by using an empirical procedure that forces the estimator of the baseline cumulative hazard to be a monotonic increasing function of time. Lin and Ying (1994) illustrate the use of the semiparametric model with a few examples. Unfortunately, software to fit this model is, at this time, not readily available in a major statistical software package. Assuming we have a model with p fixed covariates, the Lin and Ying estimator is

$$\hat{\boldsymbol{\beta}} = \left\{ \sum_{i=1}^{n} \sum_{t_j \geq t_i} \left[\mathbf{x}_i - \overline{\mathbf{x}}(t_j) \right]^{\otimes 2} \right\}^{-1} \left\{ \sum_{i=1}^{n} c_i \left[\mathbf{x}_i - \overline{\mathbf{x}}(t_i) \right] \right\}, \qquad (9.29)$$

where the expression $\mathbf{x}^{\otimes 2}$ denotes the matrix operation $\mathbf{x}\mathbf{x}'$, which is a p by p matrix, and

$$\overline{\mathbf{x}}(t_i) = \frac{\sum_{j \in R(t_i)} \mathbf{x}_j}{n_i}$$

is the arithmetic mean of the covariates among those at risk at time t_i. Klein and Moeschberger (2003) also consider the Lin and Yin model and present an example.

Aalen (1989) developed a more general additive model. He discusses issues of estimation, testing and assessment of model fit in two applied papers (Aalen 1989,1993). His model is fully additive and nonparametric and values of the regression coefficients are allowed to vary over time. We present his model in more detail than the other additive models as it provides the opportunity to fit an additive model results whose fit can be used to provide graphical descriptions that supplement fits of other models, such as the proportional hazards model.

The Aalen model, for $p+1$ fixed covariates, $\mathbf{x}' = (1, x_1, x_2, \ldots x_p)$, has hazard function at time t equal to

$$h(t, \mathbf{x}, \boldsymbol{\beta}(t)) = \beta_0(t) + \beta_1(t)x_1 + \beta_2(t)x_2 + \cdots + \beta_p(t)x_p. \qquad (9.30)$$

The coefficients in this model provide the change at time t, from the baseline hazard rate, $\beta_0(t)$, corresponding to a one-unit change in the respective covariate. Unlike any other model considered in this text, the Aalen model allows the effect of the covariate to change continuously over time. The cumulative hazard function obtained from the hazard function in (9.30) is

$$H(t, \mathbf{x}, \mathbf{B}(t)) = \int_0^t h(u, \mathbf{x}, \boldsymbol{\beta}(u)) \, du ,$$

so

$$\begin{aligned} H(t, \mathbf{x}, \mathbf{B}(t)) &= \sum_{k=0}^{p} x_k \int_0^t \beta_k(u) \, du \\ &= \sum_{k=0}^{p} x_k \mathbf{B}_k(t) , \end{aligned} \qquad (9.31)$$

where $x_0 = 1$ and $B_k(t)$ is called the *cumulative regression coefficient* for the kth covariate. It follows from (9.31) that the baseline cumulative hazard function is $B_0(t)$. Klein and Moeschberger (2003) consider the Aalen model and illustrate its use in settings in which the model contains only a few discrete covariates. Zahl and Tretli (1997) illustrate the use of the Aalen model with an analysis of data on survival of breast cancer patients in Norway, and Borgan and Langholz (1997) extend the model for use in nested case-control studies. McKeague and Sasieni (1994) consider a model that combines the time-varying coefficients of the Aalen model in (9.30) with the time-fixed coefficients in the model as illustrated in (9.28).

Aalen (1989) notes that the cumulative regression coefficients are easier to estimate than the regression coefficients themselves and present an easily computed estimator. Aalen (1993) discusses methods for estimation of the individual regression coefficients, but these involve smoothing techniques beyond the mathematical scope of this text.

We concentrate on the estimates of the cumulative regression coefficients and how they can be used to provide insight on the effect covariates have over time. Assume that we have n independent observations of time (with no tied survival times), p fixed covariates and a right-censoring indicator variable, independent of time, denoted by the usual triplet $(t_i, \mathbf{x}_i, c_i)$. Aalen's estimator of the cumulative regression coefficients is a least-squares-like estimator and is most easily presented using matrices and vectors. We let $\mathbf{X}_j$ denote an n by $p+1$ matrix, where the ith row contains the data for the ith subject, $\mathbf{x}_i'$, if the ith subject is in the risk set at time t_j, otherwise the ith row is all 0's. We let $\mathbf{y}_j$ denote a 1 by n vector, where the jth element is 1 if the jth subject's observed time, t_j, is a survival time (i.e., $c_j = 1$); otherwise all the values in the vector are 0. The estimator of the cumulative regression coefficient at time t is

$$\hat{\mathbf{B}}(t) = \sum_{t_j \leq t} \left(\mathbf{X}_j' \mathbf{X}_j\right)^{-1} \mathbf{X}_j' \mathbf{y}_j . \qquad (9.32)$$

We note that the value of the estimator changes only at observed survival times and is constant between observed survival times. Huffer and McKeague (1991) discuss weighted versions of the estimator in (9.32), but they are much more complicated to implement. The increment in the estimator is computed only when the matrix $\left(\mathbf{X}_j' \mathbf{X}_j\right)$ can be inverted. The matrix is singular, and therefore cannot be inverted, when there are fewer than $p+1$ subjects in the risk set. Other data configurations can also yield a singular matrix. For example, if the model contains a single dichotomous covariate and all subjects who remain at risk have the same value for the covariate, the matrix will be singular. Aalen's estimator of the covariance matrix of the estimator of the cumulative regression coefficients at time t is the following $(p+1)\times(p+1)$ matrix:

$$\hat{\text{Var}}\left[\hat{\mathbf{B}}(t)\right] = \sum_{t_j \leq t}\left(\mathbf{X}_j'\mathbf{X}_j\right)^{-1}\mathbf{X}_j'\mathbf{I}_j\mathbf{X}_j\left(\mathbf{X}_j'\mathbf{X}_j\right)^{-1}, \tag{9.33}$$

where $\mathbf{I}_j$ is an n by n diagonal matrix with $\mathbf{y}_j$ on the main diagonal. It follows from (9.31) and (9.32) that the estimator of the cumulative hazard function for the ith subject at time t is

$$\hat{H}\left(t,\mathbf{x}_i,\hat{\mathbf{B}}(t)\right) = \sum_{k=0}^{p}x_{ik}\hat{\mathbf{B}}_k(t) \tag{9.34}$$

and an estimator of the covariate-adjusted survivorship function is

$$\hat{S}\left(t,\mathbf{x}_i,\hat{\mathbf{B}}(t)\right) = \exp\left[-\hat{H}\left(t,\mathbf{x}_i,\hat{\mathbf{B}}(t)\right)\right]. \tag{9.35}$$

We note, as does Aalen (1989), that it is possible for an estimate of the cumulative hazard in (9.34) to be negative and to yield a value for (9.35) greater than 1.0. This is most likely to occur for small values of time, and one way to avoid this problem is to use zero as the lower bound for the estimator in (9.34). One benefit of fitting the Aalen additive model is to provide graphical evidence of the effect of a covariate over time, rather than to provide an additive covariate-adjusted survivorship function.

The graphical presentation most often used with the Aalen model is a plot of $\hat{\mathbf{B}}_k(t)$ versus t, along with the upper and lower endpoints of a pointwise confidence interval. For a 95 percent interval, one would plot

$$\hat{\mathbf{B}}_k(t) \pm 1.96\,\hat{\text{SE}}\left[\hat{\mathbf{B}}_k(t)\right],$$

where $\hat{\text{SE}}\left[\hat{\mathbf{B}}_k(t)\right]$ is the estimator of the standard error of $\hat{\mathbf{B}}_k(t)$, obtained as the square root of the kth diagonal element of the variance estimator in (9.33).

At present, there are three sources for software to fit the Aalen model. Hosmer and Royston (2002) have written a program for STATA, which we used to fit the models in the example in this Section. This program, stlh, can be obtained from the Stata Journal web site[3]. Aalen and Fekjær provide macros for use with

---

[3] The Stata Journal web site link for this program is http://www.stata-journal.com/software/sj2-4 and follow the link to the St0024 entry.

S-PLUS and R on a web site.[4] Klein and Moeschberger (2003) provide macros for use with SAS at the web site for their book.

Aalen (1989) presents a method for testing the hypotheses that the coefficients in the model are equal to zero. While tests can be made for the overall significance of the model, Hosmer and Royston (2002) choose to implement tests for the significance of individual coefficients. The individual statistics are formed from the components of the vector

$$\hat{\mathbf{U}} = \sum_{t_j} \mathbf{K}_j \hat{\mathbf{b}}(t_j). \tag{9.36}$$

The summation in (9.36) is over all non-censored times when the matrix $\left(\mathbf{X}_j'\mathbf{X}_j\right)$ is non-singular, and $\mathbf{K}_j$ is a $(p+1)\times(p+1)$ diagonal matrix of weights. Aalen (1989) suggests two choices for weights. One choice mimics the weights used by the Wilcoxon tests and is the number in the risk set at t_j, $\mathbf{K}_j = \text{diag}(m_j)$. His other choice is based on the observation that the estimator in (9.32) has the same form as the least squares estimator from linear regression. He suggests using weights equal to the square root of the inverse of a least-squares-like variance estimator, namely the inverse of the square root of the diagonal elements of $\left(\mathbf{X}_j'\mathbf{X}_j\right)^{-1}$. Lee and Weissfeld (1998) studied the performance of the Aalen's test with these two weights as well as several others. Based on simulation, results they recommend using weights based on the Kaplan-Meier estimator, $\hat{S}_{KM}(t)$, at the previous survival time, $\mathbf{K}_j = \text{diag}\left[\hat{S}_{KM}(t_{j-1})\right]$, with the convention that $\mathbf{K}_1 = \text{diag}\left[\hat{S}_{KM}(t_0) = 1\right]$ and weights equal to the product of the Kaplan-Meier weights and the Aalen's inverse standard error weights. Lee and Weissfeld (1998) found that these two weight functions were the best at detecting late and early differences, respectively. One obvious choice for weights, not previously considered, is to mimic the weights for the log-rank test and use $\mathbf{K}_j = \text{diag}(1)$. Based on experience with the log-rank and Wilcoxon tests, we expect that the tests with weights equal to 1 should also be sensitive to later effects, while the test with weights equal to the size of the risk set should be sensitive to early effects.

The Hosmer and Royston STATA command uses the inverses of the respective diagonal elements of the standard error estimator,

$$\mathbf{K}_j = \text{diag}\left\{\hat{SE}\left[\hat{\mathbf{b}}(t_j)\right]^{-1}\right\} \tag{9.37}$$

---

[4] The web site for the S-PLUS macros is http://www.med.uio.no/imb/stat/addreg/.

instead of the diagonal elements of $\left(\mathbf{X}_j'\mathbf{X}_j\right)^{-1}$.

The variance estimator of $\mathbf{U}$ in (9.36) is obtained from the variance estimator in (9.33) and is

$$
\begin{aligned}
\hat{\text{Var}}\left(\hat{\mathbf{U}}\right) &= \sum_{t_j}\mathbf{K}_j\left(\mathbf{X}_j'\mathbf{X}_j\right)^{-1}\left(\mathbf{X}_j'\mathbf{I}_j\mathbf{X}_j\right)\left(\mathbf{X}_j'\mathbf{X}_j\right)^{-1}\mathbf{K}_j \\
&= \sum_{t_j}\mathbf{K}_j\hat{\text{Var}}\left[\hat{\mathbf{b}}\left(t_j\right)\right]\mathbf{K}_j .
\end{aligned}
\tag{9.38}
$$

Bhattacharyya and Klein (2005) studied the performance of the tests when the model contains a single categorical covariate. They note the value of the test statistic obtained when using weights $\mathbf{K}_j = \text{diag}\left\{\left(\mathbf{X}_j'\mathbf{X}_j\right)^{-1}\right\}$ depends on which group is used as the reference group. They recommend using the same weights for each pairwise comparison. These include weights equal to 1.0, the size of the risk set and the Kaplan-Meier estimator. They illustrated the test with other weights as well. They conclude with the observation that choice of an optimal weight is difficult as it depends on the alternative of interest. Hence, we feel that, in the absence of a specific alternative, it is a good practice to use several different weight functions, just as we suggested in Chapter 2 for tests of the equality of survival functions; each is likely to detect a departure in a different region of the time scale.

Tests for significance of individual coefficients use the individual elements of the vector $\mathbf{U}$ and are scaled by the estimator of their standard error obtained as the square root of the appropriate element from the diagonal of the matrix in (9.38). Aalen remarks that this ratio has approximately the standard normal distribution when the hypothesis of no effect is true and the sample is sufficiently large.

To illustrate the use of the Aalen additive model, we fit this model to the GBSC data containing hormone use, grade 3 tumor (1 = Yes, 0 = No), tumor size transformed using fractional polynomials to be linear in the log hazard for the proportional hazards model and centered at its median of 25 mm and age centered at its median of 53 years. We refer you to Sauerbrei and Royston (1999) for a detailed analysis of these data using the proportional hazards model. Hosmer and Royston (2002) present a similar analysis using the data from the UMARU Impact Study described in Section 1.3.

In theory, one can estimate the cumulative regression coefficient as long as the matrix $\left(\mathbf{X}_j'\mathbf{X}_j\right)$ remains non-singular. However, even if it is non-singular, the estimate becomes unstable for the longer event times as the risk sets can become quite small. As such, it is common practice to restrict the plot of the estimated cumulative regression coefficient to less than the full range of event time. In the plots in Figure 9.4, the range is restricted to 55 months, which is about the 75th percentile of recurrence time.

Plots of the estimated cumulative regression coefficients, with 95 percent confidence bands are shown in Figure 9.4a to Figure 9.4e. The significance levels for the test of the hypothesis of no additive effect, $H_0 : \beta_k(t) = 0$ using four different weights are given in Table 9.6.

Before we discuss the five plots in Figure 9.4, we describe what the plots of the cumulative regression coefficients are expected to look like under different types of covariate effects. If a regression coefficient in (9.30) is constant over time, it follows from (9.31) that the plot of the estimated cumulative regression coefficient should look like a straight line through the origin, with slope equal to the value of the coefficient. That is, if the coefficient for x_k is $\beta_k(t) = \beta_k$ in (9.30), then $B_k(t) = t\beta_k$ in (9.31).

Deviation from a straight line in any time interval in the plot provides empirical evidence for a time-varying effect in the covariate. One form of time-varying effect is for a covariate to have a constant effect in an initial interval of time and then to have no effect at later intervals. In this situation, it follows from (9.31) that the graph of the estimated cumulative regression coefficient would be linear in the initial interval of time and would remain constant over the remaining observed time interval. For example, suppose the "true" coefficient for covariate x_k in (9.30) is 0.02 in the interval from 0 to 30 months and is zero for time greater than 30 months. We expect the graph of the estimated cumulative regression coefficient to look like the straight line $B_k(t) = 0.02t$ in the interval $[0, 30]$. Because the coefficient is equal to zero after 30 months, there is no change in the cumulative regression coefficient and we expect the graph to look constant with value $B_k(t) = 0.6$ for $t > 30$.

Another form of time-varying effect is for a covariate to have a constant effect in an initial interval of time and then to have the effect weaken over time. In this case, we expect the graph of the estimated cumulative regression coefficient to be linear in the initial interval, when the effect is constant. The shape of the plot over the remainder of the follow-up time depends on how the effect changes. For example, if the effect remains constant, but with a smaller value than in the initial interval, then the plot will still be linear but with an attenuated slope. In the previous example, if the coefficient is 0.01 for $t > 30$, we expect the plot to look like the line $B_k(t) = 0.6 + 0.01t$ for $t > 30$. On the other hand, if the coefficient is -0.02 for $t > 30$, then we expect the plot to look like $B_k(t) = 0.6 - 0.02t$ for $t > 30$.

If a covariate has no effect and its coefficient in (9.30) is equal to zero over the entire observed time interval, we expect the plot to cross back and forth over the zero line, a line with both slope and intercept equal to 0, with its pointwise confidence limits falling on either side of the zero line. After discussing the plots in Figure 9.4, we discuss the results of the tests of the hypothesis that a coefficient is equal to zero for the observed range of time over which the model can be fit.

In general, the shape of a plot provides evidence of the values of the individual regression coefficients in (9.30). It is incorrect to assume that the observed shape implies that the same type of parametric relationship with time holds in other models, such as the proportional hazards model, although the form of the plot can provide guidance on how to model a covariate (see Mau, 1986). Henderson and Milner (1991) discuss this point and suggest including in the plot an estimate of what the cumulative regression coefficient is expected to look like if the proportional hazards model is correct. As yet, this embellishment has not been added to available software fitting the Aalen model.

Figures 9.4a-e present plots of the estimated cumulative regression coefficients (solid line), the pointwise 95 percent confidence bands (short dash lines), and a reference (long dash) line at 0.0.

The plot of the estimated cumulative regression coefficient for hormone use in Figure 9.4a descends in a nearly linear fashion, supporting a constant effect over time that decreases the rate of cancer recurrence over the period of follow up.

The plot of the estimated cumulative regression coefficient for Grade 3 tumor in Figure 9.4b increases linearly for approximately the first 18 months of follow up and then remains roughly constant. This pattern is indicative of a constant increase in the rate of recurrence for the first 18 months and no effect due to grade 3 tumor after 18 months.

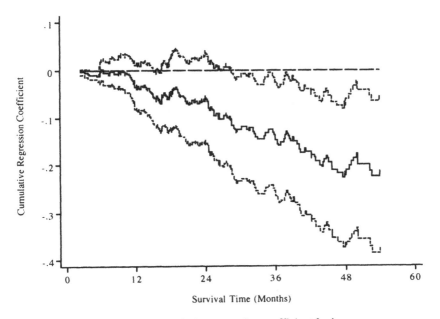

Figure 9.4a Estimated cumulative regression coefficient for hormone use

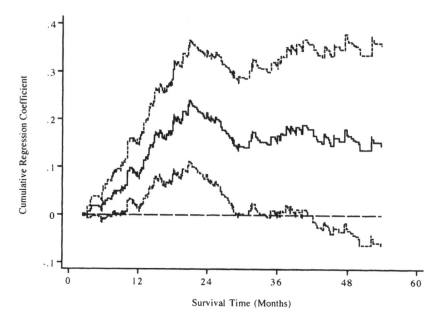

Figure 9.4b Estimated cumulative regression coefficient for grade 3 tumor

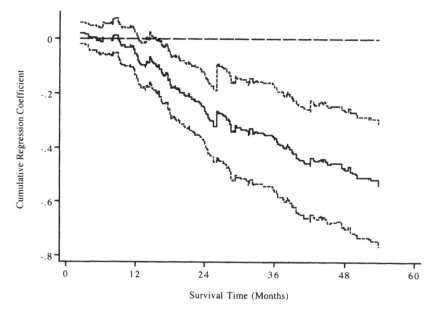

Figure 9.4c Estimated cumulative regression coefficient for $\left(10/size\right)$, centered at .4 mm^{-1}

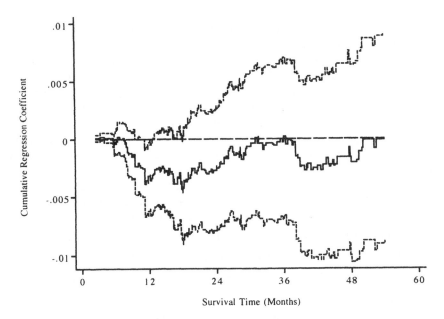

Figure 9.4d Estimated cumulative regression coefficient for age, centered at 53 years

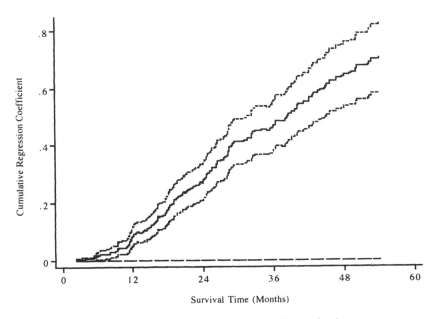

Figure 9.4e Estimated cumulative regression coefficient for the constant

The plot of the estimated cumulative regression coefficient for the inverse of tumor size in Figure 9.4c descends in a linear fashion, supporting a constant effect over time that increases the rate of cancer recurrence as tumor size increases.

The plot of the estimated cumulative regression coefficient for age in Figure 9.4d is negative and oscillates. The confidence bands contain zero through out the entire plotted range. This pattern is indicative of no overall effect due to age.

The plot of the estimated cumulative regression coefficient for the constant term Figure 9.4e ascends in a nearly linear fashion. This supports a constant increase in the rate of recurrence over the period of follow up for the baseline subject who, in this case, would be a 53 year old woman who is not using hormones and has a 25mm tumor that is not grade 3.

The significance levels of the tests for no additive effect based on each of the four weight functions are shown in Table 9.6. Based on our observations in Chapter 2 for tests of equality of survival functions and the simulations in Lee and Weissfeld (1998) we expect that the tests with weight equal to one or $\hat{S}_{KM}\left(t_{j-1}\right)$ should be more sensitive to later differences in effect, and the tests that use weights equal to the size of the risk set or $\hat{S}_{KM}\left(t_{j-1}\right)/\hat{SE}\left(\hat{b}\left(t_{j}\right)\right)$ should be more sensitive to early differences in effect.

The tests consistently reject the null hypothesis of no effect for the constant term and fail to reject the hypothesis for an age effect. These conclusions are in agreement with the results in Figures 9.4e and 9.4d.

The two tests sensitive to early differences are significant and the two tests for later differences are not significant for the effect of having a grade 3 tumor. These results are completely consistent with the plot in Figure 9.4b. The significance levels for the tests for the effect of the inverse of tumor size follow this same pattern. In this case, the results are a little puzzling because the plot in Figure 9.4c seems to indicate that the effect should be constant over time, significant both early and late.

The results for the test of the effect of hormone use are most similar to those for tumor size, indicating a significant early effect, but not so for a later effect. However, unlike tumor size, with p-values of 0.15 and 0.06, there is some indication of a possible effect at later follow up times.

In summary, the significance tests for additive effect of the four model covariates generally, though not completely, agree with their expected sensitivity to effect in regions of follow up time.

The next step in the analysis, which we leave as an exercise, is to expand the model to include a time varying covariate for the effect of a grade 3 tumor before and after 18 months.

We conclude the section with plots of the covariate adjusted (no grade 3 tumor, size 25 mm and age = 53) survival functions for the two values of hormone use, from (9.35), as follows:

Table 9.6 *p*-values for the Test of No Additive Effect, Using four Different Weights

Hypothetical Optimal Time Interval to Detect Effect	Early		Late	
Weight Function	$n(t_j)$	$\dfrac{\hat{S}_{KM}(t_{j-1})}{\widehat{SE}(\hat{b}(t_j))}$	1	$\hat{S}_{KM}(t_{j-1})$
Covariate				
Hormone Use	0.007	<0.001	0.150	0.063
Grade 3 Tumor	0.044	<0.001	0.608	0.789
Tumor Size$^\prime$	<0.001	<0.001	0.166	0.108
Age*	0.813	0.171	0.149	0.161
Constant	<0.001	<0.001	<0.001	<0.001

$\#\left(10/size\right)-0.4$

$*\ Age-53$

$$\hat{S}_A\left(t, hormone=0, grade\_3=0, size=25, age=53\right)=e^{-\hat{B}_0(t)}$$

and

$$\hat{S}_A\left(t, hormone=1, grade\_3=0, size=25, age=53\right)=e^{-\hat{B}_0(t)-\hat{B}_1(t)}.$$

For comparison purposes, we fit the proportional hazards model containing the same four covariates and computed the equivalent covariate-adjusted survival functions. All four estimated survival functions are plotted in Figure 9.5. We note that the range of the plot has been restricted to the interval $[0.5, 1.0]$.

In looking at the plots of the four estimated covariate-adjusted survival functions, two points are worth noting: First, the estimated survival curves from the Aalen linear hazards model and proportional hazards model are nearly identical. This does not imply that they will be similar in other data. However, in settings such as this where they are similar, plots like those in Figure 9.4 can provide useful diagnostic information on time-varying covariate effects that can be used to refine the fitted proportional hazards model, for example for grade 3 tumor. See Hosmer and Royston (2002) for another example of using the Aalen linear hazards models to provide guidance on time varying effects in a proportional hazards model. The second point to note is the graphical evidence of improved survival experience (i.e., longer time to recurrence) among the women using hormones.

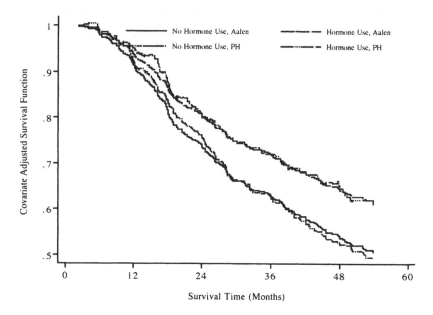

Figure 9.5 Plot of the estimated covariate adjusted survival functions from the Aalen linear hazards model and the proportional hazards model.

In general, the additive models discussed in this section should be used with some caution. While there are times when it may be clinically more meaningful to express survival experience and covariate effects in terms of an additive increase or decrease in the hazard rate, one must be sure that, if there are any iterative calculations, the program converges. In all cases, the fitted model must yield clinically plausible estimates of effect.

In the following sections, we present brief introductions to three topics: competing risks, sample-size determination, and estimation in the presence of missing values by multiple imputation. Until quite recently, each of these topics required special and not generally available statistical software. However, the situation has changed and now most users have access to the relevant methods via one or more of the major software packages.

9.6 COMPETING RISK MODELS

Competing risks or, more generally, multiple modes of failure, refers to a setting where follow up may terminate due to more than one event. For example, suppose we follow a cohort of men aged 70 years or older for five years and record the cause of death as being due to: a cardiovascular event (CVD), cancer, or other cause. The follow up time is right censored if a subject is lost to follow up or is alive at the end of the study. If no cause of death/event is of greater clinical interest than the others, then multiple modes of failure is likely the correct terminology. If one cause of death/event, for example CVD, is of primary clinical interest and the other causes/events are "competing" with the primary event, then competing risks may best describe the setting. As we show, the methods are the same, so terminology is primarily a matter of personal preference. In this section, we use the term competing risks as, in most health science applications, there is usually one primary event, with which the others compete to end follow up.

Methods for analyzing time-to-event data in the presence of competing risks are discussed and illustrated with examples in Kalbfleisch and Prentice (2002), Marubini and Valsecchi (1995). Klein and Moeschberger (2003), Lawless (2003), and Lee and Wang (2003). Pintilie (2006) has written a monograph on the topic that contains worked examples and details on how to use R and SAS to perform the calculations. Coviello and Boggess (2004) describe a Stata program that we use to perform the cumulative incidence analyses in this section.

The statistical functions presented in Chapter 2 describing the hazard, cumulative hazard and the survival function of a single event must be generalized to handle more than one event. In doing so, we show that, in the presence of competing risks, the basic descriptive statistic of event occurrence is not the survival function. Instead, it is the cumulative incidence function for each event type. Suppose we denote by the pair (T, C) the follow up time and type of event ending follow up using the convention that there are $j = 1, 2, \ldots, k$ types of events and right censoring corresponds to $C = 0$. The cause-specific hazard functions, denoted $h_j(t)$, describe the rate of failure at time t for event type j, given that the follow up time is at least t. If we assume that the k event types are mutually exclusive and that follow up terminates from one and only one event, then the overall hazard function is

$$h(t) = \sum_{j=1}^{k} h_j(t) . \tag{9.39}$$

It follows from (9.39) that the overall, event free, survival function is

$$S(t) = e^{-H(t)} , \tag{9.40}$$

where $H(t) = \sum_{j=1}^{k} H_j(t)$ is the overall cumulative hazard with

$$H_j(t) = \int_0^t h_j(u)\,du$$

denoting the cause specific cumulative hazard. The event-specific distribution function (called the *subdistribution* or *cumulative incidence function* (CIF)) is

$$F_j(t) = \Pr(T \le t, C = j) = \int_0^t h_j(u)S(u)\,du, \qquad (9.41)$$

and the overall distribution function is

$$F(t) = \sum_{j=1}^{k} F_j(t), \qquad (9.42)$$

with $S(t) = 1 - F(t)$. It follows from (9.41) that the maximum value of the subdistribution is $F_j(\infty) = \Pr(C = j)$ [5], which denotes the proportion of subjects who experience event type j.

Suppose that we have a sample of n independent observations of follow up time and event type (t_i, c_i), $i = 1, 2, \ldots, n$ where $c_i = 0$ denotes a right censored observation. The CIF is the cumulative proportion of failures due to cause j at time t. It is estimated by summing the cause-specific failure rates conditional on being at risk of failure, where the cause-specific failure rates are

$$\Pr(t \le T \le t + \Delta t, C = j) = \Pr(t \le T \le t + \Delta t, C = j \mid T \ge t)\Pr(T \ge t)$$
$$= h_j(t)S(t).$$

The sample estimator is

$$\hat{F}_j(t) = \sum_{t_{(i)} \le t} \hat{h}_j\left(t_{(i)}\right)\hat{S}(t_{(i-1)}), \qquad (9.43)$$

where $t_{(i)}$ is the ith largest event time, and $\hat{S}(t_{(i-1)})$ is the value of the Kaplan-Meier estimator of overall survival at the previous event time. The Kaplan-Meier estimator is calculated in the manner described in Chapter 2. There, $c = 1$ denoted

---

[5] A distribution function has $F(\infty) = 1$, while a subdistribution function has $F(\infty) < 1$.

follow up terminating from an event; here $c \neq 0$ denotes follow up terminating from any event. The event specific hazard estimator is

$$\hat{h}_j\left(t_{(i)}\right) = \frac{d_{ij}}{n_i},$$

where n_i is the number in the risk set and d_{ij} denotes the number of failures of type j at time $t_{(i)}$. Note that the summation in (9.43) is overall failure times, but the value only increases at observed event times as $d_{ij} = 0$ for right censored follow up times. Estimators of the variance of the event-specific estimated cumulative incidence can be obtained by using the delta method (see Appendix 1) or by a counting-process approach. In most data sets, there will be little difference between the two. The delta method estimator is a fairly complicated expression that, at time t, is

$$\hat{\text{V}}\text{ar}\left[\hat{F}_j(t)\right] = \sum_{t_i \leq t}\left\{\left[\hat{F}_j(t) - \hat{F}_j(t_i)\right]^2 \frac{d_i}{n_i\left(n_i - d_i\right)}\right\}$$

$$+ \sum_{t_i \leq t}\left\{\left[\hat{S}(t_{i-1})\right]^2 \frac{\left(n_i - d_{ij}\right)d_{ij}}{n_i^3}\right\} \qquad (9.44)$$

$$-2\sum_{t_i \leq t}\left\{\left[\hat{F}_j(t) - \hat{F}_j(t_i)\right]\left[\hat{S}(t_{i-1})\right]\frac{d_{ij}}{n_i^2}\right\}.$$

We construct confidence intervals based on the log-log transformation of the estimated cumulative incidence. The reason for using this transformation is the same as for using it in Chapter 2 for the confidence interval of the estimator for the survival function. It provides superior coverage properties over a variety of sample sizes and censoring rates. Using the results in (2.5) and (2.6), the estimator of the variance of the log-log transformation of the estimator of the cumulative incidence is

$$\hat{\text{V}}\text{ar}\left\{\ln\left[-\ln\left(\hat{F}_j(t)\right)\right]\right\} = \frac{\hat{\text{V}}\text{ar}\left[\hat{F}_j(t)\right]}{\left\{\ln\left[\hat{F}_j(t)\right] \times \hat{F}_j(t)\right\}^2} \qquad (9.45)$$

and the endpoints of the $100 \times (1-\alpha)$ percent confidence interval are

$$\ln\left[-\ln\left(\hat{F}_j(t)\right)\right] \pm z_{1-\alpha/2}\hat{\text{S}}\text{E}\left\{\ln\left[-\ln\left(\hat{F}_j(t)\right)\right]\right\}, \qquad (9.46)$$

where $\widehat{SE}(\cdot)$ denotes the square root of the variance estimator in (9.45) and $z_{1-\alpha/2}$ denotes the upper $\alpha/2$ percent point of the standard normal distribution. If we denote the lower and upper limits from (9.46) as $\hat{c}_l$ and $\hat{c}_u$ then the endpoints of the confidence interval estimator of the cumulative incidence are of the same form as those in (2.8) and are

$$\exp\left[-\exp\left(\hat{c}_u\right)\right] \text{ and } \exp\left[-\exp\left(\hat{c}_l\right)\right]. \qquad (9.47)$$

In most settings, it is good practice to present a plot of the estimated event-specific cumulative incidence, with confidence intervals, for each event type.

We begin by illustrating the calculation of the estimated cumulative incidence in a small hypothetical data set.

The data in Table 9.7 represent the follow up times for 10 hypothetical subjects. The table lists the follow up time in days and the event type. The quantities needed for the intermediate calculations required to compute the estimated cumulative incidence for each event type are shown in the first eight columns of Table 9.8. The calculated increments in the event-specific cumulative incidence are provided in columns nine and ten. The estimated event-specific cumulative incidences are presented in the last two columns.

The data in Table 9.7 and calculations in Table 9.8 are provided to allow you to verify your understanding of how the event-specific estimated cumulative incidence function in (9.43) is evaluated, but this data set is too small to provide a useful example for further analyses.

For a larger data set, we created hypothetical data for a study of factors associated with death from cardiovascular disease or other cause. Follow up time is days after admission to a hospital. Data are available for 65 subjects and cause of death was recorded as Coronary Vascular Disease (CVD), Other Cause

Table 9.7 Data for 10 Hypothetical Subjects

Id	Time	Event Type
1	9	2
2	27	0
3	18	0
4	30	1
5	10	1
6	33	2
7	13	1
8	19	2
9	24	2
10	4	1

Table 9.8 Listing of the Ordered Event Times, Event Type, Kaplan-Meier Estimate of the Overall Survival Probability, Number in the Risk Set, Number of Type 1 and Type 2 Events, Estimated Cause-Specific Hazards, Event-Specific Increment in the Estimated Cumulative Incidence, and the Event-Specific Estimated Cumulative Incidence

Time	Event Type	$\hat{S}(t_i)$	n_i	d_{i1}	d_{i2}	$h_1(t_i)$	$h_2(t_i)$	Incr. Event Type 1*	Incr. Event Type 2#	Cum. Inc. Event Type 1	Cum. Inc. Event Type 2
0		1	10	0	0	0	0	0	0	0	0
4	1	0.9	10	1	0	0.1	0	0.1	0	0.1	0
9	2	0.8	9	0	1	0	0.111	0	0.1	0.1	0.1
10	1	0.7	8	1	0	0.125	0	0.1	0	0.2	0.1
13	1	0.6	7	1	0	0.143	0	0.1	0	0.3	0.1
18	0	0.6	6	0	0	0	0	0	0	0.3	0.1
19	2	0.48	5	0	1	0	0.2	0	0.12	0.3	0.22
24	2	0.36	4	0	1	0	0.25	0	0.12	0.3	0.34
27	0	0.36	3	0	0	0	0	0	0	0.3	0.34
30	1	0.18	2	1	0	0.5	0	0.18	0	0.48	0.34
33	2	0	1	0	1	0	1	0	0.18	0.48	0.52

$* \left(d_{i1}/n_i \right) \times \hat{S}\left(t_{i-1} \right)$, $\# \left(d_{i2}/n_i \right) \times \hat{S}\left(t_{i-1} \right)$.

(OC) or right censored. There are 32 deaths from CVD, 24 from OC and 9 right censored observations. Covariates measured at admission are age (years), body mass index (kg/m^2), and gender (0 = Male, 1 = Female). We refer to the data as the CVD Risk Study, and they are available online at the web sites given in Section 1.3.

We show (in Figure 9.6) a plot of the estimated event-specific cumulative incidence function with 95 percent pointwise confidence intervals.

The estimated cumulative incidence function for both event types increases rapidly in the first 30 days, at which point the rate of increase is markedly less for other causes of death than for CVD. After 60 days, the confidence intervals do not overlap. In general, the impression is that the rate of death is much higher for CVD than for other causes in these 65 subjects.

One can test the null hypothesis that $F_{CVD}(t) = F_{OC}(t)$ and two tests are given in Pintilie (2006). We feel it is simpler to perform the test through a fitted proportional hazards model.

It is possible to extend the parametric models discussed in Chapter 8, as well as others, to fit time-to-event data in the presence of competing risks, see Lawless (2002). In this section, we focus on methods for extending the proportional hazards model to the competing risk setting. The reader is referred to Kalbfleisch and Prentice (2002) and Lunn and McNeil (1995) for details on the formulation of the partial likelihood.

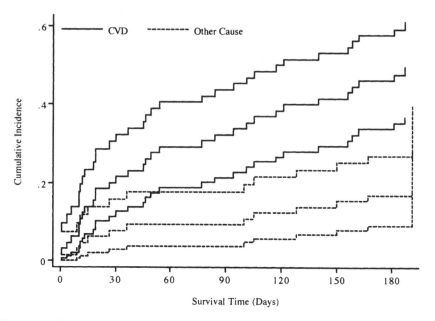

Figure 9.6 Estimated event-specific cumulative incidence functions for death from coronary vascular disease or other cause and pointwise 95 percent confidence intervals.

The most general proportional hazards model has cause-specific hazard function

$$h_{0j}(t)e^{x'\beta_j}. \tag{9.48}$$

This model allows for a cause-specific baseline hazard and cause-specific estimates of effect.

When considering regression models, it is helpful to classify the data by event type and observation within event type as $\left(t_{ji}, \mathbf{x}_{ji}, c_{ji}\right)$, $j = 1, 2, \ldots, k$ and $i = 1, 2, \ldots, n_j$. Note that, with this notation, subjects are split into event-type groups, $c_{ji} = j$, and the times are for failures of that specific type of event. The partial likelihood for this model is

$$L(\beta) = \prod_{j=1}^{k} \prod_{i=1}^{n_j} \frac{e^{x'_{ji}\beta_j}}{\sum_{l \in R(t_{ji})} e^{x'_{li}\beta_j}}, \tag{9.49}$$

where the risk set $R\left(t_{ji}\right)$ contains all subjects with follow up times greater than or equal to t_{ji} and $\boldsymbol{\beta'}=\left(\boldsymbol{\beta_1'},\boldsymbol{\beta_2'},\ldots,\boldsymbol{\beta_k'}\right)$. The partial likelihood in (9.49) can be maximized by separately maximizing

$$L\left(\boldsymbol{\beta}_j\right)=\prod_{i=1}^{n_j}\frac{e^{\mathbf{x}_{ji}'\boldsymbol{\beta}_j}}{\sum_{l\in R\left(t_{ji}\right)}e^{\mathbf{x}_{jl}'\boldsymbol{\beta}_j}}.$$

This implies that, if one is interested in fitting this model, then one may simply perform separate model fits for each event type, declaring all other event codes, other events, and censoring codes as censored observations. For example, in the CVD Risk Study, one would fit two proportional hazards models, one with event type = 1 and censoring indicated by $c\neq1$ and the other with event type = 2 and censoring indicated by $c\neq2$. In this case, one need not include the same covariates in each model. One may employ the model building methods discussed in Chapter 5 and model evaluation methods in Chapter 6. This approach presents no new challenges, so we do not consider it further. The reader is referred to Wang and Lee (2003) for an example.

A model with more structure is one where the cause-specific hazards are also proportional and is called the *proportional risks model*. Under this model the cause-specific hazard is

$$h_0\left(t\right)e^{\beta_{j0}+\mathbf{x}'\boldsymbol{\beta}_j},\tag{9.50}$$

where $\beta_{j0}, j=1,2,\ldots,k$ denote a set of design variables for the event types with the convention that $\beta_{10}=0$ (i.e., event type 1 is the reference event type).

This model provides an easy approach to testing, albeit with proportional hazards assumptions, the equality of event-specific cumulative-incidence functions. This is accomplished by fitting a model containing only the design variables for event type.

The partial likelihood for this model uses an expanded data set that contains k copies of each subject's data, with the data being entered into the model as zero for replicates corresponding to the events other than the observed value. A new failure variable is created and is equal to 1 for the replicate for the event and zero otherwise.

The data structure is most easily seen with an example. In Table 9.9, we present the expanded data for three subjects: subject 5 died at 121 months from CVD, subject 7 died at 100 months from other causes and subject 72 was censored at 186 months. The new event variable is denoted as "status" in the table and equals 1 on the first record if the subject died from CVD, event 1, is equal to 1 on the second record if the subject died due to other causes, event 2, and is always zero if the

Table 9.9 Example of the Expanded Data Needed to Fit the Proportional Risks Model with Two Competing Risks

Id	Time	Event Type	Status	Delta	Age	Age1	Age2
5	121	1	1	0	88	88	0
5	121	1	0	1	88	0	88
7	100	2	0	0	56	56	0
7	100	2	1	1	56	0	56
72	186	0	0	0	74	74	0
72	186	0	0	1	74	0	74

$age2 = \delta \times age$ and $age1 = (1 - \delta) \times age$.

subject's follow up time was censored. The indicator variable "delta" is used to model the cause-specific hazard as well as to create event specific covariate values denoted in the table as Age1 and Age2. One fits the proportional hazards model using "time" as the time to event, "status" as the event / censoring indicator and includes "delta" and both age covariates. The coefficient for delta is β_{20} in (9.50). The two age coefficients provide cause-specific estimates of age effects. The partial likelihood for the expanded set of data using sample size $N = n \times k$ is

$$L(\beta_j) = \prod_{i=1}^{N} \left[\frac{e^{\beta_{j0} + \mathbf{x}_i'\beta_{ji}}}{\sum_{j=1}^{k} \sum_{l \in R(t_i)} e^{\beta_{j0} + \mathbf{x}_l'\beta_j}} \right]^{d_i},$$

where β_{ji} is the appropriate event-specific set of coefficients, $\beta_{10} = 0$ and $d_i = 1$ if any event occurs at time t_i and is zero otherwise.

Table 9.10 Estimated Coefficients, Standard Errors, z-Scores, Two-Tailed p-values, and 95% Confidence Interval Estimates for the Proportional Risks Model for the CVD Risk Study ($n = 65$)

	Coef.	Std. Err.	z	$p>z$	95% CIE
delta	0.617	0.4776	1.29	0.196	−0.319, 1.553
age_1	0.067	0.0137	4.91	<0.001	0.040, 0.094
age_2	−0.028	0.0149	−1.86	0.063	−0.057, 0.002
bmi_1	0.105	0.0376	2.80	0.005	0.032, 0.179
bmi_2	−0.148	0.0577	−2.56	0.011	−0.261, −0.035
gender_1	0.428	0.4018	1.06	0.287	−0.360, 1.215
gender_2	0.181	0.5613	0.32	0.748	−0.919, 1.281

The results of fitting the proportional risks model to the CVD Risk data containing the covariates age, centered at 70 years, body mass index, centered at 25 kg/m², and gender are shown in Table 9.10. In the table, the coefficients for covariates that end with "_1" provide estimates of effect for death from CVD and those that end with "_2" provide estimates of effect for death from other causes. The estimate for "delta" provides the shift in the log baseline hazard for other causes of death relative to CVD. Here the baseline subject is a 70-year old male with a bmi of 25 kg/m².

The estimate for delta is not significant, which suggests that the cause-specific baseline hazard functions are within sampling variation of each other[6]. The estimates of the effect of age and body mass index are both significant and positive for the cause-specific hazard for CVD death. Thus, increasing age and body mass index significantly increase the rate of death from CVD in the presence of risk of death from other causes. Estimators for hazard ratios for clinically meaningful increments in these covariates may be computed using the method described for continuous covariates in Chapter 3. The estimates of effect for age and body mass index are negative for death from other causes, with the estimated coefficient for age being significant at the 10 percent but not the 5 percent level of significance. This implies that increasing age and body mass index decrease the rate of death from other causes in the presence of risk of death from CVD. Of note, these are hypothetical data, and results should not be interpreted as real effects. The estimates of effect for female gender are not significant for either cause of death. We note that a fit of the cause-specific hazard model in (9.48), left as an exercise, showed that the estimated coefficient for age was positive and marginally significant for CVD death, and the estimated coefficient for body mass index was negative and significant for other cause of death.

The proportional risks model is fit using standard statistical software for the proportional hazards model and, as a result, the full range of model building methods discussed in Chapter 5 are available, in particular, those for selecting variables, examining the scale of continuous covariates, and selecting interactions. Except for the Grønnesby-Borgan goodness-of-fit test, which has not been extended to the competing risk setting, the model assessment techniques discussed in Chapter 6 may also be employed. These are left as an exercise.

Following the fit of the proportional risks model, it is possible to compute covariate-adjusted estimated cumulative-incidence functions. One must obtain the estimated baseline survival function for the first event type, denoted $\hat{S}_1(t)$, from

---

[6] To test the equality of the two unadjusted cumulative incidence functions, one fits the model containing only delta. In results not shown, $\hat{\beta}_{30} = -0.288$, with Wald test p-value of 0.287. This is somewhat at odds with earlier observations about similarity of the plotted functions in Figure 9.6.

the fit. This is the usual estimated baseline survival function described in Chapter 3. It follows from (9.50) that the estimated baseline cumulative hazard for event type 1 is

$$\hat{H}_1(t) = -\ln\left[\hat{S}_1(t)\right]$$

and for event type j it is

$$\hat{H}_j(t) = \hat{H}_1(t) \times \exp\left(\hat{\beta}_{j0}\right).$$

The estimated baseline overall survival function is

$$\hat{S}_0(t) = \prod_{j=1}^{k} e^{-\hat{H}_{j0}(t)}.$$

The estimated baseline cumulative incidence functions are obtained from (9.43) as follows:

$$\hat{F}_{j0}(t) = \sum_{t_{(i)} \leq t} \hat{h}_{j0}\left(t_{(i)}\right) \hat{S}_0(t_{(i)-1}), \tag{9.51}$$

where the estimator of the baseline hazard function for event type j is

$$\hat{h}_{j0}\left(t_{(i)}\right) = \frac{d_{ji} e^{\hat{\beta}_{j0}}}{\displaystyle\sum_{l \in R(t_{(i)})} e^{x_l \hat{\beta}_j}}, \tag{9.52}$$

with the convention that $\hat{\beta}_{10} = 0$.

We plot the estimated baseline cumulative incidence functions obtained from the fitted model in Table 9.10 in Figure 9.7. The plot is restricted to the first 180 days of follow up as the estimators of the baseline event-specific hazard functions in (9.52) are unstable when the number of subjects in the risk set becomes small. The adjusted baseline estimate for other cause of death is larger than the adjusted baseline estimate for CVD death, as the coefficient for delta in Table 9.10 is positive. However, the difference is judged not to be significant as $p = 0.20$.

One may obtain estimators of the event-specific cumulative-incidence functions adjusted to a specific covariate, x_0, by using the following estimator of the covariate-specific hazard function in (9.51)

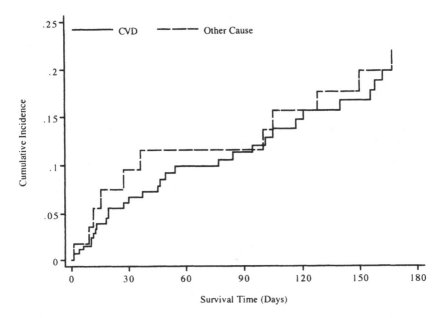

Figure 9.7 Estimated covariate-adjusted cumulative incidence for death from coronary vascular disease or other causes from the fitted model in Table 9.10.

$$\hat{h}_j\left(t_{(i)}, \mathbf{x}_0\right) = \frac{d_{ji} e^{\mathbf{x}_0'\hat{\boldsymbol{\beta}}_j}}{\displaystyle\sum_{l \in R\left(t_{(i)}\right)} e^{\mathbf{x}_l'\hat{\boldsymbol{\beta}}_j}}.$$

For example, the value of the vector of covariates for 70-year old males with a body mass index of 25 is $\mathbf{x}_0' = (\delta, 0, 0, 1)$ and $\delta = 0$ for CVD death and $\delta = 1$ for other causes of death.

In summary, recent contributions to statistical software make it relatively easy to fit proportional hazards models in the presence of competing risks. Model building follows the same general methods described in Chapter 5 and model assessment follows the methods described in Chapter 6. Estimated coefficients can be used to provide event-specific estimated hazard ratios in the same manner as illustrated in Chapter 6. The fitted model can also provide the basis for covariate-adjusted estimators of the event-specific cumulative incidence functions.

9.7 SAMPLE SIZE AND POWER

We assume that readers of this text have had some experience with or exposure to methods for selecting a sample size designed to test a specified statistical hypothesis with stated Type I and Type II errors in settings where the test is not based on a time-to-event analysis. For example, in the case of the two sample t-test, where $H_0 : \mu_1 = \mu_2$ (or in the case of a test of equality of two proportions, $H_0 : \pi_1 = \pi_2$) the method for sample size determination yields a total sample size, n, which most often is equally allocated to the two groups. In these settings, one assumes that it is possible to obtain the value of the particular outcome variable on each of the n subjects. That is, there are no partially observed values. For example, if we are measuring height of adult males, t we assume that the measuring device can accommodate the entire expected range of heights. This is not likely to be the case when the outcome variable is the time to an event. Much of this text has dealt with methods for handling data that contain censored, most often right censored, observations. We describe in Chapter 2 how the information in right-censored observations contributes to the analysis. While not stated explicitly, it should be clear to you that there can be no analysis unless there are uncensored observations and that the power of the statistical methods depends on the number of events, m, observed and not necessarily the total sample size n.

We show in this section that determining the sample size when the outcome is time-to-event is really a two-step process. We first determine the total number of events required and then we determine the total number of subjects who must be followed to obtain the requisite number of events. The methods for determining the number of events are quite similar to methods for selecting a total sample size in settings like the test for the equality of two proportions. This requires that we state the hypothesis in terms of statistical parameters in the model, their estimators and their variance, specify a clinically important change in the parameters, specify the two error probabilities, and then combine these quantities into a probabilistic statement that can be inverted to yield an expression for the sample size. For example, Fleiss, Levin ad Paik (2003) work through these details for the test of the equality of two proportions. There is considerably more guesswork in the second step. In a time-to-event study in human populations, there is likely to be an enrollment period and then an additional period of follow up. The lengths of these two periods are usually dictated by practical considerations such as the accrual rate of patients and the total length of the study. Other factors influence the study size: We know that not all subjects enrolled will experience the event, and a certain proportion of subjects will be lost to follow up by the end of the study. Hence, we have to inflate the number of subjects to accommodate the sources of incomplete information.

Sample size methods for testing the equality of the hazard for two groups that account for censoring are discussed and illustrated with examples in several texts (Collett, 2003; Chow, Shao and Wang, 2003; Parmar and Machin, 1995; and Therneau and Grambsch, 2000). Recently Barthel, Babiker, Royston and Parmar

(2006) developed an approach that extends the simple two-group method to settings with more than two groups, accounts for censoring, losses to follow up, non-proportional hazards and allows for treatment cross over. Barthel, Royston and Babiker (2005) provide a Stata program called ART[7] (Analysis of Resources for Trails) that implements the extended methods. Software to perform sample size calculations similar to those demonstrated here is available in a number of other packages. Barthel, Babiker, Royston and Parmar (2006) list the packages available at the time the paper was published and compare their capabilities. Recently, SAS, Version 9.1, has added a procedure to estimate power and sample size, but it has limited capabilities in the area of time-to-event analyses. We begin by describing the simple two-group approach to estimating the number of events first proposed by Schoenfeld (1983) and then use the approach ART to illustrate sample size estimation for a hypothetical study design.

The method proposed by Schoenfeld (1983) is based on the log-rank test which, as noted in Chapter 3, is equivalent to the score test in a univariable proportional hazards model. Schoenfeld shows [also see Collett (2003) Section 10.2.1 for the mathematical details], that the number of events needed in a two-group trial for a two-sided log rank test to detect a log hazard ratio of θ (i.e., $HR = \exp(\theta)$) at the α level of significance and power $1 - \beta$ is

$$m = \frac{\left(z_{\alpha/2} + z_\beta\right)^2}{\theta^2 \pi (1 - \pi)}, \tag{9.53}$$

where $z_{\alpha/2}$ and z_β are the corresponding percentage points from the standard normal distribution and π is the fraction of subjects allocated to the first group. Note that under equal allocation, $\pi = 0.5$, the result in (9.53) simplifies to

$$m = \frac{4\left(z_{\alpha/2} + z_\beta\right)^2}{\theta^2}.$$

As an example, suppose a two-group randomized trial is investigating a new treatment that study clinicians think could provide a 25 percent reduction in the rate of death (i.e., $HR = 0.75$). If the trial allocates subjects equally to the two treatments and uses $\alpha = 0.05$ and 80 percent power, $\beta = 0.2$, then the required number of events is

---

[7] The link for the web site is http://www.stata-journal.com/software/sj5-1/, use the st0013_1 entry to download the ART program.

$$379.5 = \frac{4(-1.96 - 0.842)^2}{\left[\ln(0.75)\right]^2},$$

which one would round up to 380. This is the required sample size only in a setting where we begin at time zero with 380 subjects randomized to the two groups and then follow these subjects until each has experienced the event of interest, death. This is never the case. In particular, the rate of failure of most clinical conditions or diseases is rarely high enough that all subjects fail within a reasonable time span for a clinical study. Some observations are certain to be right-censored. To take censoring into account, we need to adjust m by dividing it by an estimate of the overall probability of death by the end of the study. If the condition or disease has been studied in the past, you may have an estimate of its survival function, $\hat{S}_0(t)$, for example, the Kaplan-Meier estimate from an earlier study. This estimate can be used to approximate the survival function under the new treatment and a proportional hazards model as

$$\hat{S}_1(t) = \left[\hat{S}_0(t)\right]^{\exp(\theta)}.$$

Schoenfeld shows [also see Collett (2003) Section 10.3.1] that, under a model where subjects are recruited uniformly in the first a "years" and then are followed for an additional f "years", an estimate of the probability of death at the end of the study, $a + f$ "years", is

$$\bar{F}(a+f) = 1 - \frac{1}{6}\left[\bar{S}(f) + 4\bar{S}(0.5a + f) + \bar{S}(a + f)\right],$$

where

$$\bar{S}(t) = \pi \times \hat{S}_0(t) + (1 - \pi) \times \hat{S}_1(t),$$

and π is the proportion of subjects allocated to the standard (0) treatment. The estimated number of subjects that must be followed is

$$\begin{aligned} n &= \frac{m}{\bar{F}(a+f)} \\ &= \frac{\left(z_{\alpha/2} + z_\beta\right)^2}{\bar{F}(a+f)\theta^2 \pi(1-\pi)}. \end{aligned} \tag{9.54}$$

Suppose our hypothetical study plans to enroll subjects for $a = 2$ years and then follow them for an additional $f = 3$ years. Furthermore, suppose that we are able to determine from our own previous research or the literature that,

$$\hat{S}_0(3) = 0.7, \ \hat{S}_0(4) = 0.65 \text{ and } \hat{S}_0(5) = 0.55.$$

It follows that

$$\hat{S}_1(3) = 0.765 = [0.7]^{0.75},$$

$$\hat{S}_1(4) = 0.724 = [0.65]^{0.75},$$

and

$$\hat{S}_1(5) = 0.639 = [0.55]^{0.75}.$$

If we allocate subjects equally, the average survival probabilities at these three time points are

$$\bar{S}(3) = 0.733, \ \bar{S}(4) = 0.687 \text{ and } \bar{S}(5) = 0.595,$$

and the average probability of death at the end of the study is estimated to be

$$\bar{F}(5) = 0.321 = 1 - \frac{1}{6}[0.733 + 4 \times 0.687 + 0.595].$$

This implies that the total number of subjects that must be enrolled is

$$n = 1,183.8 = \frac{380}{0.321}$$

or, rounded to a number divisible by two, $n = 1,184$. With this total number of subjects, the study would need to enroll, on average, 49-50 subjects per month for the two-year enrollment period. We note that, when we use these values of $\hat{S}_0(t)$, HR $= 0.75$ and use the extended method in the ART program, we obtain $m = 383$ and $n = 1,174$. The small difference is caused by the fact that the ART program uses a piecewise exponential distribution and a more exact estimate of the probability of death by the end of the study that involves calculating the number of subjects in the risk set at each time point, indicating the beginning of specified periods of accrual and follow up.

One additional problem not accounted for in (9.54) is the effect that lost-to-follow up has on the number of subjects in the risk sets. Suppose we assume that the hazard for lost-to-follow up is approximately constant and equal to $0.0513 = -\ln(0.95)$ (i.e., 5 percent are lost in the first year). Using the ART program in Stata, we find that this increases the number of subjects needed to 1,227, rounded to 1,228 to be divisible by 2.

At the study design stage it is unusual to make only a single sample size calculation. Typically, we vary the factors that affect the sample size to get an idea of the sensitivity of the sample size to each. In a time-to-event analysis, there is the usual factor of effect size, but the baseline survival distribution, the length of the recruitment and follow up periods and the loss to follow up also have an effect on the sample size. To illustrate this, we repeated the sample size calculation at various levels of these factors and display the results in Table 9.11. We did not change the baseline survival function, $\hat{S}_0(t)$, from the values given above. If one had access to pilot data or data from prior studies, then logical alternatives would be the distributions corresponding to the upper and lower Greenwood confidence bands for the Kaplan-Meier estimator. Each would give rise to a table like Table 9.11. The calculations were performed using ART and assuming the total length of the study is five years.

Table 9.11 Total Sample Size and Required Number of Subjects to be Recruited per Month (n, r), Necessary to Detect the Stated Hazard Ratio Using a Two-Sided Log-Rank Test with a Significance Level of 5 Percent and 80 Percent Power for a Total Length of Study of 5 Years

Percent Lost (per year)	Length of Recruitment Period	Hazard Ratio		
		0.75	0.5	0.25
		Required Number of Events		
		0.75	0.5	0.25
5	1	1114, 92.8	278, 18.9	78, 6.5
	2	1228, 51.1	252, 10.5	88, 3.6
	3	1358, 37.7	280, 7.8	98, 2.7
	4	1552, 32.3	320, 6.7	112, 2.3
10	1	1176, 98.0	238, 19.8	82, 6.8
	2	1288, 53.6	262, 10.9	90, 3.8
	3	1418, 39.4	290, 8.1	100, 2.8
	4	1614, 33.6	332, 6.9	116, 2.4
15	1	1250, 104.1	252, 20.9	86, 7.1
	2	1358, 56.6	276, 11.5	94, 3.9
	3	1488, 41.3	302, 8.4	104, 2.9
	4	1688, 35.1	344, 7.2	119, 2.5

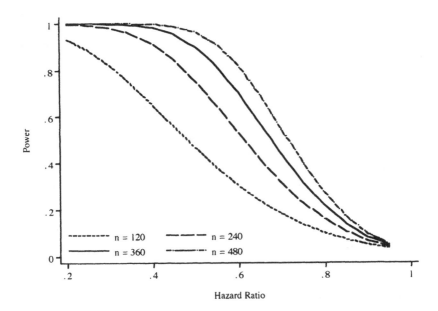

Figure 9.8 Estimated power of a two-sided 5 percent level of significance log-rank test to detect the hazard ratio using the stated sample size.

The results in Table 9.11 show that the number of events depends only on the magnitude of the hazard ratio. The sample size depends most heavily on the hazard ratio and the length of the recruitment period. It is relatively less sensitive to the percentage of lost-to-follow up. If the results in Table 9.11 were part of an actual study design exercise, the next step would be to make a realistic assessment of subject accrual and examine in more detail the power various sample sizes would have to detect a range of possible hazard ratios.

Suppose that the study team decides that they can only recruit subjects for one year, with four additional years follow up and they think that enrolling 20 subjects per month is quite realistic. Furthermore, they feel that loss to follow up is likely to be about 10 percent per year. To explore the effect of sample size on power, we calculated it, not only for 20 subjects per month, but also for 10, 30, and 40 per month for hazard ratios ranging from 0.2 to 0.95. The calculated values of the power obtained from ART are plotted in Figure 9.8. The power exceeds 80 percent for a sample size of 240 (20/month) for hazard ratios less than approximately 0.5. If 30 subjects per month are possible, the study can detect hazard ratios less than 0.65 with 80 percent power or higher. These calculations can be repeated, varying any of the design factors, and would add to the overall understanding of factors affecting the study design. With this information, the study team could make an informed decision on the best overall design for their particular study.

The calculations of sample size and power presented in this section have used equal allocation of subjects to groups. This is most often the case in a randomized trial. In a purely observational study, one has little or no control over the distribution of subjects in groups. The methods illustrated, for example (9.53), are easily modified to accommodate other allocation ratios/proportions to study the same issues of sample size and power for key study covariates.

In summary, methods for determining sample size in a survival analysis are similar to other statistical models in that they require the usual model and testing specifications, but are different in that you are required to specify a period for accrual of subjects, a period of follow up and the underlying survival experience in a control group.

9.8 MISSING DATA

Until now, all data sets we have used have had no missing data. This is the case in virtually all texts where the primary focus is on development and application of statistical methods for the analysis of data. One of the primary reasons is that, until relatively recently, none of the major software packages had easy-to-use routines to implement statistical methods for replacing missing data. The situation has changed and both SAS and Stata have routines that can be used with missing data in survival analysis. Other more specialized software is also available (see Horton and Lipsitz, 2001). The goal of this Section is to briefly introduce the reader to the basic issues and assumptions and illustrate them with an application to a modified version of the WHAS100 data.

A great deal of work has been done on missing data and, in particular, multiple imputation (Little and Rubin, 2002, and Schafer, 1997). For an introductory level presentation see Allison (2001), Schafer (1999) or Schafer and Graham (2002). Harle and Zhou (2007) provide an extensive list of references on the topic and an overview of the methods and available software. They do not, however, mention the user-supplied program for Stata that we use in this Section. Our primary focus is on the approach described in Van Buuren, Boshuizen and Knook (1999) as implemented in Stata by Royston (2004, 2005a, 2005b)[8].

The basis of all the methods for replacing missing data is their use of the information in the observed values of the covariates to predict the missing values. One of the main differences between the methods is how they use the known values. Key to this are the assumptions about the missing data. The strongest of these is called *Missing Completely At Random* (MCAR) (Rubin, 1976). Under

---

[8] We refer the reader to a helpful tutorial on using the Stata routine ice at
http://www.ats.ucla.edu/stat/stata/library/ice.htm.

MCAR one assumes that the probability that a value is missing does not depend on the outcome or on any of the covariates that are measured. Its estimator is

$$\Pr(M = 1) = \frac{n_{mis}}{n},$$

where M denotes the variable recording if an observation is missing, n_{mis} denotes the number of missing values out of n for a particular covariate. Under most settings this is not likely to be a realistic assumption. As an alternative, under *Missing At Random* (MAR), one assumes that the probability that a value is missing depends on the observed values of the covariates through a model for

$$\Pr(M = 1 \mid \mathbf{X}_{obs}, \boldsymbol{\theta}),$$

where $\mathbf{X}_{obs}$ denotes the observed values of the covariates and $\boldsymbol{\theta}$ is a vector of parameters for the model. Under MAR, it is assumed that the probability of being missing does not depend on the unobserved values of measured covariates. These are the assumptions that software packages use when implementing multiple imputation. One practical point to remember is that the imputation process can be improved by including as many covariates as possible (i.e., ones with missing data as well as others with no missing data). Missing values are said to be *Not Missing At Random* (NMAR) if the probability that a value is missing depends on both the observed and unmeasured missing values, i.e.,

$$\Pr(M = 1 \mid \mathbf{X}_{mis}, \mathbf{X}_{obs}, \boldsymbol{\theta}).$$

Under NMAR, additional external information about the distribution of $\mathbf{X}_{mis}$ is required for imputation.

To implement multiple imputation, one must specify the three models: a model that predicts the missing values from observed covariate values, the model for missing values (MAR usually), and the statistical model for complete data. These models are used to impute all missing values for each covariate, resulting in a "complete" set of data. This process is repeated m times, and the results of the m analyses are combined. SAS and Stata use different methods for the imputation. SAS uses a method called *Markov Chain Monte Carlo* (MCMC) that models the full multivariate distribution of the missing values, which is usually assumed to be multivariate normal. The Stata routine performs imputation by a series of univariable regression models for the conditional, not the joint distribution, of the missing values. This approach is able to handle continuous and discrete covariates by using different regression models (e.g., the linear regression model for continuous covariates and the logistic regression model for dichotomous covariates). We discuss this point further in the example. The disadvantage is that the conditional univariate distributions used may be incompatible with the joint distribution.

Once the imputed complete data sets are created and analyzed, the results are combined using rules proposed by Rubin (1987). Denote the estimator of a particular regression coefficient from the fit to the m multiple imputation data sets as $\hat{\beta}^i, i = 1, 2, \ldots, m$ and the estimator of its variance as $\hat{V}^i, i = 1, 2, \ldots, m$. The combined multiple imputation estimator of the regression coefficient is

$$\bar{\beta} = \frac{1}{m} \sum_{i=1}^{m} \hat{\beta}^i \qquad (9.55)$$

and the estimator of the variance of $\bar{\beta}$ is

$$\bar{T} = \bar{V} + \left(1 + \frac{1}{m}\right) B, \qquad (9.56)$$

where

$$\bar{V} = \frac{1}{m} \sum_{i=1}^{m} V^i$$

and

$$B = \frac{1}{m-1} \sum_{i=1}^{m} \left(\hat{\beta}^i - \bar{\beta}\right)^2.$$

Inferences are based on a t-distribution with degrees of freedom

$$v = (m-1) \times \left[1 + \frac{\bar{V}}{\left(1 + \frac{1}{m}\right) B}\right]^2.$$

Both SAS and Stata have routines to perform the calculations in (9.55) and (9.56). The results are displayed in the tabular convention of the particular model (i.e., the proportional hazards model in our case).

To illustrate the methods, we modified the WHAS100 data by randomly deleting approximately 20 percent of the values for age, gender, and body mass index. The replacement of observed with missing values was done separately for each covariate. This resulted in a data set with only 58 complete cases. We list, in Table 9.12, the hypothetical newly observed data for three subjects with missing values, denoted by "•". We used both the chained regression equation approach from Stata and the MCMC method in SAS's MI procedure to do five imputations of the missing data; these values are also listed. As suggested by Van Buuren, Boshuizen and Knook (1999) we included both the log of the follow up time and the follow up status as predictor covariates for the regression models. We note that, for the continuous covariates, age, and body mass index, the imputed values from the two packages are not the same. However, the correlations over all 500 values (100 subjects and 5 imputations) are high, with correlations of 0.92 for age and 0.82 for body mass index. Because SAS assumes that gender is continuous, its imputed values lie between user-specified minimum and maximum values of zero and one. Stata, on the other hand correctly imputes the value as zero or one

Table 9.12 Listing of Three Subjects with Missing Data (Obs) and the Five Imputations from Stata and SAS.

Package		Id	Age	Gender	Body Mass Index
	Obs	5	•	•	30.7
	1	5	48	0	30.7
	2	5	74	0	30.7
Stata	3	5	65	1	30.7
	4	5	73	1	30.7
	5	5	61	1	30.7
	1	5	72.1	0.50	30.7
	2	5	63.8	0.90	30.7
SAS	3	5	66.7	0.07	30.7
	4	5	59.9	0.26	30.7
	5	5	53.4	0.54	30.7
	Obs	14	58	0	•
	1	14	58	0	32.1
	2	14	58	0	34.8
Stata	3	14	58	0	28.0
	4	14	58	0	32.6
	5	14	58	0	31.6
	1	14	58	0	33.4
	2	14	58	0	30.8
SAS	3	14	58	0	32.3
	4	14	58	0	24.5
	5	14	58	0	32.2
	Obs	33	81	•	•
	1	33	81	1	36.7
	2	33	81	1	28.0
Stata	3	33	81	1	26.5
	4	33	81	1	24.8
	5	33	81	0	35.7
	1	33	81	0.22	30.6
	2	33	81	0.55	24.9
SAS	3	33	81	0.24	20.8
	4	33	81	0.27	22.1
	5	33	81	0.37	22.8

from its fitted logistic model. SAS also has the capability to use a logistic model, but only when the pattern of missing values in the covariates is monotone. A pattern would be monotone in Table 9.12 for the following pattern of missing values: if age is missing, then gender and body mass index are also missing, and if gender is missing, then body mass index is also missing. This does not hold in the example data, no matter in what order the three covariates are listed.

We fit the proportional hazards model to the imputed data sets produced by SAS and Stata in Stata and the results are given in the bottom two panels of Table 9.13. The results from the fit of the model to the WHAS100 data are shown in the top panel, and the results from the fit to the complete cases in the modified data set are shown in the second panel.

The results from the fit of the model to the complete cases illustrate the loss of efficiency and increased standard errors, when compared with the complete case analysis and analyses based on the imputed data. In particular, age is no longer significant and body mass index is marginally significant. The estimated standard errors from the fit of the model to the imputed data sets are much closer to those from the complete data analysis. The estimated coefficients from the fit to Stata's imputed data are closer to the estimates from the complete data than to those obtained from the fit to SAS's imputed data. The results for age and body mass index are reasonably close. However, the results are substantially different for the coefficient gender. We suspect that this may be caused by the fact that SAS imputed gender as if it was continuous. In any analysis of multiple imputation data, the results may depend on the number of imputations. We repeated the analyses in Table 9.13 using 10, 20, and 50 imputations. The results were similar to those

Table 9.13 Results of Fitting the Proportional Hazards Model to the Complete Data ($n = 100$), the Complete Cases in the Modified Data ($n = 58$), and the Imputed Data from Stata and SAS

		Coeff.	Std. Err.	z	p	95% CIE
Complete Data $n = 100$	age	0.037	0.0127	2.92	0.004	0.012, 0.062
	gender	0.145	0.3060	0.47	0.637	−0.455, 0.744
	bmi	−0.071	0.0361	−1.96	0.05	−0.141, 0.000
Complete Case Analysis $n = 58$	age	0.019	0.0169	1.11	0.266	−0.014, 0.052
	gender	−0.108	0.3870	−0.28	0.779	−0.867, 0.650
	bmi	−0.091	0.0505	−1.81	0.071	−0.190, 0.008
Stata MI Data, $n = 100$	age	0.034	0.0142	2.41	0.016	0.006, 0.062
	gender	0.149	0.3275	0.46	0.649	−0.493, 0.791
	bmi	−0.063	0.0450	−1.40	0.163	−0.151, 0.025
SAS MI Data, $n = 100$	age	0.029	0.0151	1.94	0.052	0.000, 0.059
	gender	0.324	0.3299	0.98	0.326	−0.323, 0.970
	bmi	−0.046	0.0362	−1.28	0.201	−0.117, 0.025

reported in the table using five imputations. This is not surprising, because Rubin (1987) showed that, unless the rates of missing information are unusually high, not much precision is gained beyond five to ten imputations.

Both SAS and Stata provided useful multiple imputation data sets in this example. In this analysis, multiple imputation completed 42 percent of the data, near the upper bound of 50 percent suggested by Royston (2004). For the multiple imputations, we assumed a specific model that includes the covariates age, gender, and BMI. Aspects of model building can become complex when using multiple imputations. Conceptually, values could be imputed before or after the model-building process. On the one hand, when imputing values before the model-building process, biased estimates can arise if certain features of the model are not incorporated into the imputation process because they might only be known after model-building is complete (e.g., interactions or non-linear functional forms for continuous covariates). On the other hand, when imputing values after the model-building process, the model-building process is restricted to observations with complete data. This can also result in biased estimates. There is no simple solution to this problem, and we recommend that you do not attempt model-building and multiple imputations without a thorough understanding of both techniques.

In summary, application of methods for multiple imputation of missing data in the covariates can provide more efficient and consistent estimates of model parameters and is likely worth doing when there is a moderate, but not an extreme, amount of missing data in the covariates. However, one must pay close attention to the assumptions about randomness of missing values, the proportion of values that are imputed, and the issues involved in combining model building and multiple imputations.

EXERCISES

1. Consider the following hypothetical study of two treatment modalities to reduce the occurrence of muscle soreness among middle-aged men beginning weight training. Study participants were 400 middle-aged men who joined a health club for the specific purpose of weight training. Subjects were randomized into one of two instructional programs designed to prevent muscle soreness. The control treatment consisted of the standard written brochures and instructions used by the health club to explain proper technique, including suggestions for frequency and duration of training. The new method included one hour with a personal trainer as well as the brochures. Subjects were followed and the dates on which muscle soreness limited the prescribed workout were recorded. The dates were converted into the number of days between soreness episodes.

   The data may be found on the statistical data set web site at the University of Massachusetts/Amherst and the John Wiley web site discussed in Section 1.3. The data are in a file called RECUR.DAT. The variables are: ID (1–400), AGE (years), TREAT (0 = NEW, 1 = CONTROL), TIME0 (day of the previous episode), TIME1 (day of new episode), CENSOR (1 = muscle soreness episode occurred at TIME1, 0 = subject left the study or the study ended at TIME1) and EVENT (1–4 muscle soreness episodes). The maximum number of episodes observed was four.

Every study subject had one episode, 386 had two, 324 had three, and 186 had four. Thus, the data file has 1296 records and is in the form shown for the counting process recurrent-event model shown in Table 9.1. The data for this hypothetical study were generated to have sufficient power to detect particular differences in the models. A careful analysis will uncover these differences.

(a) Fit the AG counting process recurrent event model to these data obtaining both the information matrix-based estimates and the robust estimates of the standard errors of the estimated coefficients for AGE and TREAT.

(b) Repeat problem 1(a) fitting the PWP-CP recurrent event model. Does the effect of the covariates depend on the episode number?

(c) Repeat problem 1(a) fitting the PWP-GT recurrent event model. Does the effect of the covariates depend on the episode number?

(d) Repeat problem 1(a) fitting the TT-R recurrent event model. Does the effect of the covariates depend on the episode number?

(e) Prepare a table of estimated hazard ratios, with 95 percent confidence intervals, comparing the new method to the control method, corresponding to a 10-year change in age, for each of the four models fit. Compare and contrast the point and interval estimates under the four models. Compare and contrast the interpretation of the four sets of point and interval estimates.

2. None of the data sets used in the text have correlated observations; for this problem, we suggest repeating the type of analysis done with the GBCS Study data in Section 9.3 by creating groups of size 2 and 5 after sorting on age.

(a) Fit the shared frailty models containing hormone use, tumor size and progesterone receptors using the newly created group variable based on age to define subjects with a shared frailty. Is there evidence of significant heterogeneity?

(b) Fit the stratified proportional hazards models. Compare the estimates of the coefficients from the two different model fits, the shared frailty models in 2(a), and the stratified model.

(c) Refit the model with group size 2, centering size at 25mm and progesterone receptors at 30, and save the estimated frailties and baseline survival function following the fit of the model. Plot the estimated covariate adjusted survival functions at the two levels of hormone use at baseline ($z = 1$) and using the 10th and 90th percentiles of the estimated frailties. The resulting plot should be similar to Figure 9.1.

3. To provide a data set for applying methods to analyze a nested case-control study, we created a small data set from the main WHAS data (this is not the subset of the WHAS data described in Section 1.3). Before performing the

case control sampling, we broke ties in survival times by subtracting a uniform (0,1) random variable from each value of LENFOL corresponding to a death, and censored values were not changed. The modified version of LENFOL is denoted as T. The sampling procedure selected five controls for each case. These data are in the file WHASNCC.DAT found on the web sites containing the data sets from this text. The variables are SET, CASE, T, LENFOL, FSTAT, AGE, SEX, BMI, CHF and MIORD, and NR. The variable describing the set of one case and five controls is SET where CASE = 1 for the indexed death time and NR is the number of subjects in the risk set in the original cohort.

(a) Use the methods for the analysis of nested case control studies to fit the proportional hazards model to these data.

(b) Following the fit of the model in problem 4(a), prepare a table of estimated hazard ratios with corresponding 95 percent confidence intervals.

(c) Graph the estimated covariate-adjusted survivorship functions, comparing the survival experience of those with and without heart complications (i.e., CHF = 0 vs. CHF = 1).

4. Fit the Aalen model to the WHAS100 data using a model containing AGE, SEX, and BMI.

(a) Do the plots from the estimated cumulative regression coefficients from a fit of the Aalen additive model suggest possible time-varying effects in AGE and BMI? If the plots indicate that the effects may change over time, then fit the proportional hazards model containing the time-varying covariates.

(b) Compute and then plot the covariate adjusted survival functions from the fit in 4(a) for 72 -year old males and females with a body mass index of 25.

5. A data set similar to the one used in Section 9.6 is COMPRISK and is available on the two web sites. The variables are ID, AGE, GENDER, BODY MASS INDEX, TIME and EVENT TYPE.

(a) Compute and plot the estimated cumulative incidence function for each event type, with its 95 percent confidence bands.

(b) Fit the marginal competing risk model for each event type containing the three covariates.

(c) Repeat problem 5(b) using the proportional risk model.

(d) Compare the coefficient estimates from the model in 5(a) and 5(b).

(e) Compute and plot the covariate-adjusted (70-year old females with a body mass index of 30 kg/m^2) cumulative incidence functions for the two event types.

6. Suppose you consulted on the design of a randomized trial being proposed to determine whether a new treatment reduces the rate of death by 35 percent over the existing treatment. Due to circumstances out of your control, the study can be no longer than 24 months. Assume, to a close approximation, that the sur-

vival function for the existing treatment is well approximated by the exponential function $S_0(t) = \exp(-0.03 \times t)$.

(a) If the clinicians can recruit subjects for 6 months and then follow them for an additional 18 months, how many events are needed and what total sample size for the two-sided log-rank test to have 90 percent power with a 5 percent level of significance?

(b) Provide a power curve for the sample size in 6(a) and one-half of that in 6(a).

APPENDIX 1

The Delta Method

Deriving an expression for an estimator of the variance of the estimator is one problem faced by statisticians when developing an estimator of a parameter. Both estimators are needed for confidence interval estimation and/or hypothesis testing.

Statisticians use a procedure commonly called the delta method to obtain an estimator of the variance when the estimator is not a simple sum of observations. The basic idea is to use a method from calculus called a *Taylor series expansion* to derive a linear function that approximates the more complicated function. We refer the reader to any introductory calculus text for a discussion of the Taylor series expansion.

To apply the delta method, the function must be one that can be approximated by a Taylor series and, in general, this means that it is a "smooth" function, with no "corners." Consider such a function of a random variable X denoted as $f(X)$. To apply the delta method, we use the first two terms of a Taylor series expansion about the mean of the variable to approximate the value of the function as

$$f(X) \cong f(\mu) + (X - \mu) f'(\mu), \tag{A.1}$$

where

$$f'(\mu) = \frac{\partial f(X)}{\partial X}\Big|_{X=\mu}$$

is the derivative of the function with respect to X evaluated at the mean of X. It follows from (A.1) that the variance of the function is approximately

$$\begin{aligned} \mathrm{Var}\big[f(X)\big] &\cong \mathrm{Var}(X - \mu) \times \big[f'(\mu)\big]^2 \\ &\cong \sigma^2 \times \big[f'(\mu)\big]^2, \end{aligned} \tag{A.2}$$

where σ^2 is the variance of X. The delta method estimator of the variance of the function is obtained when we use the estimators of μ and σ^2 in (A.2) as follows

$$\hat{\mathrm{Var}}\big[f(x)\big] \cong \hat{\sigma}^2 \times \big[f'(\hat{\mu})\big]^2. \tag{A.3}$$

As an example, consider the function $\ln(X)$. The expansion from (A.1) is

$$\ln(X) \cong \ln(\mu) + (X - \mu)\frac{1}{\mu}. \tag{A.4}$$

The delta method estimator of the variance from (A.3) is

$$\hat{\mathrm{Var}}\big[\ln(X)\big] \cong \hat{\sigma}^2 \frac{1}{\hat{\mu}^2},$$

where $\hat{\sigma}^2$ and $\hat{\mu}$ denote estimators of σ^2 and μ.

As a second example, we provide the details for the development of the delta method estimator of the variance of the log of the Kaplan–Meier estimator of the survival function shown in (2.3) and that of the Kaplan–Meier estimator itself in (2.5). The estimator as shown in (2.1) is

$$\hat{S}(t) = \prod_{t_{(i)} \leq t} \frac{n_i - d_i}{n_i},$$

and its log is

$$\ln\big[\hat{S}(t)\big] = \sum_{t_{(i)} \leq t} \ln\left(\frac{n_i - d_i}{n_i}\right)$$
$$= \sum_{t_{(i)} \leq t} \ln(\hat{p}_i),$$

where $\hat{p}_i = (n_i - d_i)/n_i$. The first key assumption in the development of the variance estimator is that the observations of survival among the n_i subjects at risk are independent Bernoulli trials with constant probability, p_i. Under this assumption, the estimator of the constant probability is $\hat{p}_i$ with variance estimator $\hat{p}_i(1 - \hat{p}_i)/n_i$. The Taylor series expansion for the log function in (A.4) yields

$$\ln(\hat{p}_i) \cong \ln(p_i) + (\hat{p}_i - p_i)\frac{1}{\hat{p}_i},$$

and from (A.3) the delta method variance estimator is

$$\widehat{\text{Var}}\left[\ln(\hat{p}_i)\right] \cong \frac{1}{\hat{p}_i^2}\frac{\hat{p}_i(1-\hat{p}_i)}{n_i}$$

$$\cong \frac{d_i}{n_i(n_i-d_i)}\,.$$

The second key assumption is that observations in different risk sets are independent. Thus the delta method estimator of the variance of the log of the Kaplan–Meier estimator, as shown in (2.3) is

$$\widehat{\text{Var}}\left\{\ln\left[\hat{S}(t)\right]\right\} \cong \sum_{t_{(i)}\leq t}\widehat{\text{Var}}\left[\ln(\hat{p}_i)\right]$$

$$\cong \sum_{t_{(i)}\leq t}\frac{d_i}{n_i(n_i-d_i)}\,.$$

The estimator of the variance of the Kaplan–Meier estimator comes from a second application of the delta method. In this application the function is

$$f(X) = \exp(X),$$

e.g., $\hat{S}(t) = \exp\left\{\ln\left[\hat{S}(t)\right]\right\}$. It follows from (A.1) that the series expansion is

$$\exp(X) \cong \exp(\mu) + (X-\mu)\exp(\mu)$$

and, from (A.2) the approximate variance is

$$\widehat{\text{Var}}\left[\exp(X)\right] \cong \sigma^2\left[\exp(\mu)\right]^2. \tag{A.5}$$

Application of the approximation in (A.5) yields the Greenwood estimator in (2.5), namely

$$\widehat{\text{Var}}\left[\hat{S}(t)\right] \cong \left[\hat{S}(t)\right]^2 \sum_{t_{(i)}\leq t}\frac{d_i}{n_i(n_i-d_i)}\,.$$

The confidence interval estimator for the Kaplan–Meier estimator discussed in Chapter 2 is based on the log-log survival function, that is, $\ln\left\{-\ln\left[\hat{S}(t)\right]\right\}$. The variance estimator of this function requires a second application of the expansion of the log function. In this case, $X = \ln\left[\hat{S}(t)\right]$ and application of the approximation to the variance of the log of a random variable yields the estimator shown in (2.6),

$$\hat{\text{Var}}\left\{ \ln\left[-\ln\left(\hat{S}(t) \right) \right] \right\} \cong \frac{1}{\left[\ln\left(\hat{S}(t) \right) \right]^2} \sum_{t_{(i)} \le t} \frac{d_i}{n_i \left(n_i - d_i \right)}$$

The results presented in this appendix provide a brief introduction to the use of the delta method within the specific context of deriving an estimator of the variance of the Kaplan–Meier estimator, or functions of it. The technique is quite general and has been used in a variety of settings [see Agresti (1990) for applications in general categorical data models].

APPENDIX 2

An Introduction to the Counting Process Approach to Survival Analysis

We refer to the counting process approach to the analysis of survival time throughout the text. This method has been the source of many new developments in the field since it was first used by Aalen [(1975) and (1978)]. Two texts document the mathematical details of this powerful method in a thorough manner. Fleming and Harrington (1991) and Andersen, Borgan, Gill and Keiding (1993). Fleming and Harrington (1991) focus primarily on the analysis of survival time while Andersen et al. (1993) consider analysis of survival time as well as other, more general statistical problems. We encourage readers of this text to see Andersen et al. (1993, Chapter 1) for an excellent overview of the types of statistical problems that can be formulated as counting processes. Fleming and Harrington (1991, Chapter 0) and Andersen et al. (1993, Section II.1) provide nontechnical mathematical introductions to the approach. This appendix introduces a few of the key ideas and constructs used in the counting process approach to the analysis of survival time. For this reason, many of the more technical mathematical assumptions and details will not be discussed.

Suppose we follow a single subject from time of enrollment, $t = 0$, in a study of a particular cancer until the subject dies from this cancer. Furthermore, we assume it is a 5-year study and that this subject is enrolled on the first day of the study. Thus the maximum length of follow-up for this subject is 60 months. We denote the survival time random variable as X. A common approach to modeling the possibility of right censoring is to assume that there is a second random variable, independent of X, which records the time until observation terminates from anything other than the event of interest, for example, death from another cause or loss to follow-up for reasons unrelated to any study factor. We denote this random variable as Z. The actual observed time random variable is $T = \min(X, Z)$ and the available data for a subject consists of T and an indicator variable C whose value is

1 if $T = X$ and 0 if $T = Z$. Thus the variable T records follow-up time and C is the censoring indicator variable.

Three functions of time central to the counting process approach are: the counting process

$$N(t) = I(T \leq t, C = 1),$$

the at-risk process

$$Y(t) = I(T \geq t),$$

and the intensity process

$$\lambda(t)dt = Y(t)h(t)dt,$$

where

$$h(t)dt = \Pr(t \leq T < t + dt, C = 1 | T \geq t)$$

is the hazard function for survival time. The function $I(\cdot)$ is the indicator function whose value is 1 if the argument is true and 0 otherwise.

The counting process records, in our example, whether death from cancer occurs at time t. The function "counts" this by jumping from a value of 0 to a value of 1. Suppose our hypothetical subject died from cancer after being in the study 32 months, $(T = 32, C = 1)$. The counting process function for this subject is equal to zero until 32 months. At exactly 32 months, the function jumps to a value of 1. The function is equal to 1 for the remaining 28 months of follow-up time. If the subject's follow-up time is right censored, $C = 0$, then a death is not counted and the counting process is equal to 0 for all values of t. If our hypothetical subject was removed from the study at 32 months for reasons unrelated to the cancer, $(T = 32, C = 0)$, then the counting process for this subject is equal to zero over the 60 months of follow-up.

The at-risk process indicates whether the subject is still being followed, at risk for death, at time t. This function jumps from a value of 1 to a value of 0 when follow-up ends because of death or censoring. For a hypothetical subject with follow-up time of 32 months, the at-risk process is equal to 1 from the beginning of follow-up until 32 months. The function jumps/drops to a value of zero just after 32 months because the subject is no longer at risk for the remaining 28 months of the study.

The intensity process may be viewed as an "expected number of deaths" at time t. This follows from the fact that the function is of the form "$n \times p$" (i.e., the expected number of events in a binomial distribution). The at-risk process corresponds to "n" and the hazard function to "p".

The process of following the hypothetical subject from time zero to time t may be thought of as an accumulation of many conditional independent steps, much like the argument used to construct the Kaplan–Meier estimator in Chapter 2. The total expected number of deaths up to time t is obtained from the intensity process in the same manner as the cumulative hazard is obtained from the hazard function, namely by integrating the intensity process over time to obtain

$$\Lambda(t) = \int_0^t \lambda(u) \, du$$
$$= \int_0^t Y(u)h(u) \, du,$$

and this function is called the cumulative intensity process.

Thus one may think of the counting process as the total number of observed events and the cumulative intensity process as the total number of expected events up to time t. The difference between these two quantities is a residual-like quantity called the *counting process martingale*,

$$M(t) = N(t) - \Lambda(t).$$

This function is the basis for the martingale residuals that play a central role in model evaluation methods in Chapter 6. Another way to express the relationship between the counting, intensity, and martingale processes is via a linear-like model

$$N(t) = \Lambda(t) + M(t).$$

When expressed in this way, we see that the counting process, the observed part of the model, is the sum of a systematic component, the cumulative intensity process and a residual, the martingale process. In our hypothetical example, death or censoring can occur only one time and at the actual follow-up time, T, the value of the martingale is

$$M(T) = \begin{cases} 1 - \Lambda(T) & \text{if } C = 1 \\ 0 - \Lambda(T) & \text{if } C = 0 \end{cases}.$$

It is well beyond the scope of this appendix to explain what makes a process a martingale and what gives $M(t)$ this quality. We refer the interested reader to the texts cited above for these technical details. It suffices for the purposes of this appendix and text to think of $M(t)$ as being similar to a residual.

Now suppose we have observations of follow-up time and censoring indicator variable on n subjects in our hypothetical cancer study. We assume that observations of time are independent and identically distributed. We denote the actual observed times and right censoring indicator variables in the usual way as (t_i, c_i), $i = 1, 2, \ldots, n$. In this setting, a basic result from counting process theory is that the estimator of the cumulative intensity process for the ith subject at time t is

$$\hat{\Lambda}_i(t) = Y_i(t)\hat{H}(t),$$

where

$$Y_i(t) = I(t_i \geq t)$$

$$\hat{H}(t) = \sum_{t_j \leq t} \frac{c_j}{n_j}$$

is the Nelson–Aalen estimator of the cumulative hazard at t and

$$n_j = \sum_{i=1}^{n} Y_i(t_j)$$

is the number at risk at time t_j. The estimator of the martingale residual for the ith subject at his/her follow-up time is

$$\begin{aligned}\hat{M}(t_i) &= c_i - \hat{\Lambda}(t_i) \\ &= c_i - Y_i(t_i)\hat{H}(t_i) \\ &= c_i - \hat{H}(t_i)\end{aligned}$$

because $Y_i(t_i) = I(t_i \geq t_i) = 1$. We denote this martingale residual as $\hat{M}_i$. We note that, like residuals from most regression models, $\Sigma \hat{M}_i = 0$.

Assume that we have, in addition to follow-up time and censoring indicator variables, observations on p fixed (not time-varying) covariates. Assume that we fit a proportional hazards regression model. The estimator of the cumulative intensity process for the ith subject at time t is

$$\hat{\Lambda}(t, \mathbf{x}_i, \hat{\boldsymbol{\beta}}) = -Y_i(t)e^{\mathbf{x}\hat{\boldsymbol{\beta}}}\ln\left[\hat{S}_0(t)\right].$$

Thus the value of the martingale residual for the ith subject at his/her follow-up time is

$$\hat{M}_i = c_i - e^{x_i'\hat{\beta}} \ln\left[\hat{S}_0(t_i)\right].$$

The estimated martingale residuals are the basis for many of the diagnostic methods for assessing various aspects of the fitted model described in Chapters 5 and 6.

One, if not the, major theoretical benefit derived from formulating a survival analysis as a counting process is that a number of theorems from martingale theory may be used to prove many of the distributional results cited in this text. For example, this theory may be used to prove that the maximum partial likelihood estimators of the coefficients in a proportional hazards model are asymptotically normally distributed with a covariance matrix that may be estimated by the observed information matrix (Chapter 3). A second example involves the proof that the Kaplan–Meier estimator and functions of it are asymptotically normally distributed (Chapter 2). The list of applications of this theory in survival analysis is quite long. The central theme in all of the applications involves proving that a particular scaled and centered estimator, such as the Kaplan–Meier estimator, $\sqrt{n}\left[\hat{S}(t) - S(t)\right]$, is a martingale.

In summary, we feel that it is important for anyone using the regression methods for the analysis of survival time described in this text to have at least a superficial knowledge of the basics of the counting process paradigm.

APPENDIX 3

Percentiles for Computation of the Hall and Wellner Confidence Band

$1-\alpha$	$\hat{a} = n\hat{\sigma}^2(t_{(m)})/\left[1+n\hat{\sigma}^2(t_{(m)})\right]$							
	0.1	0.25	0.40	0.50	0.60	0.75	0.90	1.0
0.90	0.599	0.894	1.062	1.133	1.181	1.217	1.224	1.224
0.95	0.682	1.014	1.198	1.273	1.321	1.354	1.358	1.358
0.99	0.851	1.256	1.470	1.552	1.600	1.626	1.628	1.628

$$\hat{\sigma}^2(t_{(m)}) = \sum_{t_{(i)}} \frac{d_i}{n_i(n_i - d_i)}$$

REFERENCES

Aalen, O.O. (1975). *Statistical inference for a family of country processes*. Ph.D. Thesis, University of California, Berkeley.

Aalen, O.O. (1978). Non parametric inference for a family of counting processes. *Annals of Statistics*, **6**:701–726.

Aalen, O.O. (1989). A linear regression model for the analysis of life times. *Statistics in Medicine*, **8**:907–925.

Aalen, O.O. (1993). Further results on the non-parametric linear regression model in survival analysis. *Statistics in Medicine*, **12**:1509–1588.

Aalen, O.O. (1994). Effects of frailty in survival analysis. *Statistical Methods in Medical Research*, **3**:227–243.

Agresti, A. (1990). *Categorical Data Analysis*. John Wiley & Sons, Inc. New York.

Akaike, H. (1974). A new look at statistical model identification. *IEEE Transactions on Automatic Control*, **19**:716–723.

Alioum, A. and Commenges, D. (1996). A proportional hazards model for arbitrarily censored and truncated data. *Biometrics*, **52**:512–524.

Allison P. (1995) Survival Analysis Using the SAS System: A Practical Guide.SAS Institute Inc., Cary, North Carolina.

Allison, P.D. (2001). *Missing Data*, Sage Publications, Thousand Oaks, CA.

Altshuler, B. (1970). Theory for the measurement of competing risks in animal experiments. *Math Bioscience*, **6**:1–11.

Ambler, G. and Royston, P. (2001). Fractional polynomial model selection procedures: investigating type I error rate. *Journal of Statistical Simulation and Computation*, **69**:89-108.

Andersen, P.K. (1992). Repeated assessment of risk factors in survival analysis. *Statistical Methods in Medical Research*, **1**:297–315.

Andersen, P.K. and Gill, R.D. (1982) Cox's regression model for counting processes: A large sample study. *Annals of Statistics*, **10**:1100–1120.

Andersen, P.K., Borgan, Ø., Gill, R.D. and Keiding, N. (1993). *Statistical Models Based on Counting Processes*. Springer–Verlag, New York.

Andersen, P.K., Klein, J.P., Knudsen, K.M., and Tabanera y Palacios, R. (1997). Estimation of variance in Cox's regression model with shared gamma frailties. *Biometrics*, **53**:1475–1484.

Arjas, E. (1988). A graphical method for assessing goodness–of–fit in Cox's proportional hazards model. *Journal of American Statistical Association*, **83**:204–212.

Barlow, W.E. and Prentice, R.L. (1988). Residuals for relative risk regression. *Biometrics*, **75**:65–74.

Barthel, F. M.-S., Babiker, A., Royston, P. and Parmar, M.K.B. (2006) Evaluation of sample size and power for multi-arm survival trials allowing for non-uniform accrual, non-proportional hazards, loss to follow-up and cross-over. *Statistics in Medicine*, **25**:2521–2542.

Barthel, F. M.-S., Royston, P. and Babiker, A. (2005) A menu driven facility for complex sample size calculation in randomized controlled trials with a survival or binary outcome. *Stata Journal*, **5**:123–129.

Bendel, R.B. and Afifi, A.A. (1977). Comparison of stopping rules in forward regression. *Journal of American Statistical Association*, **72**:46–53.

Bhattacharyya, M. and Klein, J.P. (2005) A note on testing in Aalen's additive regression models. *Statistics in Medicine*, **24**:223–2240.

BMDP Statistical Software (1992). BMDP Classic 7.0 for DOS. SPSS, Inc. Chicago.

Borgan, Ø. and Langholz, B. (1993). Nonparametric estimation of relative mortality from nested case-control studies. *Biometrics*, **49**:593–602.

Borgan, Ø. and Langholz, B. (1997). Estimation of excess risk from case–control data using Aalen's linear regression model. *Biometrics*, **53**:690–697.

Borgan, Ø., Goldstein, L. and Langholz, B. (1995). Methods for the analysis of sampled cohort data in the Cox proportional hazards model. *Annals of Statistics*, **23**:1749–1778.

Borgan, Ø. and Leistøl. K. (1990). A note on confidence bands for the survival curve based on transformations. *Scandanavian Journal of Statistics*, **17**:35–41.

Breslow, N.E. (1970). A generalized Kruskal–Wallace test for comparing *K* samples subject to unequal patterns of censorship. *Biometrika*, **57**:579–594.

Breslow, N.E. (1974). Covariance analysis of censored survival data. *Biometrics*, **30**:89–100.

Breslow, N.E. and Day, N.E. (1980). *Statistical Methods in Cancer Research. Volume I: The Analysis of Case-Control Studies.* Oxford University Press, Oxford, U.K.

Breslow, N.E. and Day N.E. (1987). *Statistical Methods in Cancer Research. Volume II: The Design and Analysis of Cohort Studies.* Oxford University Press, Oxford, U.K.

Brookmeyer, R. and Crowley, J.J. (1982). A confidence interval for the median survival time. *Biometrics*, **38**:29–41.

Bryson, M.C. and Johnson, M.E. (1981). The incidence of monotone likelihood in the Cox model. *Technometrics*, **23**:381–384.

Cain, K.C. and Lange, N.T. (1984). Approximate case influence for the proportional hazards regression model with censored data. *Biometrics*, **40**:493–499.

Cain, L.E. and Cole, S. E. (2005). Letter to the Editor on Survival analysis for recurrent event data: an application to childhood diseases. *Statistics in Medicine*, **25**:1431-1433.

Carstensen, B. (1996). Regression models for interval censored data: application to HIV infection in Danish homosexual men. *Statistics in Medicine*, **15**:2177–2189.

Chappell, R. (1992). A note on linear rank tests and Gill and Schumacher's test of proportionality. *Biometrika*, **79**:199–201.

Chiriboga, D., Yarzebeski, J., Goldberg, R.J., Gore, J.M. and Alpert, J.S. (1994). Temporal trends (1975–1990) in the incidence and case-fatality rates of primary ventricular fibrillation complicating acute myocardial infarction: a community wide perspective. *Circulation*, **89**:998–1003.

Chow, S-C., Jun Shao, J. and Wang, H. (2003) *Sample Size Calculations in Clinical Research*, Taylor & Francis, Boca Raton.

Clayton, D. (1994). Some approaches to the analysis of recurrent event data. *Statistical Methods in Medical Research*, 3:244–262.

Clayton, D.G. and Hills, M. (1993). *Statistical Models in Epidemiology*, Oxford University Press, Oxford, U.K.

Clayton D.G. and Hills M. (1997). Analysis of follow-up studies with Stata 5.0. *Stata Technical Bulletin Number 40*. Stata Corporation, College Station, TX.

Cleveland, W.S. (1993). *Visualizing Data*, Hobart Press, Summit, NJ.

Collett, D. (2002). *Modelling Binary Data, Second Edition*. Chapman Hall, London, U.K.

Collett, D. (2003). *Modelling Survival Data in Medical Research Second Edition*. Chapman Hall, London, U.K.

Commenges, D. and Andersen, P.K. (1995). A score test of homogenity for survival data. *Life Time Data Analysis*, 1:145–160.

Costanza, M.C. and Afifi, A.A. (1979). Comparison of stopping rules in forward stepwise discriminant analysis. *Journal of the American Statistical Association*, 74:777–785.

Coviello, V. and Boggess, M. (2004). Cumulative incidence estimation in the presence of competing risks. *Stata Journal* 4 103–112.

Cox, D.R. (1972). Regression models and life tables (with discussion). *Journal of Royal Statistical Society*: Series B, 34:187–220.

Cox, D.R. and Oakes, D. (1984). *Analysis of Survival Data*. Chapman Hall, London, U.K.

Cox, D.R. and Snell, E.J. (1968). A general definition of residuals with discussion. *Journal of Royal Statistical Society*: Series A, 30:248–275.

Crowder, M.J., Kimber, A.C., Smith, R.L. and Sweeting, T.J. (1991). *Statistical Analysis of Reliability Data*. Chapman Hall, London, U.K.

Crowley, J. and Hu, M. (1977). Covariance analysis of heart transplant survival data. *Journal of American Statistical Association*, 78:27–36.

DeGruttola, V. and Lagakos, S.W. (1989). Analysis of doubly–censored survival data with application to AIDS. *Biometrics*, **45**:1–12.

Dempster, A.P., Laird, N.M. and Rubin, D.R. (1977). Maximum likelihood estimation from incomplete data via the EM algorithm (with discussion). *Journal of the Royal Statistical Society*: Series B, **39**:1–38.

Efron, B. (1977). The efficiency of Cox's likelihood function for censored data. *Journal of American Statistical Association*, **72**:557–565.

Elandt–Johnson, R.C. and Johnson, N.L. (1980). *Survival Models and Data Analysis*. John Wiley & Sons, Inc. New York.

Evans, M., Hastings, N. and Peacock, B. (1993). *Statistical Distributions*. 2nd edition. Wiley–Interscience, John Wiley & Sons, Inc. New York.

Farrington, C.P. (1996). Interval censored survival data: A generalized linear modeling approach. *Statistics in Medicine*, **15**:283–292.

Fleiss, J., Levin, B. and Paik, M.C. (2003) *Statistical methods for Rates and Proportions: Third Edition*. John Wiley & Sons, Inc., New York

Finkelstein, D.M. (1986). A proportional hazards model for interval censored failure time data. *Biometrics*, **42**:845–854.

Fisher, L.L. (1992). Discussion of Session 1: Clinical trials, survival analysis. *Statistics in Medicine*, **11**:1881–1885.

Fisher L.D. and Lin D.Y. (1999) Time-dependent Covariates in the Cox Proportional-hazards regression model. *Annual Review of Public Health*, **20**:145-157.

Fleming, T.R. and Harrington, D.P. (1984). Nonparametric estimation of the survival distribution in censored data. *Communication in Statistics: Theory and Methods*, **13**:2469–2486.

Fleming, T.R. and Harrington, D.P. (1991). *Counting Process and Survival Analysis*. John Wiley & Sons, Inc. New York.

Fleming, T.R., Harrington, D.P. and O'Sullivan, M. (1987). Supremium versions of the logrank and generalized Wilcoxon statistics. *Journal of the American Statistical Association*, **82**:312–320.

Gehan, E.A. (1965). A generalized Wilcoxon test for comparing arbitrarily singly–censored samples. *Biometrics*, **52**:203–223.

Gill, R. and Schumacher, M. (1987). A simple test of the proportional hazards assumption. *Biometrika*, **75**:289–300.

Goldberg, R.J., Gore, J.M., Alpert, J.S. and Dalen, J.E. (1986). Recent changes in the attack rates and survival of acute myocardial infarction (1975–1981): The Worcester Heart Attack Study. *Journal of the American Medical Association*, **255**:2774–2779.

Goldberg, R.J., Gore, J.M., Alpert, J.S. and Dalen, J.E. (1988). Incidence and case fatality rates of acute myocardial infarction (1975–1984): The Worcester Heart Attack Study. *American Heart Journal*, **115**:761–767.

Goldberg, R.J., Gore, J.M., Gurwitz, J.H., Alpert, J.S, Brady, P., Stohsnitter, W., Chen, Z. and Dalen, J.E. (1989). The impact of age on the incidence and prognosis of initial myocardial infarction: The Worcester Heart Attack Study. *American Heart Journal*, **117**:543–549.

Goldberg, R.J., Gore, J.M., Alpert, J.S., Osganian, V., de Groot, J., Bade, J., Chen, Z., Frid, D. and Dalen, J. (1991). Cardiogenic shock after acute myocardial infarction: Incidence and mortality from a community wide perspective, 1975–1988. *New England Journal of Medicine*, **325**:1117–1122.

Goldberg, R.J., Gorak, E.J., Yarzebski, J., Hosmer, D.W., Dalen, P., Gore, J.M. and Dalen, J.E. (1993). A community-wide perspective of gender differences and temporal trends in the incidence and survival rates following acute myocardial infarction and out-of-hospital deaths due to coronary heart disease. *Circulation*, **87**:1997–1953.

Goldberg, R.J., Ciu, J., Olendzki, R.D., Spencer, F. Yarzebski, J., Lessard, D. and Gore, J. (2005). Excess body weight, clinical profile, management practices and hospital prognosis in men and women after acute myocardial infarction, *American Heart Journal*, **151**:1297–1304.

Grambsch, P.M. and Therneau, T.M. (1994). Proportional hazards tests in diagnostics based on weighted residuals. *Biometrika*, **81**:515–526.

Grambsch, P.M., Therneau, T.M. and Fleming, T.R. (1995). Diagnostic plots to reveal functional form for covariates in multiplicative intensity models. *Biometrics*, **51**:1469–1482.

Granger, C.B., Goldberg, R.J., Dabbous, O., Pieper, K.S., Eagle, K.A., Cannon, C.P., Van de Werf, F., Avezum, Á., Goodman, S.G., Flather, M.D., Fox, K.A.A., for the Global Registry of Acute Coronary Events Investigators (2003). Predictors of hospital mortality in the Global Registry of Acute Coronary Events. *Archives of Internal Medicine*, **163**:2345–2353.

Gray, R.J. (1992). Flexible methods for analyzing survival data using splines, with applications to breast cancer prognosis. *Journal of the American Statistical Association*, **87**:942–951.

Greenwood, M. (1926). The natural duration of cancer. *Reports on Public Health and Medical Subjects*. **33**:1–26. Her Majesty's Stationery Office, London.

Gross, A.J. and Clark, V.A. (1975). *Survival Distributions: Reliability Applications in the Biomedical Sciences*. John Wiley & Sons, Inc. New York.

Grønnesby, J.K. and Borgan, Ø. (1996). A method for checking regression models in survival analysis based on the risk score. *Lifetime Data Analysis*, **2**:315–328.

Gutierrez, R.G. Carter, S.L., and Drukker, D.M. (2001). On boundary-value likelihood ratio tests. *Stata Technical Bulletin*, **60**:15-18.

Hald, A. (1990). *A History of Probability and Statistics and Their Applications Before 1750*. John Wiley & Sons, Inc. New York.

Hall, W.J. and Wellner, J.A. (1980). Confidence bands for a survival curve from censored data. *Biometrika*, **67**:133–143.

Hall, W.J., Rogers, W.H. and Pregibon, D. (1982). Outliers matter in survival analysis. *Rand Corporation Technical Report P*-6761. Santa Monica, CA.

Hammer, S. M., K. E. Squires, M. D. Hughes, J. M. Grimes, L. M. Demeter, J. S. Currier, J. J. Eron, Jr., J. E. Feinberg, H. H. Balfour, Jr., L. R. Deyton, J. A. Chodakewitz and M. A. Fischl, for the AIDS Clinical Trials Group 320 Study Team (1997). A controlled trial of two nucleoside analogues plus indinavir in persons with human immunodeficiency virus infection and CD4 cell counts of 200 per cubic millimeter or less. *New England Journal of Medicine*, **337**: 725-33.

Harle, O. and Zhou, X-H. (2007) Multiple Imputation: Review of theory, implementation and software. *Statistics in Medicine*, **26**:3057-3077.

Harrell, F.E. (2001). *Regression Modeling Strategies with Applications to Linear Models, Logistic Regression and Survival Analysis,* Springer, New York.

Harrell, F.E., Lee, K.L. and Mark, D.B. (1996). Tutorial in biostatistics. Multivariable models: issues in developing models, evaluating assumptions and adequacy and measuring and reducing errors. *Statistics in Medicine,* **15**:361–387.

Harrington, D.P. and Fleming, T.R. (1982). A class of rank test procedures for censored survival data. *Biometrika,* **69**:553–566.

Henderson, R. and Milner, A. (1991). Aalen plots under proportional hazards. *Applied Statistics,* **40**:401–409.

Horton, N.J. and Lipsitz, S.R. (2001). Multiple imputation in practice: Comparison of software packages for regression models with missing values. *The American Statistician,* **55**: 244–254.

Hosmer, D.W. and Lemeshow, S. (1999). *Applied Survival Analysis: Regression Modeling of Time to Event Data,* John Wiley & Sons, Inc. New York.

Hosmer, D.W. and Lemeshow, S. (2000). *Applied Logistic Regression,* Second Edition. John Wiley & Sons, Inc. New York.

Hosmer, D.W. and Royston, P. (2002) Using Aalen's linear hazards model to investigate time-varying effects in the proportional hazards model. *Stata Journal,* **2**:331-350.

Hougaard, P. (1995). Frailty models for survival data. *Lifetime Data Analysis,* **1**:255–274.

Hougaard, P. (2000). *Analysis of Multivariate Survival Data,* Springer, New York.

Huffler, F.W. and McKeague, I.W. (1991). Weighted least squares estimation for Aalen's additive risk model. *Journal of the American Statistical Association,* **86**:114–129.

Jenkins, S.P. (1997). Discrete time proportional hazards regression. *Stata Technical Bulletin,* **39**:17–32.

Jewell, N.P. (1994). Non-parametric estimation and doubly-censored data: General idea and applications to AIDS. *Statistics in Medicine,* **13**:2081-2095.

Johnson, N.L. and Kotz, S. (1997). *Discrete Multivariate Distributions*. John Wiley & Sons, Inc. New York.

Kabat–Zinn, J., Wheeler, E., Light, T., Skillings, A., Scharf, M.J., Cropley, T.G., Hosmer, D. and Bernhard, J.D. (1998). Influence of a mindfulness meditation-based stress reduction intervention on rates of skin clearing in patients with moderate to severe psoriasis undergoing phototherapy (UVB) and photochemotherapy (PUVA). *Psychosomatic Medicine*, **60**:625–632.

Kalbfleisch, J.D. and Prentice, R.L. (2002). *The Statistical Analysis of Failure Time Data*. Second Edition. John Wiley & Sons, Inc. New York.

Kaplan, E.L. and Meier, P. (1958). Nonparametric estimation from incomplete observations. *Journal of the American Statistical Association*, **53**:457–481.

Kelly, P.J. and Lim, L.L-Y. (2000). Survival analysis for recurrent event data: an application of Childhood infectious Diseases. *Statistics in Medicine*, **19**:13-33.

Kim, M.Y., DeGruttola, V.G. and Lagakos, S. (1993). Analyzing doubly censored data with covariates, with application to AIDS. *Biometrics*, **45**:1-11.

Klein, J.P. and Moeschberger, M.L. (2003). *Survival Analysis Techniques for Censored and Truncated Data: Second Edition*. Springer–Verlag, New York.

Kleinbaum, D.G. and Klien, M. (2005) *Survival Analysis: A Self–Learning Text*. Second Edition. Springer–Verlag, New York.

Kleinbaum, D.G., Kupper, L.L., Muller, K.E. and Nizam, A. (1998). *Applied Regression Analysis and Multivariable Methods*. 3rd edition. Duxbury Press. Pacific Grove, CA.

Kuk, A.Y.C. (1984). All subsets regression in a proportional hazards model. *Biometrika*, **71**:587–592.

Langholz, B. and Borgan, Ø. (1995). Counter-matching: A stratified nested case–control sampling method. *Biometrika*, **82**:69–79.

Lawless, J.F. (2003). *Statistical Models and Methods for Lifetime Data* Second Edition. John Wiley & Sons, Inc. New York.

Lawless, J.F. and Singhal, K. (1978). Efficient screening of non-normal regression models. *Biometrics*, **34**:318–327.

Le, C.T. (1997). *Applied Survival Analysis*. John Wiley & Sons, Inc., New York.

Lee, E.T. and Wang J.W. (2003). *Statistical Methods for Survival Data Analysis*. Third Edition, John Wiley & Sons, Inc., New York.

Liang, K.Y. and Zeger, S.L. (1986a). Longitudinal data analysis, using generalized linear models. *Biometrika*, **73**:13–22.

Liang, K.Y. and Zeger, S.L. (1986b). Longitudinal data analysis for discrete and continuous models. *Biometrics*, **42**:121–130.

Liang, K.Y., Self, S.G., Bandeen–Roche, K.J. and Zeger, S. (1995). Some recent developments for regression analysis of multivariate failure time data. *Lifetime Data Analysis*, **1**:403–416.

Lin, X. and Wang, H. (2004). A new testing approach for comparing the overall homogeneity of survival curves. *Biometrical Journal*, **46**:489-496.

Lin, D.Y. and Wei, L.J. (1989). The robust inference for the Cox proportional hazards model. *Journal of the American Statistical Association*, **84**:1074–1078.

Lin, D.Y. and Ying, Z. (1994). Semiparametric analysis of the additive risk model, *Biometrika*, **81**:61–71.

Lin, D.Y., Wei, L.J. and Ying, Z. (1993). Checking the Cox model with cumulative sums of Martingale based residuals. *Biometrika*, **80**:557–572.

Little, R.J.A. and Rubin, D.B. (2002). *Statistical Analysis with Missing Data*, 2nd ed. Wiley, New York.

Lunn, M. and McNeil, D. (1995). Applying the Cox regression to competing risks. *Biometrics* **51**:524–532.

McCullagh, P. and Nelder, J.A. (1989). *Generalized Linear Models*. 2nd edition. Chapman Hall, London, U.K.

McCusker, J., Vickers–Lahti, M., Stoddard, A.M., Hindin, R., Bigelow, C., Garfield, F., Frost, R., Love, C. and Lewis, B.F. (1995). The effectiveness of alternative planned durations of residential drug abuse treatment. *American Journal of Public Health*, **85**:1426–1429.

McCusker, J., Bigelow, C., Frost, R., Garfield, F., Hindin, R., Vickers–Lahti, M. and Lewis, B.F. (1997a). The effects of planned duration of residential drug abuse treatment on recovery and HIV risk behavior. *American Journal of Public Health*, **87**:1637–1644.

McCusker, J., Bigelow, C., Vickers–Lahti, M., Spotts, D., Garfield, F. and Frost, R. (1997b). Planned duration of residential drug abuse treatment: efficacy versus treatment. *Addiction*, **92**:1467–1478.

McKeague, I.W. and Sasieni, P.D. (1994). A partly parametric additive risk model. *Biometrika*, **81**:501–514.

Makuch, R.W. (1982). Survival curve estimation using covariates. *Journal of Chronic Diseases*, **3**:437–443.

Mallows, C. (1973). Some Comments on Cp. *Technometrics*, **15**:661–676.

Mann, N., Schaefer, R.E. and Singparwalla, N.D. (1974). *Methods for Statistical Analysis of Reliability and Life Data*. John Wiley & Sons, Inc., New York.

Mantel, N. (1966). Evaluation of survival data and two new rank order statistics arising in its consideration. *Cancer Chemotherapy Reports*, **50**:163–170.

Marubini, E. and Valsecchi, M.G. (1995). *Analyzing Survival Data from Clinical Trials and Observational Studies*. John Wiley & Sons, Ltd., Chichester, U.K.

MathType[5]: Mathematical Equation Editor (2004). Design Sciences, Inc. Long Beach, CA 90803.

Mau, J. (1986). On a graphical method for the detection of time-dependent effects of covariants in survival data. *Applied Statistics*, **35**:245–255.

May, S. and Hosmer, D.W. (1998). A simplified method for calculating a goodness-of-fit test for the proportional hazards model. *Lifetime Data Analysis*, **4**:109–120.

May, S. and Hosmer, D. W. (2004). A cautionary note on the use of the Grønnesby and Borgan goodness-of-fit test for the Cox proportional hazards model. *Lifetime Data Analysis*, **10**:283–291.

Mickey, J. and Greenland, S. (1989). A study of the impact of confounder selection criteria on effect estimation. *American Journal of Epidemiology*, **129**:125–137.

Miller, R.G. (1981). *Survival Analysis*. John Wiley & Sons, Inc., New York.

Nelson, W. (1969). Hazard plotting for incomplete failure data. *Journal of Quality Technology*, 1:27–52.

Nelson, W. (1972). Theory and application of hazard plotting for censored failure data. *Technometrics*, **14**:945–965.

Nelson, W. (2004). *Applied Life Data Analysis*, Second Edition. John Wiley & Sons, Inc., New York.

Nelson, W. (1990). *Accelerated Testing, Statistical Models, Test Plans, and Data Analysis*. John Wiley & Sons, Inc., New York.

Nagelkerke, N. J. D. (1991). A note on a general definition of the coefficient of determination. *Biometrika* **78**: 691–692.

Neuhaus, J. (1992). Statistical methods for longitudinal and clustered designs with binary outcomes. *Statistical Methods in Medical Research*, 1:249–273.

Nielsen, G.G., Gill, R.D., Andersen, P.K. and Sørensen, T.I.A. (1992). A counting process approach to maximum likelihood estimation in frailty models. *Scandinavian Journal of Statistics*, **19**:25–43.

Ng'andu, N.H. (1997). An empirical comparison of statistical tests for assessing the proportional hazards assumption of Cox's model. *Statistics in Medicine*, **16**:611–626.

Oakes, D. (1981). Survival times: Aspects of partial likelihood (with discussion). *International Statistical Review*, **49**:235–264.

Pintilie, M. (2006). *Competing Risks, A Practical Perspective*. John Wiley & Sons Ltd. Chichester, West Sussex, England.

O'Quigley, J. and Pessione, F. (1989). Score tests for homogenity of regression effect in the proportional hazards model. *Biometrics*, **45**:135–144.

O'Quigley. J. and J. Stare (2002) Proportional hazards models with frailties and random effects. *Statistics in Medicine*, **21**:3219–3233.

O'Quigley, J., R. Xu, and J. Stare (2005) Explained randomness in proportional hazards models. *Statistics in Medicine*, **24**: 479–489.

Parmar, M.K.B. and Machin, D. (1995). *Survival Analysis: A Practical Approach.* John Wiley & Sons, Ltd., Chichester, U.K.

Parzen, M. and Lipsitz, S. R. (1999) A global goodness-of-fit statistic for Cox regression models,. *Biometrics,* **55**:580 – 584.

Peterson, A.V. (1977). Expressing the Kaplan–Meier estimation as a function of empirical subsurvival functions. *Journal of the American Statistical Association,* **72**:854–858.

Peto, R. and Peto, J. (1972). Asymptotically efficient rank invariance test procedures (with discussion). *Journal of the Royal Statistical Association. Series A,* **135**:185–206.

Pettitt, A.N. and Bin Daud, L. (1989). Case–weighted measures of influence for proportional hazards regression. *Applied Statistics,* **38**:51–67.

Pettitt, A.N. and Bin Daud, L. (1990). Investigating time dependence in Cox proportional hazards model. *Applied Statistics,* **39**:313–329.

Pickels, A., Crouchley, R., Simonoff, E.L., Meyer, J., Rutter, M., Hewitt, J. and Silbery, J. (1994). Survival models for developmental genetic data: Age at onset of puberty and antisocial behavior in twins. *Genetic Epidemiology,* **11**:155–170.

Prentice R.L. (1978). Linear rank tests with right censored data. *Biometrika,* **65**:167–179, Correction **70**:304 (1983).

Prentice, R.L. and Gloecker, L.A. (1978). Regression analysis of grouped survival data with application to breast cancer data. *Biometrics,* **34**:57–67.

Prentice, R.L., Williams, J. and Peterson, A.V. (1981). On the regression analysis of multivariate failure time data. *Biometrika,* **68**:373–379.

Quantin, C., Moreau, T., Asselain, B., Maccario, J. and Lellouch, J. (1996). A regression survival model for testing the proportional hazards hypothesis. *Biometrics,* **52**:874–885.

Rothman, K.J. and Greenland, S. (1998). *Modern Epidemiology.* 3rd edition. Lippincott–Raven., Philadelphia, PA.

Royston, P (2001). Flexible parametric alternatives to the Cox model and more. *The Stata Journal,* **1**(1): 1- 28.

Royston, P. (2004). Multiple imputation of missing values. *The Stata Journal* **4**(3):227–241.

Royston, P. (2005a). Multiple imputation of missing values: Update. *The Stata Journal* **5**(2):188–201.

Royston, P. (2005b) Multiple imputation of missing values: Update of ice. *The Stata Journal* **5**(4):527–536.

Royston, P. (2006). Explained variation for survival models. *The Stata Journal*, **6**(1): 83–96.

Royston, P. and Altman, D.G. (1994). Regression using fractional polynomials of continuous covariates: parsimonious parametric modeling (with discussion). *Applied Statistics*, **43**:429–467. Reprinted in *Stata Technical Bulletin Reprints*, **8**:123-132.

Royston, P. and Ambler, G. (1998). Multivariable fractional polynomials, *Stata Technical Bulletin*, **43**:24-32.

Royston, P. and Sauerbrei, W. (2007). Improving the robustness of fractional polynomials by preliminary covariate transformation; A pragmatic approach. *Computational Statistics & Data Analysis*, **51**:4240–4253.

Rubin, D.B. (1976). Inference and Missing data, *Biometrika* **63**: 581–592.

Rubin, D.B. (1987) *Multiple Imputation for Nonresponse in Surveys*. John Wiley & Sons. Inc., New York

Ryan, T. (1997). *Modern Regression Methods*. John Wiley & Sons, Inc., New York.

SAS Institute Inc. (2003). SAS/STAT®, SAS Institute, Cary, NC.

SAS Institute Inc. (2004). *Base SAS® 9.1 Procedures Guide*. Cary, NC: SAS Institute Inc.

SAS Institute Inc. (2004). *SAS/STAT® 9.1 User's Guide*. Cary, NC: SAS Institute Inc.

SAS Institute Inc. (2004). *Getting Started with the SAS® Power and Sample Size Application*. Cary, NC: SAS Institute Inc.

Sauerbrei, W., Meier-Hirmer, C., Benner, A. and Royston, P. (2006). Multivariable regression model building by using fractional polynomials: description of SAS, STATA and R programs. *Computational Statistics and Data Analysis,* **50**:3464–3485.

Sauerbrei, W and Royston, P. (1999) Building multivariable prognostic and diagnostic models: transformation of the predictors using fractional polynomials. *Journal of the Royal Statistical Society Series A,* **162** part 1, 71-94.

Savage, I.R. (1956). Contributions to the theory of rank-order statistics — the two sample case. *Annals of Mathematical Statistics,* **27**:590–615.

Schafer, J.L. (1997), *Analysis of Incomplete Multivariate Data,* Chapman & Hall, New York.|

Schafer, J.L. (1999), Multiple imputation: A primer, *Statistical Methods in Medical Research,* **8**: 3–15|

Schafer, J.L. and Graham, J.W. (2002), Missing data: Our View of the State of the Art, *Phychological Methods,* **7**:147–177.

Schmoor, C. Olschweski, M. and Schumacher, M. (1996). Randomized and non-randomized patients in clinical trials: experiences with comprehensive cohort studies. *Statistics in Medicine,* **15**: 263-271.

Schemper, M. and Stare, J. (1996). Explained variation in survival analysis. *Statistics in Medicine,* **15**:1999–2012.

Schoenfeld, D. (1980). Chi-squared goodness-of-fit tests for the proportional hazards regression model. *Biometrika,* **67**:145–153.

Schoenfeld, D. (1982). Partial residuals for the proportional hazards regression model. *Biometrika,* **69**:239–241.

Schoenfeld, D. (1983) Sample-size formula for the proportional-hazards regression model. *Biometrics,* **39**:499–503.

Schumacher, M. Bastert, G., Bojar, H., Hübner, K., Olschweski M., Sauerbrei, W. Schmoor, C., Beyerle, C. Newmann,, R.L.A. and Rauschecker, H.F. (1994). Randomized 2x2 trail evaluating hormonal treatment and the duration of chemotherapy in node positive beast cancer patients. *Journal of Clinical Oncology,* **12**: 2086-2093

StataCorp (2005). *Stata Statistical Software: Release 9.0,*. Stata Corporation, College Station, TX.

Sun, J. (2006). *The Statistical Analysis of Interval-censored Failure Time Data*, Springer, New York.

Tarone, R.E. and Ware, J. (1977). On distribution free tests of the equality of survival distributions. *Biometrika*, **64**:156–160.

The 3C Study Group (2003). Vascular factors and risk of dementia: design of the Three-City Study and baseline characteristics of the study population. *Neuroepidemiology*: **22**:316-325

Therneau, T.M. and Grambsch, P.M (2000). *Modeling Survival Data: Extending the Cox Model.* Springer, New York.

Therneau, T.M., Grambsch, P.M. and Fleming, T.R. (1990). Martingale–based residuals for survival models. *Biometrika*, **77**:147–160.

Thomsen, B.L., Keiding, N. and Altman, D.G. (1991). A note on the calculation of expected survival, illustrated by the survival of liver transplant patients. *Statistics in Medicine*, **10**:733–738.

Tsiatis, A.A. (1980). A note on a goodness–of–fit test for the logistic regression model. *Biometrika*, **67**:250–251.

Van Buuren, S. Boshuizen, H.C. and Knook, D.L. (1999) Multiple imputation of missing blood pressure covariates in survival analysis. *Statistics in Medicine* **18**:681–694.

Vaupel, J.W., Manton, K.G. and Stallard, E. (1979). The impact of heterogenity in individual frailty on the dynamics of mortality. *Demography*, **16**:439–454.

Ware, J.H. and DeMets, D.L. (1976). Reanalysis of some baboon descent data. *Biometrics*, **32**:459–463.

Wei, L.J. (1992). The accelerated failure time model: a useful alternative to the Cox regression model in survival analysis. *Statistics in Medicine*, **11**:1871–1879.

Wei, L.J., Lin, D.Y. and Weissfeld (1989). Regression analysis of multivariate incomplete failure time data by modeling marginal distributions. *Journal of the American Statistical Association*, **84**:1065–1073.

White, H. (1980). A heteroskedasticity consistent covariance matrix estimator and a direct test for heteroskedasticity. *Econometrika*, **48**:817–838.

White, H. (1982). Maximum likelihood estimation of misspecified models. *Economterika*, **50**:1–26.

Yashin, A.I., Vaupel, J.W. and Jachine, I.A. (1995). Correlated individual frailty: an advantageous approach to survival analysis of bivariate data. *Mathematical Population Studies*, **5**:145–149.

Yuan, S.-Sh. (1993). *Prediction of length of oxygen use in BPD babies*, Masters Thesis, School of Public Health, University of Massachusetts, Amherst, MA.

Zahl, P.H. and Tretli S. (1997). Long-term survival of breast cancer patients in Norway by age and clinical stage. *Statistics in Medicine*, **13**:1435–1450.

Zhou, M. (2001). Understanding the Cox regression models with time-change covariates. *The American Statistician*, **55**:153-155.

INDEX

WILEY SERIES IN PROBABILITY AND STATISTICS
ESTABLISHED BY WALTER A. SHEWHART AND SAMUEL S. WILKS

Editors: *David J. Balding, Noel A. C. Cressie, Nicholas I. Fisher,*
Iain M. Johnstone, J. B. Kadane, Geert Molenberghs, David W. Scott,
Adrian F. M. Smith, Sanford Weisberg
Editors Emeriti: *Vic Barnett, J. Stuart Hunter, David G. Kendall,*
Jozef L. Teugels

The *Wiley Series in Probability and Statistics* is well established and authoritative. It covers many topics of current research interest in both pure and applied statistics and probability theory. Written by leading statisticians and institutions, the titles span both state-of-the-art developments in the field and classical methods.

Reflecting the wide range of current research in statistics, the series encompasses applied, methodological and theoretical statistics, ranging from applications and new techniques made possible by advances in computerized practice to rigorous treatment of theoretical approaches.

This series provides essential and invaluable reading for all statisticians, whether in academia, industry, government, or research.

† ABRAHAM and LEDOLTER · Statistical Methods for Forecasting
  AGRESTI · Analysis of Ordinal Categorical Data
  AGRESTI · An Introduction to Categorical Data Analysis, *Second Edition*
  AGRESTI · Categorical Data Analysis, *Second Edition*
  ALTMAN, GILL, and McDONALD · Numerical Issues in Statistical Computing for the
    Social Scientist
  AMARATUNGA and CABRERA · Exploration and Analysis of DNA Microarray and
    Protein Array Data
  ANDĚL · Mathematics of Chance
  ANDERSON · An Introduction to Multivariate Statistical Analysis, *Third Edition*
* ANDERSON · The Statistical Analysis of Time Series
  ANDERSON, AUQUIER, HAUCK, OAKES, VANDAELE, and WEISBERG ·
    Statistical Methods for Comparative Studies
  ANDERSON and LOYNES · The Teaching of Practical Statistics
  ARMITAGE and DAVID (editors) · Advances in Biometry
  ARNOLD, BALAKRISHNAN, and NAGARAJA · Records
* ARTHANARI and DODGE · Mathematical Programming in Statistics
* BAILEY · The Elements of Stochastic Processes with Applications to the Natural
    Sciences
  BALAKRISHNAN and KOUTRAS · Runs and Scans with Applications
  BALAKRISHNAN and NG · Precedence-Type Tests and Applications
  BARNETT · Comparative Statistical Inference, *Third Edition*
  BARNETT · Environmental Statistics
  BARNETT and LEWIS · Outliers in Statistical Data, *Third Edition*
  BARTOSZYNSKI and NIEWIADOMSKA-BUGAJ · Probability and Statistical Inference
  BASILEVSKY · Statistical Factor Analysis and Related Methods: Theory and
    Applications
  BASU and RIGDON · Statistical Methods for the Reliability of Repairable Systems
  BATES and WATTS · Nonlinear Regression Analysis and Its Applications

*Now available in a lower priced paperback edition in the Wiley Classics Library.
†Now available in a lower priced paperback edition in the Wiley–Interscience Paperback Series.

BECHHOFER, SANTNER, and GOLDSMAN · Design and Analysis of Experiments for Statistical Selection, Screening, and Multiple Comparisons

BELSLEY · Conditioning Diagnostics: Collinearity and Weak Data in Regression

† BELSLEY, KUH, and WELSCH · Regression Diagnostics: Identifying Influential Data and Sources of Collinearity

BENDAT and PIERSOL · Random Data: Analysis and Measurement Procedures, *Third Edition*

BERRY, CHALONER, and GEWEKE · Bayesian Analysis in Statistics and Econometrics: Essays in Honor of Arnold Zellner

BERNARDO and SMITH · Bayesian Theory

BHAT and MILLER · Elements of Applied Stochastic Processes, *Third Edition*

BHATTACHARYA and WAYMIRE · Stochastic Processes with Applications

BILLINGSLEY · Convergence of Probability Measures, *Second Edition*

BILLINGSLEY · Probability and Measure, *Third Edition*

BIRKES and DODGE · Alternative Methods of Regression

BISWAS, DATTA, FINE, and SEGAL · Statistical Advances in the Biomedical Sciences: Clinical Trials, Epidemiology, Survival Analysis, and Bioinformatics

BLISCHKE AND MURTHY (editors) · Case Studies in Reliability and Maintenance

BLISCHKE AND MURTHY · Reliability: Modeling, Prediction, and Optimization

BLOOMFIELD · Fourier Analysis of Time Series: An Introduction, *Second Edition*

BOLLEN · Structural Equations with Latent Variables

BOLLEN and CURRAN · Latent Curve Models: A Structural Equation Perspective

BOROVKOV · Ergodicity and Stability of Stochastic Processes

BOULEAU · Numerical Methods for Stochastic Processes

BOX · Bayesian Inference in Statistical Analysis

BOX · R. A. Fisher, the Life of a Scientist

BOX and DRAPER · Response Surfaces, Mixtures, and Ridge Analyses, *Second Edition*

* BOX and DRAPER · Evolutionary Operation: A Statistical Method for Process Improvement

BOX and FRIENDS · Improving Almost Anything, *Revised Edition*

BOX, HUNTER, and HUNTER · Statistics for Experimenters: Design, Innovation, and Discovery, *Second Editon*

BOX and LUCEÑO · Statistical Control by Monitoring and Feedback Adjustment

BRANDIMARTE · Numerical Methods in Finance: A MATLAB-Based Introduction

† BROWN and HOLLANDER · Statistics: A Biomedical Introduction

BRUNNER, DOMHOF, and LANGER · Nonparametric Analysis of Longitudinal Data in Factorial Experiments

BUCKLEW · Large Deviation Techniques in Decision, Simulation, and Estimation

CAIROLI and DALANG · Sequential Stochastic Optimization

CASTILLO, HADI, BALAKRISHNAN, and SARABIA · Extreme Value and Related Models with Applications in Engineering and Science

CHAN · Time Series: Applications to Finance

CHARALAMBIDES · Combinatorial Methods in Discrete Distributions

CHATTERJEE and HADI · Regression Analysis by Example, *Fourth Edition*

CHATTERJEE and HADI · Sensitivity Analysis in Linear Regression

CHERNICK · Bootstrap Methods: A Guide for Practitioners and Researchers, *Second Edition*

CHERNICK and FRIIS · Introductory Biostatistics for the Health Sciences

CHILÈS and DELFINER · Geostatistics: Modeling Spatial Uncertainty

CHOW and LIU · Design and Analysis of Clinical Trials: Concepts and Methodologies, *Second Edition*

CLARKE and DISNEY · Probability and Random Processes: A First Course with Applications, *Second Edition*

* COCHRAN and COX · Experimental Designs, *Second Edition*

---

*Now available in a lower priced paperback edition in the Wiley Classics Library.

†Now available in a lower priced paperback edition in the Wiley–Interscience Paperback Series.

---

*Now available in a lower priced paperback edition in the Wiley Classics Library.
†Now available in a lower priced paperback edition in the Wiley–Interscience Paperback Series.

*Now available in a lower priced paperback edition in the Wiley Classics Library.

†Now available in a lower priced paperback edition in the Wiley–Interscience Paperback Series.

HURD and MIAMEE · Periodically Correlated Random Sequences: Spectral Theory and Practice

HUSKOVA, BERAN, and DUPAC · Collected Works of Jaroslav Hajek—with Commentary

HUZURBAZAR · Flowgraph Models for Multistate Time-to-Event Data

IMAN and CONOVER · A Modern Approach to Statistics

† JACKSON · A User's Guide to Principle Components

JOHN · Statistical Methods in Engineering and Quality Assurance

JOHNSON · Multivariate Statistical Simulation

JOHNSON and BALAKRISHNAN · Advances in the Theory and Practice of Statistics: A Volume in Honor of Samuel Kotz

JOHNSON and BHATTACHARYYA · Statistics: Principles and Methods, *Fifth Edition*

JOHNSON and KOTZ · Distributions in Statistics

JOHNSON and KOTZ (editors) · Leading Personalities in Statistical Sciences: From the Seventeenth Century to the Present

JOHNSON, KOTZ, and BALAKRISHNAN · Continuous Univariate Distributions, Volume 1, *Second Edition*

JOHNSON, KOTZ, and BALAKRISHNAN · Continuous Univariate Distributions, Volume 2, *Second Edition*

JOHNSON, KOTZ, and BALAKRISHNAN · Discrete Multivariate Distributions

JOHNSON, KEMP, and KOTZ · Univariate Discrete Distributions, *Third Edition*

JUDGE, GRIFFITHS, HILL, LÜTKEPOHL, and LEE · The Theory and Practice of Econometrics, *Second Edition*

JUREČKOVÁ and SEN · Robust Statistical Procedures: Aymptotics and Interrelations

JUREK and MASON · Operator-Limit Distributions in Probability Theory

KADANE · Bayesian Methods and Ethics in a Clinical Trial Design

KADANE AND SCHUM · A Probabilistic Analysis of the Sacco and Vanzetti Evidence

KALBFLEISCH and PRENTICE · The Statistical Analysis of Failure Time Data, *Second Edition*

KARIYA and KURATA · Generalized Least Squares

KASS and VOS · Geometrical Foundations of Asymptotic Inference

† KAUFMAN and ROUSSEEUW · Finding Groups in Data: An Introduction to Cluster Analysis

KEDEM and FOKIANOS · Regression Models for Time Series Analysis

KENDALL, BARDEN, CARNE, and LE · Shape and Shape Theory

KHURI · Advanced Calculus with Applications in Statistics, *Second Edition*

KHURI, MATHEW, and SINHA · Statistical Tests for Mixed Linear Models

KLEIBER and KOTZ · Statistical Size Distributions in Economics and Actuarial Sciences

KLUGMAN, PANJER, and WILLMOT · Loss Models: From Data to Decisions, *Second Edition*

KLUGMAN, PANJER, and WILLMOT · Solutions Manual to Accompany Loss Models: From Data to Decisions, *Second Edition*

KOTZ, BALAKRISHNAN, and JOHNSON · Continuous Multivariate Distributions, Volume 1, *Second Edition*

KOVALENKO, KUZNETZOV, and PEGG · Mathematical Theory of Reliability of Time-Dependent Systems with Practical Applications

KOWALSKI and TU · Modern Applied U-Statistics

KVAM and VIDAKOVIC · Nonparametric Statistics with Applications to Science and Engineering

LACHIN · Biostatistical Methods: The Assessment of Relative Risks

LAD · Operational Subjective Statistical Methods: A Mathematical, Philosophical, and Historical Introduction

LAMPERTI · Probability: A Survey of the Mathematical Theory, *Second Edition*

---

*Now available in a lower priced paperback edition in the Wiley Classics Library.

†Now available in a lower priced paperback edition in the Wiley–Interscience Paperback Series.

LANGE, RYAN, BILLARD, BRILLINGER, CONQUEST, and GREENHOUSE · Case Studies in Biometry

LARSON · Introduction to Probability Theory and Statistical Inference, *Third Edition*

LAWLESS · Statistical Models and Methods for Lifetime Data, *Second Edition*

LAWSON · Statistical Methods in Spatial Epidemiology

LE · Applied Categorical Data Analysis

LE · Applied Survival Analysis

LEE and WANG · Statistical Methods for Survival Data Analysis, *Third Edition*

LePAGE and BILLARD · Exploring the Limits of Bootstrap

LEYLAND and GOLDSTEIN (editors) · Multilevel Modelling of Health Statistics

LIAO · Statistical Group Comparison

LINDVALL · Lectures on the Coupling Method

LIN · Introductory Stochastic Analysis for Finance and Insurance

LINHART and ZUCCHINI · Model Selection

LITTLE and RUBIN · Statistical Analysis with Missing Data, *Second Edition*

LLOYD · The Statistical Analysis of Categorical Data

LOWEN and TEICH · Fractal-Based Point Processes

MAGNUS and NEUDECKER · Matrix Differential Calculus with Applications in Statistics and Econometrics, *Revised Edition*

MALLER and ZHOU · Survival Analysis with Long Term Survivors

MALLOWS · Design, Data, and Analysis by Some Friends of Cuthbert Daniel

MANN, SCHAFER, and SINGPURWALLA · Methods for Statistical Analysis of Reliability and Life Data

MANTON, WOODBURY, and TOLLEY · Statistical Applications Using Fuzzy Sets

MARCHETTE · Random Graphs for Statistical Pattern Recognition

MARDIA and JUPP · Directional Statistics

MASON, GUNST, and HESS · Statistical Design and Analysis of Experiments with Applications to Engineering and Science, *Second Edition*

McCULLOCH and SEARLE · Generalized, Linear, and Mixed Models

McFADDEN · Management of Data in Clinical Trials, *Second Edition*

* McLACHLAN · Discriminant Analysis and Statistical Pattern Recognition

McLACHLAN, DO, and AMBROISE · Analyzing Microarray Gene Expression Data

McLACHLAN and KRISHNAN · The EM Algorithm and Extensions, *Second Edition*

McLACHLAN and PEEL · Finite Mixture Models

McNEIL · Epidemiological Research Methods

MEEKER and ESCOBAR · Statistical Methods for Reliability Data

MEERSCHAERT and SCHEFFLER · Limit Distributions for Sums of Independent Random Vectors: Heavy Tails in Theory and Practice

MICKEY, DUNN, and CLARK · Applied Statistics: Analysis of Variance and Regression, *Third Edition*

* MILLER · Survival Analysis, *Second Edition*

MONTGOMERY, PECK, and VINING · Introduction to Linear Regression Analysis, *Fourth Edition*

MORGENTHALER and TUKEY · Configural Polysampling: A Route to Practical Robustness

MUIRHEAD · Aspects of Multivariate Statistical Theory

MULLER and STOYAN · Comparison Methods for Stochastic Models and Risks

MURRAY · X-STAT 2.0 Statistical Experimentation, Design Data Analysis, and Nonlinear Optimization

MURTHY, XIE, and JIANG · Weibull Models

MYERS and MONTGOMERY · Response Surface Methodology: Process and Product Optimization Using Designed Experiments, *Second Edition*

MYERS, MONTGOMERY, and VINING · Generalized Linear Models. With Applications in Engineering and the Sciences

*Now available in a lower priced paperback edition in the Wiley Classics Library.

†Now available in a lower priced paperback edition in the Wiley–Interscience Paperback Series.

† NELSON · Accelerated Testing, Statistical Models, Test Plans, and Data Analyses
† NELSON · Applied Life Data Analysis
NEWMAN · Biostatistical Methods in Epidemiology
OCHI · Applied Probability and Stochastic Processes in Engineering and Physical Sciences
OKABE, BOOTS, SUGIHARA, and CHIU · Spatial Tesselations: Concepts and Applications of Voronoi Diagrams, *Second Edition*
OLIVER and SMITH · Influence Diagrams, Belief Nets and Decision Analysis
PALTA · Quantitative Methods in Population Health: Extensions of Ordinary Regressions
PANJER · Operational Risk: Modeling and Analytics
PANKRATZ · Forecasting with Dynamic Regression Models
PANKRATZ · Forecasting with Univariate Box-Jenkins Models: Concepts and Cases
* PARZEN · Modern Probability Theory and Its Applications
PEÑA, TIAO, and TSAY · A Course in Time Series Analysis
PIANTADOSI · Clinical Trials: A Methodologic Perspective
PORT · Theoretical Probability for Applications
POURAHMADI · Foundations of Time Series Analysis and Prediction Theory
POWELL · Approximate Dynamic Programming: Solving the Curses of Dimensionality
PRESS · Bayesian Statistics: Principles, Models, and Applications
PRESS · Subjective and Objective Bayesian Statistics, *Second Edition*
PRESS and TANUR · The Subjectivity of Scientists and the Bayesian Approach
PUKELSHEIM · Optimal Experimental Design
PURI, VILAPLANA, and WERTZ · New Perspectives in Theoretical and Applied Statistics
† PUTERMAN · Markov Decision Processes: Discrete Stochastic Dynamic Programming
QIU · Image Processing and Jump Regression Analysis
* RAO · Linear Statistical Inference and Its Applications, *Second Edition*
RAUSAND and HØYLAND · System Reliability Theory: Models, Statistical Methods, and Applications, *Second Edition*
RENCHER · Linear Models in Statistics
RENCHER · Methods of Multivariate Analysis, *Second Edition*
RENCHER · Multivariate Statistical Inference with Applications
* RIPLEY · Spatial Statistics
* RIPLEY · Stochastic Simulation
ROBINSON · Practical Strategies for Experimenting
ROHATGI and SALEH · An Introduction to Probability and Statistics, *Second Edition*
ROLSKI, SCHMIDLI, SCHMIDT, and TEUGELS · Stochastic Processes for Insurance and Finance
ROSENBERGER and LACHIN · Randomization in Clinical Trials: Theory and Practice
ROSS · Introduction to Probability and Statistics for Engineers and Scientists
ROSSI, ALLENBY, and McCULLOCH · Bayesian Statistics and Marketing
† ROUSSEEUW and LEROY · Robust Regression and Outlier Detection
* RUBIN · Multiple Imputation for Nonresponse in Surveys
RUBINSTEIN and KROESE · Simulation and the Monte Carlo Method, *Second Edition*
RUBINSTEIN and MELAMED · Modern Simulation and Modeling
RYAN · Modern Engineering Statistics
RYAN · Modern Experimental Design
RYAN · Modern Regression Methods
RYAN · Statistical Methods for Quality Improvement, *Second Edition*
SALEH · Theory of Preliminary Test and Stein-Type Estimation with Applications
* SCHEFFE · The Analysis of Variance
SCHIMEK · Smoothing and Regression: Approaches, Computation, and Application
SCHOTT · Matrix Analysis for Statistics, *Second Edition*
SCHOUTENS · Levy Processes in Finance: Pricing Financial Derivatives

*Now available in a lower priced paperback edition in the Wiley Classics Library.
†Now available in a lower priced paperback edition in the Wiley–Interscience Paperback Series.

*Now available in a lower priced paperback edition in the Wiley Classics Library.

†Now available in a lower priced paperback edition in the Wiley–Interscience Paperback Series.

WELSH · Aspects of Statistical Inference

WESTFALL and YOUNG · Resampling-Based Multiple Testing: Examples and Methods for *p*-Value Adjustment

WHITTAKER · Graphical Models in Applied Multivariate Statistics

WINKER · Optimization Heuristics in Economics: Applications of Threshold Accepting

WONNACOTT and WONNACOTT · Econometrics, *Second Edition*

WOODING · Planning Pharmaceutical Clinical Trials: Basic Statistical Principles

WOODWORTH · Biostatistics: A Bayesian Introduction

WOOLSON and CLARKE · Statistical Methods for the Analysis of Biomedical Data, *Second Edition*

WU and HAMADA · Experiments: Planning, Analysis, and Parameter Design Optimization

WU and ZHANG · Nonparametric Regression Methods for Longitudinal Data Analysis

YANG · The Construction Theory of Denumerable Markov Processes

YOUNG, VALERO-MORA, and FRIENDLY · Visual Statistics: Seeing Data with Dynamic Interactive Graphics

ZELTERMAN · Discrete Distributions—Applications in the Health Sciences

* ZELLNER · An Introduction to Bayesian Inference in Econometrics

ZHOU, OBUCHOWSKI, and McCLISH · Statistical Methods in Diagnostic Medicine

*Now available in a lower priced paperback edition in the Wiley Classics Library.
†Now available in a lower priced paperback edition in the Wiley–Interscience Paperback Series.

CPSIA information can be obtained at www.ICGtesting.com
Printed in the USA
BVOW08*0047110714

358511BV00001B/1/P